Psychological Factors in
Cardiovascular Disorders

Psychological Factors in Cardiovascular Disorders

ANDREW STEPTOE

St George's Hospital Medical School
University of London

1981

ACADEMIC PRESS

A Subsidiary of Harcourt Brace Jovanovich, Publishers
LONDON   NEW YORK   TORONTO   SYDNEY   SAN FRANCISCO

Academic Press Inc. (London) Ltd
24–28 Oval Road
London NW1

US edition published by
Academic Press Inc.
111 Fifth Avenue,
New York, New York 10003

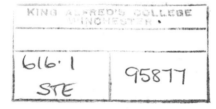
British Library Cataloguing in Publication Data

Steptoe, A
    Psychological factors in cardiovascular disorders.
    1. Cardiovascular system – Diseases – Psychological aspects
    I. Title
    616.1'0019   RC667   80-49721

ISBN 0-12-666450-1

Typesetting by Kelmscott Press Ltd., 30 New Bridge Street, London EC4
Printed and Bound by T. J. Press (Padstow) Ltd., Padstow, Cornwall

For my mother and father

Preface

The link between psychological factors and cardiovascular disorders has fostered a wide-ranging clinical and research literature. Firm conclusions about the nature of the connection remain elusive however. Emotional and behavioural responses are frequently invoked as contributing to disorders such as essential hypertension, while psychological stress is popularly accepted as one cause of the prevalence of ischaemic heart disease in Western societies. Yet at the same time there is considerable scepticism amongst clinicians as to whether the study of these aspects adds to understanding of aetiology, or assists in the treatment of cardiovascular complaints.

This volume presents an argument on the role of psychological factors in the development and maintenance of cardiovascular disease. The term "psychological" has been interpreted broadly in this context to include not only personal or social pressures and disturbances, but all forms of environmental stimulation that do not result directly in tissue damage. Essential hypertension and ischaemic heart disease are the principal disorders under scrutiny, although a certain amount of material related to stroke is also presented. The thrust of the argument is that the influence of behaviour and emotion can be documented experimentally and clinically, both in the precipitation of symptoms in the physically predisposed individual, and in the pathological processes underlying dysfunction. Furthermore, interventions resulting in changes of behaviour are valuable in the management of cardiovascular risk factors and manifest disease.

Several types of evidence, marshalled from diverse fields of research, are relevant to these claims. The book is accordingly divided into four sections. Section 1 outlines the mechanisms that might translate higher nervous stimulation into cardiovascular pathology. The primary focus is on autonomic and neuroendocrine pathways, and the manner in which these interact with other components of disease processes. However, the fact that such mechanisms are present does not mean that they are necessarily involved in the mediation of emotional and behavioural effects on the circulation.

In Section 2, the experimental approach to the problem is described. Such experiments not only demonstrate that autonomic and neuro-endocrine pathways are sensitive to psychological stimulation; they may also illustrate the severe pathological sequelae of psychological disturbance in animals, telescoping processes that take many years to operate in man. In addition, laboratory investigations of humans permit close analysis of those components of environmental stimulation and personal coping resource that are crucial in modulating cardiovascular responses.

Ultimately, the mechanisms and processes detailed in the laboratory have to be confirmed in the clinical context. The data relevant to this enterprise are outlined in Section 3. Although much psychosocial epidemiology and clinical experience is consistent with experimental observations, many of the connections are tentative. As far as essential hypertension and ischaemic heart disease are concerned, the influence of different psychological factors does not appear to be uniform. Rather, varying forms of cardiovascular dysfunction may be consequent on different aspects of behaviour or social experience. Finally in Section 4, the implications of these theories for behavioural management and intervention are outlined.

I am very happy to be able to express my gratitude to a number of colleagues who were kind enough to read and comment on various portions of the manuscript; errors, omissions and opinions are, of course, entirely my own responsibility. From St George's Hospital Medical School, Professors Michael Davies, Andrew Mathews and Brian Robinson all assisted me with their expertise in different aspects of the subject matter. Elsewhere, I am pleased to acknowledge the constructive suggestions of Professor Peter Sleight, and Drs Michael Marmot and David Woodman. I am also greatly in the debt of Dr Derek Johnston from the Department of Psychiatry at Oxford University, who selflessly ploughed through the entire manuscript, and gave his valuable help. Lastly, the assistance and encouragement of my wife Jane remain inestimable.

October, 1980   ANDREW STEPTOE

Contents

ix

SECTION 3

SECTION 4

1
Cardiovascular Disease: Risks and Mechanisms

This book is concerned with the role of psychological factors in the development of atherosclerotic disorders and high arterial pressure. Although atherosclerosis (or atheroma) occurs in most major arteries, health is threatened principally by occlusions of the coronary vessels, and the arteries serving the brain. Atherosclerosis is not a new disease —signs of arterial stenosis are found even in Egyptian mummies—but only in the twentieth century have cardiovascular disorders become the commonest cause of death in industrialised nations (McGill, 1977).

Some 45 per cent of deaths in Britain during 1975 were cardiovascular in origin, with ischaemic (coronary) heart disease alone accounting for 26 per cent (DHSS, 1976). Over the same year heart disease caused 37·8 per cent of deaths in the USA, while a further 10·3 per cent were due to strokes (National Heart, Lung and Blood Institute, 1977). To put these figures into perspective, cancers led to 19·3 per cent of deaths in the USA over the same year. The problem is thus of major proportions, despite the fact that cardiovascular mortality has actually been falling over recent years. Between 1970 and 1976, the rate for ischaemic heart disease was reduced by 15·7 per cent in the USA, while the number of fatal strokes also declined. The decreases are proportionally greater than the changes in non-cardiovascular death rates, and may reflect both improvements in coronary care, and vigorous treatment of risk factors such as high blood pressure.

Nevertheless, mortality rates are a crude index of the severity and prevalence of cardiovascular disease. A distinction can be made between latent atheroma and its clinical endpoints. Atherosclerotic lesions develop progressively with age in most peoples in the world, even though many will never manifest serious symptoms (McGill, 1968). An extensive autopsy study of men and women dying from non-cardiovascular diseases was carried out in five European towns by the

1

World Health Organisation (Kagan *et al.*, 1976a). Fibrous athero-sclerotic plaques were found in the aortae and coronary arteries of 80–90 per cent of males aged 40, and in the same proportion of females by the age of 50. Complicated and calcified lesions appeared even in 20-year-olds, increasing markedly in middle age. Much coronary disease is thus undetected, coming to medical attention only when the patient complains of episodic chest pain (angina pectoris), or suffers a myocardial infarction. Occasionally it may be discovered through the identification of cardiac arrhythmias, electrocardiographic abnormali-ties, or heart failure. Sudden cardiac death is another endpoint; definitions of this phenomenon vary, but it is generally considered to be death within a few minutes or hours of symptom onset. As will be seen later in the chapter, however, many cases of sudden cardiac death are not straightforward manifestations of ischaemic heart disease.

The pattern of cerebrovascular accidents is even more complicated, since only a proportion are due to atherosclerosis. Consequently the epidemiology is not consistent, and some of the factors associated with ischaemic heart disease are less strongly related to stroke.

This chapter is concerned with the physiological and biochemical parameters that contribute to the risk of ischaemic heart disease and stroke. These risk factors will be considered not only as statistical indices of vulnerability, but also in terms of their functional significance. Some may be related to the underlying disease processes, while others affect the onset of clinical symptoms. Many risks were first identified in retrospective and cross-sectional surveys. Several prospective investi-gations have now been reported in which examinations were carried out before the appearance of disease. The relationships with cardio-vascular disease are not identical in each population that has been studied. However, a corpus of evidence has been built up confirming the relevance of arterial blood pressure, serum cholesterol and cigarette smoking in ischaemic heart disease. These factors will thus be discussed separately, using data from the National Pooling Project (1978).

Arterial blood pressure

The Pooling Project (1978) combined results from five longitudinal studies of middle-aged white US males, including groups in Framing-ham, Chicago and Tecumseh. More than 8300 subjects were incorpor-ated into the Project, and followed up for an average of 8·6 years. Over this period, some 650 originally disease-free men suffered either a fatal or non-fatal myocardial infarction, or sudden cardiac death; the diagnostically softer end-point of angina pectoris was not considered in this analysis.

Figure 1.1 summarises the risk associated with systolic blood pressure level. Pressures have been divided into quintiles (20 per cent segments) of the whole range, rather than arbitrary normotensive and hypertensive categories. Vulnerability increases progressively with rising pressure level, so that men with readings over 150 mmHg are more than twice as likely to sustain severe clinical heart disease than those in the lowest quintile. Moderate pressures result in an intermediate level of risk, since raised morbidity is not confined to cases of clinically defined hypertension. A similar relationship has been recorded for diastolic pressure, and there is little support for the common belief that women "tolerate" high pressure better than men (**Kannel** *et al.*, 1971).

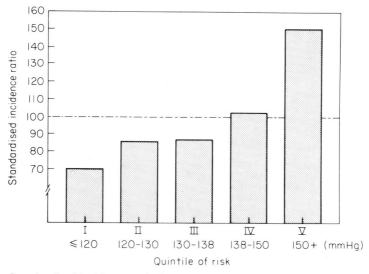

FIG. 1.1. Standardised incidence ratio for occurrence of sudden cardiac death or first myocardial infarction in middle-aged men, categorised according to initial level of systolic blood pressure (Pooling Project, 1978).

The risk of stroke also varies with arterial pressure. Figure 1.2 is derived from the Framingham study, and confirms that the incidence of cerebrovascular events grows with pressure level in both men and women. When these data were analysed by multivariate techniques, so that the contribution of arterial pressure could be evaluated independently, the correlations between systolic pressure and atherothrombotic brain infarction remained highly significant (**Kannel**, 1976).

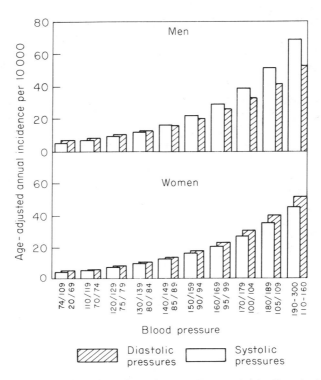

FIG. 1.2. Incidence of atherothrombotic brain infarction in the Framingham Study, categorised by sex and initial blood pressure level. Adults aged 45–74 included. (Kannel, 1976.)

These data from the USA have been substantiated by surveys in other countries (Miall and Chinn, 1974; Goldbourt *et al.*, 1975). The management of high arterial pressure is central to the prevention of morbid cardiovascular events. Antihypertensive medication has become a major preoccupation and expense in industrialised nations; in 1975, over $380 million were spent in the USA alone. Clinical trials indicate that pressure can be reduced with drugs, and that these modifications may be associated with reductions in fatal and non-fatal myocardial events (Fries, 1967, 1970; Berglund *et al.*, 1978). However, the importance of blood pressure as a risk factor should not be confused with questions about the efficacy of treatment, or the cost-effectiveness of management with drugs (Short, 1975; Weinstein and Stason, 1977). Much of this book is committed to examining the role of psychological factors in the development and maintenance of high arterial pressure. In order to do justice to the condition, it will be necessary to describe some features in the aetiology of essential hypertension, focusing on the involvement of the neocortex and central nervous system. Arterial pressure is therefore discussed in more detail in Chapter 3.

Serum cholesterol

The contribution of cholesterol concentration in the blood to ischaemic heart disease incidence has been consistently documented prospectively. Data from the Pooling Project are illustrated in Fig. 1.3; apart from the unexpectedly low incidence amongst men in the second quintile, morbidity increases with lipid concentration. There appears to be no safe cholesterol level, and the relative risk between quintiles V and I is 2·19.

The position with respect to stroke is less clear, since the epidemiological evidence is inconsistent. Kannel (1976) reported that serum cholesterol and β-lipoproteins were significantly related to stroke only in men under 55, while Paul (1971) found no general association. However, the comparison with heart disease is compromised by the

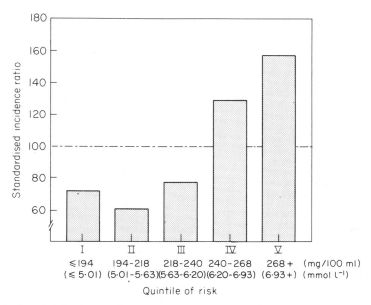

Fig. 1.3. Standardised incidence ratio for experience of sudden cardiac death or first myocardial infarction in middle-aged men, categorised according to initial level of serum cholesterol (Pooling Project, 1978).

relatively small numbers of stroke cases, and by the different types of cerebral pathology.

While the significance of serum cholesterol is generally accepted, the relevance of dietary habits and fat intake remains controversial (Sirtori *et al.*, 1975). Keys (1970) studied heart disease in seven countries, and showed positive correlations between the proportion of calories derived from saturated fatty acids in different populations, and their mean serum cholesterol concentrations. These cohort figures are shown in Table 1.1; populations with a higher proportion of saturated fatty acids have greater serum lipid values. It has consequently been argued that ·major efforts in heart disease prevention should be focused on diet and eating habits (Stamler, 1978).

TABLE 1.1

Relations between serum cholesterol concentration and percentage of total calories derived from saturated fatty acids in the diet (Keys, 1970)

Saturated fatty acids in diet (%)	Geographical region	Serum cholesterol	
		mg/100 ml	mmol l^{-1}
3	Rural Japan	170	4·39
7	Corfu	198	5·11
8	Crete	202	5·21
9	Dalmatia	186	4·81
9–10	Rural Italy	200	5·17
14	Slavonia	198	5·11
19	West Finland	253	6·54
19	Netherlands	230	5·94
22	East Finland	265	6·85

Note. Populations for which fatty acid values were estimated from dietary records rather than being determined directly are not included.

Yet it is doubtful that differences between populations may be taken as causal evidence; almost invariably, disparities can be found. For example, the Samburu tribe in Kenya eat a diet rich in saturated fats, but have low serum lipid and heart disease rates (Shaper, 1962). The samples from Corfu and Slavonia included in Table 1.1 have identical cholesterol levels, yet the saturated fats in their diets differ by a factor of two. Furthermore, the correlations between serum cholesterol and diet of individuals within populations are generally low (Keys, 1970). Stamler (1978) has argued that this may be due to inadequate data collection, so that true values of cholesterol and fat intake are not established. Others doubt the sufficiency of cross-sectional approaches to the problem (Jacobs *et al.*, 1979). Nevertheless, the lack of association within populations remains an uncomfortable fact for proponents of dietary change (Oster, 1980).

The discrepancies between fat intake and serum lipid may be due to the processes of cholesterol metabolism. Only a small proportion of the total body cholesterol circulates in the serum, the distribution being affected by the amounts synthesised, equilibration between serum and tissues, and the rate of catabolysis (Oliver, 1976). The influence of variations in diet may thus be limited, and this is consistent with experiments on diet manipulation. Vergroesen (1975) studied the effects of replacing saturated fats with the unsaturated linoleic acid. Increasing the proportion of calories derived from unsaturated fats from 20 to 35 per cent led to a significant reduction in serum cholesterol; but a further rise to 50 per cent had no added effect. Connor and Connor (1977) measured lipid levels in 25 people on cholesterol-free diets, and then when they were eating 1000 mg per day of egg yolk cholesterol. Even this gross change raised average plasma concentrations only from 211 to 247 mg/100 ml (5·45 to 6·38 mmol l^{-1}). Considering this experimental diet was well above the population average for lipids (400 to 600 mg per day), the data suggest that serum levels are heavily buffered against variations in dietary intake.

Trials of ischaemic heart disease prevention through lowering serum cholesterol with drugs or diet have yielded inconclusive results. A Finnish study of primary prevention through diet has been criticised for non-randomisation and other problems (Meittinen *et al.*, 1972; Fejfar, 1975). On the other hand, the prospective trial using clofibrate on men with relatively high serum cholesterol showed a significant reduction in non-fatal infarcts, but not in the incidence of fatal attacks and angina (Oliver, 1978). The effects of clofibrate in secondary prevention amongst patients with ischaemic heart disease are apparently minimal (Coronary Drug Project, 1975). One difficulty is that many manipulations fail to produce substantial decreases in cholesterol concentrations (Buchwald *et al.*, 1977). Thus, except in cases where saturated fat intake is very high, the effects of dietary restriction are uncertain.

Cigarette smoking

Cigarette smoking has been increasingly recognised as a major influence on heart disease. The pioneering study of smoking habits in British physicians revealed 30 per cent higher cardiac mortality amongst self-reported cigarette smokers (Doll and Hill, 1964). The association has subsequently been confirmed for men in prospective and retrospective surveys (Paffenbarger and Wing, 1969; Goldbourt *et al.*, 1975). Data from the Pooling Project are illustrated in Fig. 1.4. The relative risk for heavy smokers in comparison with non-smokers is 3·39, while light smokers sustain an intermediate rate.

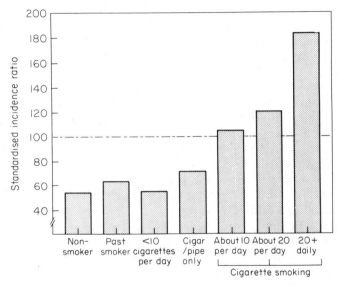

FIG. 1.4. Standardised incidence ratio for occurrence of sudden cardiac death or first myocardial infarction in middle-aged men, categorised according to smoking habits (Pooling Project, 1978).

The link is less clear for women, although this may be due in part to the size of the cohorts that have been investigated. Smoking was not an important risk in Framingham women, either for heart disease or brain infarct (Kannel *et al.*, 1971; Kannel, 1976). The effects of modifications in smoking behaviour on morbidity have yet to be tested directly; however, the data in Fig. 1.4 indicate that ex-smokers do not remain at the risk levels of those currently smoking.

Other risk factors

A number of additional characteristics, such as obesity, impaired glucose tolerance and ECG abnormalities, are linked with cardiovascular disease, and consequently figure in prospective studies of predisposing factors. Weight may be important because of its association with blood pressure, although body mass has been identified as an independent long-term element of risk (Rabkin *et al.*, 1977) (Striking differences in coronary disease are found between individuals reporting high and low levels of physical exercise (Morris *et al.*, 1973).) This factor has been explored prospectively in the longshoremen of San Francisco (Brand *et al.*, 1979) ; the incidence of fatal heart attacks was significantly greater in those with low physical work rates, after adjustment for age, race, smoking, body mass and ECG disturbances. It is possible that lack of exercise impairs haemodynamic function, and contributes to chronic caloric imbalance.

It should be emphasised that epidemiological surveys are concerned with identifying the factors that best predict the incidence of cardio-vascular disease. This does not necessarily mean that these indices are directly involved in the disease process, or that they should be the primary targets of intervention or prevention. From this brief summary, it is apparent that behaviour contributes directly to cardiovascular disorders in several important ways. Cigarette smoking, fatty diet and inadequate exercise are all problems of behaviour, not illnesses or organic dysfunctions. The most fruitful approaches to their modification may be through changing behaviour, and not medical interventions. Thus even before the possibility of an independent psychological influence is discussed, the behavioural dimensions of cardiac problems are clear.

However, psychosocial vulnerability need not even be considered, if the known biological risks account for all cases. The prevalence and interaction between factors should therefore be considered.

The prevalence of risk factors

People are more likely to suffer from some atherosclerotic disease when they are at risk on more than a single dimension. Although the indices described in earlier sections are independent of each other, they combine to produce much greater chances of illness. The pattern varies with different cardiovascular dysfunctions. Thus the association between stroke and blood pressure may be unaffected by cholesterol, while arterial pressure, cholesterol and smoking all interact in the case of ischaemic heart disease (Paul, 1971). Figure 1.5, derived from the Pooling Project, divides the population into quintiles of combined risk on diastolic pressure, cholesterol and smoking. People in the highest 20 per cent are nearly six times more vulnerable than those in quintile 1.

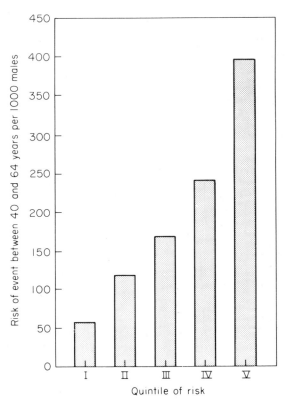

F<small>IG</small>. 1.5. Risk of coronary disease (sudden cardiac death, fatal and non-fatal first myocardial infarction) in middle-aged men, according to combined status on diastolic blood pressure, serum cholesterol and smoking. Rate per 1000 individuals. (Pooling Project, 1978.)

Incidence has been plotted in terms of the number of first events occurring in men aged between 40 and 64; an excess of 337·8 cases per 1000 men over 24 years is attributable to these factors.

Prospective epidemiological studies indicate that it is quite rare for an individual who does not score high on two or three factors to develop ischaemic heart disease. In the Pooling Project, the 20 per cent in the highest multiple risk quintile sustained 40 per cent of major first coronary events. However, a substantial number of cases are not completely accounted for by known factors. For example, the incidence of coronary disease in Framingham is twice as high as that in Honolulu and Puerto Rico, even after allowing for cholesterol, blood pressure and smoking (Gordon *et al.*, 1974).

Another point about cardiovascular vulnerability should be emphasised; ischaemic heart disease is far from universal, even in the presence of risks. It can be estimated from Fig. 1.5 that some 60 per cent of men in the highest quintile will remain disease-free over the 24-year period. Using a different data base, Oliver (1976) calculated that although people at risk on the three major factors sustain eight times more cardiac disease over a decade than those not displaying these characteristics, the incidence is still only 17 per cent; thus 83 per cent of "high risk" subjects survive throughout that time. Tibblin (1969) studied 834 men born in Gothenburg during 1913, 23 of whom later suffered myocardial infarction. All the victims scored positively on at least one of four major risk factors, but then so did 771 of the remainder.

There are two implications of these patterns. Firstly, additional chronic influences may make independent contributions, combining with known risks to potentiate the danger to certain individuals. Secondly, the elements that provoke or trigger clinical symptoms may be different from those involved in atheroma. Since atherosclerosis is itself widespread in the population, it is possible that acute processes are superimposed on the long-term mechanisms in people who develop diagnosed heart disease. These alternatives can be clarified by identifying the ways in which risk factors operate.

Risk factors and atherogenesis

The evidence already outlined points to associations between risks and cardiovascular morbidity. While some of the linkages may be purely correlational, other parameters are significant in the disease process itself. The principal component of atheroma is the raised plaque, an irregular thickening of the intimal layer of the vessel wall, projecting into the lumen. Plaques are characterised by connective tissue, extra and intracellular lipid accumulation, and smooth muscle cells. They cause stenosis and narrowing of the lumen, and when complicated by thrombus, may actually occlude an artery.

A number of years ago it was hypothesised that the non-raised fatty streaks present in the arterial vessel walls from childhood onwards were precursors of atheroma. Their association with later pathology is not certain, however. The distribution of fatty streaks in the arterial tree is different from that of raised plaques, as is the pattern of lipid deposition. Fatty streaks are not consistently related to diet, serum

lipids or other factors linked with atheroma (McGill, 1977). Furthermore, there are ethnic variations in plaques that are not associated with
the frequency of fatty streaks (Mitchell and Schwartz, 1965).

The lipid deposits in atheroma are thought to derive from the
"insudation" of circulating lipoproteins. Support for this theory comes
from several sources, including chemical analysis of arterial extracts,
the detection of specific antigens by immunofluoresence, and the injection of autologous labelled lipoproteins (Walton, 1975). Lipid
enters the arterial wall in low density (β) and very low density (VLD)
lipoprotein fractions, and is shed by these unstable molecules. Once in
the deposit, cholesterol metabolism is extremely slow, so that equilibration with the plasma does not occur, and lipid is accumulated.
Lipid deposition is coupled with smooth muscle proliferation in the
lesion. These cells are apparently monoclonal in character, although
the significance of this finding is unclear (Benditt, 1976).

The other important process that may act in concert with lipid insudation in atherogenesis and the development of arterial stenosis is
thrombus formation. The thrombus is an aggregation of platelets,
fibrin strands and leucocytes. While there has been much controversy
over the significance of the mechanism, it is probable that thrombi,
developing in response to localised injury, may be incorporated into
plaque. This is reflected in the stratified appearance of plaques, which
suggests repeated deposition of thrombus elements (Chandler and
Pope, 1975). The role of platelets in the initiation of thrombogenesis
will be described in Chapter 2.

Coronary atheroma is not inevitably followed by symptoms of
ischaemia. When the disease is expressed clinically, it may emerge as
angina, myocardial infarction or sudden cardiac death. The pattern is
further complicated by the different forms of infarction. A regional or
segmental infarction results from reduction in flow through one major
coronary artery. According to animal experiments, deprivation of
blood for as little as 10 minutes can cause myocardial necrosis (Davies,
1977). Some authorities argue that severe stenosis alone can precipitate
a regional infarct, while others consider that total occlusion by a combination of thrombus and atheroma is required. The reported incidence
of occlusive thrombi in acute infarction varies widely between laboratories, probably reflecting variations of definition and research technique (Davies *et al.*, 1976). Certainly, thromboemboli are important
complications in the period immediately following infarction, being
particularly common amongst patients with elevated plasma fibrinogen
levels (Fulton and Duckett, 1976). In contrast to the regional infarct,
subendocardial necrosis may follow reduction in overall coronary flow,

and failure to perfuse subendocardial tissue. This type of infarct is associated with triple vessel disease, and lesions are diffuse. Factors that impair myocardial perfusion, such as left ventricular failure and aortic valve disease, may also promote subendocardial necrosis. The different forms of infarct are, however, commonly found in combination (Davies, 1977).

The serum cholesterol concentration is directly involved in atherogenesis through its relationship with lipid insudation. Smith and Slater (1973) analysed blood samples taken during the week before death, and were able to demonstrate high positive correlations between intimal lipoprotein and serum cholesterol levels. The VLD lipoproteins are secreted from the liver parenchyma at a rate directly dependent on the output of hepatic triglycerides, and free fatty acid (FFA) availability; hence, high levels of triglycerides in the plasma are also associated with ischaemic heart disease (Brown *et al.*, 1965). Serum cholesterol has an additional role as an intimal irritant, promoting connective tissue responses and fibrous thickening in the plaque.

Arterial pressure, too, is implicated functionally in atherogenesis, and it is not simply a correlational risk. The endothelial surface is sensitive to blood flow sheer, and may be damaged by the stress of high arterial pressures. This mechanical effect is reflected in the distribution of atheroma through the arterial tree, since lesions are more common in regions exposed to high pressure (Mitchell and Schwartz, 1965). The endothelial damage promotes atheroma, since it increases the permeability of the vessel wall, facilitating the flux of lipoproteins (Fry, 1973). With extremes in arterial pressure, actual separation of endothelial cells can occur. Intimal damage also allows platelets to adhere on exposed basement membrane, initiating thrombus formation.

The mechanism by which cigarette smoking influences atherogenesis has been less easy to identify. Nicotine releases catecholamines, which have powerful effects on platelet aggregation and adhesion, as will be seen in Chapter 2. Carbon monoxide acts to increase endothelial permeability, and carboxyhaemoglobin concentration has been associated with risk of atherosclerotic disease in smokers (Wald *et al.*, 1973; Kjeldson, 1975). Thus it is possible that carbon monoxide also contributes to the association between smoking and cardiovascular disorders.

These data indicate that the major risk factors are involved in the atherosclerotic disease process itself. However, it is evident that clinical symptoms are not an inevitable consequence of atheroma. In the case of sudden cardiac death, there may be functional irregularities superimposed on the vulnerable diseased state of the myocardium.

Sudden cardiac death

Sudden cardiac death represents a major problem in its own right, accounting as it does for a considerable proportion of fatalities each year. It is associated with ischaemic heart disease, since advanced stenosis is almost universal amongst victims (Lovegrove and Thompson, 1978). Freisinger *et al.* (1970) were able to demonstrate a direct relationship between the extent of coronary occlusion identified angiographically in cardiac patients and subsequent mortality.

However, sudden cardiac death cannot be considered simply as the last stage of progressive heart disease, when the coronary arteries are finally occluded completely by plaque and thrombi, leading to ischaemia and infarction. In a large proportion of cases, no acute infarction or occlusion is found (Davies, 1977). The incidence of acute pathological events varies between series. Thus Baroldi (1969) identified coronary occlusions in less than 50 per cent of cases, and stenosis derived from old plaque rather than fresh deposits. Others have reported occlusive thrombi in as few as 20 per cent of sudden cardiac deaths (Kuller *et al.*, 1975). Similarly, acute regional infarcts are the exception rather than the rule, with a frequency near 20 per cent (Reichenbach *et al.*, 1977; Lovegrove and Thompson, 1978). Patients who are resuscitated from sudden death commonly show no signs of infarction (Cobb *et al.*, 1975).

The absence of acute lesions in many cases suggests that the event precipitating death is functional in origin, and not necrosis or a change in the geometry of coronary arteries. Both in the presence and absence of acute occlusions, the most common immediate cause of sudden death is ventricular fibrillation (Verrier and Lown, 1978; Crampton and Schwartz, 1978). Ventricular fibrillation is an electrical phenomenon which rarely occurs in the absence of ischaemia, but is at the same time not primarily dependent on structural changes to the myocardium. Consequently electrical disturbances, reflected in ECG abnormalities such as the long QT syndrome and ST segment deviation, predict sudden cardiac death in survivors of ventricular fibrillation. Coronary patients with ventricular arrhythmias are at special risk for early death (Kitchin and Pocock, 1977). There is also evidence that asymptomatic ventricular disturbances, detected for example during screening, may increase the individual's vulnerability (Hinkle *et al.*, 1969; Fisher and Tyroler, 1973; Calvert *et al.*, 1977).

Thus cardiac morbidity does not directly reflect the degree of arterial disease, and the mechanisms that provoke electrical instability and ventricular fibrillation have a special importance. Functional disturbances, which have no effect on atheroma, may be involved in the manifestation of ischaemic heart disease.

Cerebrovascular disease

The aetiology of cerebrovascular diseases, and its relation to risk factors is complicated by the range of disorders that can provoke damage. While brain infarctions may result from atheroma and embolisms of either intra- or extra-cranial origin, other cases of stroke do not involve arterial stenosis at all. Thus, cerebral haemorrhage is thought to be due to the rupture of microaneurysms developing on the small arterial branches of the cerebrum. These aneurysms are independent of atheroma, so that the risks associated with intracerebral haemorrhage differ from those predicting infarction. Only high arterial pressure and age, from amongst the standard factors, are linked with haemorrhage (Cole and Yates, 1967). Although infarctions with thrombosis predominate in most populations, there are wide variations in the proportion of strokes due to haemorrhage and other disorders (Kagan *et al.*, 1976b; Kurtzke, 1976).

Arterial pressure is the one risk factor that is associated strongly with most forms of stroke, since it increases vulnerability to non-sclerotic disorders as well as to infarction. Microaneurysms contain deposits of fats and fibrin, and accumulations are promoted by the mechanical distensions generated by high pressures (Ross Russell, 1975). In animals, lesions in the blood–brain barrier can be provoked experimentally by hypertension, leading to regional cerebral damage (Dinsdale *et al.*, 1976). Hypertensive vascular spasms or encephalopathy may be due to breakdowns in cerebral vascular regulatory mechanisms, following phases of high arterial pressure (Meyer *et al.*, 1976). Hypertension may also facilitate the mechanisms of platelet aggregation, and these are receiving increased attention in stroke pathology (Agnoli and Fazio, 1977).

Brain infarctions are frequently associated with thrombi. An arterial mural thrombus may fragment, producing emboli of platelets and fibrin that travel to smaller vessels and block the cerebral microcirculation; cases have been reported in which thrombi at the carotid bifurcation were dislodged, causing transient ischaemia and temporary blindness (Gunning *et al.*, 1964). But the comparatively low incidence of strokes has prevented identification of multiple risk factors with any precision, and prospective surveys have to be supplemented by retrospective and single case reports (Bell and Symon, 1979). As in the case of sudden cardiac death, cerebrovascular events may be related to long-term atheroma, while having a number of distinctive immediate causes.

Summary and conclusions

The gravity of the problem of cardiovascular disease in the world today has been outlined. Blood pressure, serum cholesterol concentration and cigarette smoking are among the factors linked to ischaemic heart disease and stroke. Research into atherogenesis suggests that the role of these risks is not simply correlative, but functional.

However, the factors identified in epidemiological research do not account for all cases; furthermore, many people at high risk remain free of coronary disease. A distinction must be drawn between latent atheroma, and the processes eliciting clinical manifestations and symptoms. Atherogenesis may continue undetected in an individual, unless sudden cardiac death, myocardial infarction or anginal pain develop; the mechanisms triggering these disease states are distinct, and superimposed on those promoting atheroma.

Psychological and behaviour factors may contribute to this complex pattern in several ways:

a. They may have indirect effects through the standard risk factors. Many of the subsequent chapters are concerned with essential hypertension, since arterial pressure has persistently been revealed as a crucial element of cardiovascular disturbance. Some risks, such as cigarette smoking and lack of exercise, are themselves behaviours, while psychological interventions may be appropriate for dealing with others — including diet and weight.

b. The psychosocial environment, behaviour or personality may influence the disease process directly, and a great deal of research has been focused on this possibility. The link may be chronic — affecting the development of progressive vascular disease, or acute — triggering the crisis that provokes clinical symptoms in an individual already at risk through stenosis.

The roles of emotion and behaviour are evaluated in later chapters. Higher nervous factors are likely to be mediated by neural, humoral and endocrine mechanisms. Chapters 2 and 3 therefore identify cerebral influences on cardiovascular regulation, and outline the pathways that might modulate pathological dysfunctions.

2
Neural and Endocrine Factors in Cardiovascular Control

The regulation of arterial pressure and tissue blood flow

A full description of the factors involved in the maintenance of an adequate circulation has not been attempted here, since the interactions between structural, humoral and nervous elements are highly complex. The discussion is focused on the pathways that might mediate psychological influences on the heart and circulation; the role of the central nervous system in regulation, and in the release of vasoactive humoral agents, has therefore been emphasised.

Guyton (1978) summarised the principle goals of cardiovascular regulation as the maintenance of arterial pressure, and the control of local tissue blood supply. The flow to each vascular bed must be sufficient to satisfy metabolic requirements, and remove waste products. The need for oxygen and other fuels is not constant, but depends on the rate of cellular metabolism, and the activity level in each tissue.

Demands on the circulation are consequently integrated into the overall programme of actions, and vary with sleeping, eating, fighting and other behaviours.

Tissues themselves are able to maintain constant blood flow in the face of changes in perfusion pressure through an intrinsic capacity for "autoregulation". This response of the vascular smooth muscle to local conditions involves both physical and metabolic factors. Thus a rise in blood flow increases delivery of oxygen, and removes vasodilator metabolites at a faster rate, precipitating compensatory vasoconstriction. The physical component operates through properties inherent in the cells of vessel walls, since in order to sustain a constant tension in the wall, elevations of distending pressure are countered by reductions in vessel diameter (Law of Laplace). The power of autoregulation is demonstrated in cases of coarctation of the aorta, where an obstruction in the aorta causes relatively high arterial pressures in the upper part of the body, and low or normal pressure below the constriction. Wakim *et al.* (1948) found that flow in the arms and legs of patients was within normal limits, despite pressure in the upper limbs being some 50 per cent higher than the lower limbs; autoregulatory vaso-constriction had adjusted flow in the face of differing perfusion pressures.

In some vascular beds, these local factors determine flow almost entirely, so that blood supply is relatively unaffected by neural tone. This appears to be true of the brain, although the role of vasomotor nerves in the control of cerebral flow may be more significant than generally acknowledged (Purves, 1978). Local properties predominate in the regulation of flow through other tissues only under certain con-ditions. Thus blood supply to resting striate muscle beds is modulated by extrinsic neural and humoral influences. However, during heavy exercise, increased flow is prompted in large measure by the metabolic demands of the tissues, and the importance of vasoconstrictor tone diminishes.

The sympathetic branch of the autonomic nervous system is widely involved in cardiovascular control. Noradrenaline is the transmitter at sympathetic terminals, but adrenergic receptors are conventionally categorised into two groups on the basis of pharmacological evidence. The α receptors are distributed in the smooth muscle of blood vessel walls, and stimulation promotes vasoconstriction. Phenylephrine sel-ectively stimulates α-receptor sites, while traffic is inhibited by the competitive antagonist phentolamine. In contrast, β-adrenergic stimulation results in dilatation of skeletal and coronary arterioles, in-creases in the rate and force of cardiac activity, and augmentation of lipolysis and insulin release. The numerous β antagonists include propranolol, and isoproterenol is an antagonist with relatively pure adrenergic action.

Sympathetic stimulation may also lead to discharge of the catecho-lamines adrenaline and noradrenaline from the adrenal medulla. The medulla comprises about 10 per cent by weight of the adrenal glands, and consists almost entirely of catecholamine-secreting chromaffin cells. On stimulation, stored catecholamines are released, while syn-thesis is augmented by increasing the production of catalysing enzymes. These enzymes, in particular dopamine-β-hydroxylase (DβH), and phenylethanolamine-N-methyltransferase (PNMT), are therefore sometimes measured as incides of sympathetic activity (Noth and Mulrow, 1976; Perlman and Chalfie, 1977). Some 80 per cent of adrenomedullary secretions in man are in the form of adrenaline, while the remainder is noradrenaline; the precise proportions of the two depend however on the species studied.

The catecholamines mirror and extend the circulatory responses to sympathetic stimulation. Noradrenaline has the more profound pressor effect, since it produces vasoconstriction in most vascular beds, while adrenaline dilates skeletal muscle vessels. Both agents may increase myocardial contractility and heart rate. Nevertheless, the pattern of cardiovascular response varies with the rate and duration of secretion. Thus while circulating noradrenaline causes vasoconstriction directly, it induces a secondary dilatation by promoting local metabolism.

Since some noradrenaline overflows from sympathetic terminals into the plasma, it is difficult to distinguish adrenal medullary responses from those due to direct nervous inputs. When the agent 6-hydroxydopamine (6-OHDA) is injected, peripheral noradrenergic terminals are destroyed without affecting the adrenal medulla. After such treatment, the adrenal output of catecholamines is augmented; however under basal conditions, vascular competence is maintained primarily by sympathetic traffic (de Champlain and von Ameringen, 1973).

It is relevant to later discussions of psychological factors to note that catecholamine release and action are partially dependent on the output of corticosteroids from the adrenal cortex. The interaction takes two forms. Firstly, the metabolism of the medullary enzymes DβH and PNMT is modulated permissively by glucocorticoids (Ciaranello *et al.*, 1976). In the second place, corticosteroids play a part in maintaining vascular reactivity to catecholamines; following adrenalectomy, responsiveness is reduced, but can be restored by injecting corticosteroids (Drew and Leach, 1971). Thus two of the major pathways sensitive to psychological influence are mutually dependent (see also p. 34).

In many species, vascular innervation is not restricted to adrenergic vasoconstrictor fibres, since active dilatation in muscle beds is facilitated cholinergically. The evidence for active neurogenic vasodilatation in the skeletal muscles of man is largely indirect, as these tracts have been difficult to isolate in primates (Greenfield, 1966). Yet cholinergic vasodilatation may be important in the response to psychosocial stimulation, influencing the pattern of blood flow distribution.

Apart from the catecholamines, other humoral agents are also involved in the control of peripheral vascular tone. Renin is synthesised in the kidney, and stored in granules within the juxtaglomerular cells that surround the renal afferent arteriole. On secretion from the kidney, renin acts on the renin substrate in the plasma to form angiotensin I. Although inactive itself, angiotensin I is converted into angiotensin II, a potent vasoconstrictor, and the stimulant of aldosterone from the adrenal cortex.

The renin–angiotensin system is partially governed by negative feedback loops in the periphery; thus circulating angiotensin suppresses juxtaglomerular activity. However, the central nervous system is also crucially involved in renin release (Davis and Freeman, 1976). This influence takes several forms. Sympathetic vasoconstrictor tone, mediated α adrenergically, modulates pressure in the afferent arterioles, which in turn stimulates renal vascular receptors. The sympathetic nervous system also acts directly (via β-adrenergic mechanisms) on the juxtaglomerular apparatus, while receptors in the macula densa may be sensitive to glomerular filtration rate (Bühler *et al.*, 1972).

The kidney is concerned in cardiovascular dynamics in another important way. The overall fluid balance of the body is maintained by pressure diuresis, which in turn regulates blood volume. A rise in renal pressure above the normal level causes an increase in water and electrolyte output, while excretion is reduced after a fall in pressure. The mechanism is extremely sensitive, so that a change of only a few millimeters in arterial pressure will lead to an alteration of more than 50 per cent in urinary excretion (Thompson and Pitts, 1952). Although the effects of pressure diuresis are clouded by autoregulatory compensation, the kidney is inevitably involved in sustaining lasting changes in arterial pressure (Guyton *et al.*, 1972).

Autonomic nervous influences on the heart

The vascular control mechanisms discussed in the last section depend on the maintenance of a pressure head sufficient to drive blood into the smaller vessels. Arterial pressure is in turn affected by regional flow, as vascular resistance in each tissue contributes to the total peripheral resistance, while pressure diuresis modulates blood volume. The third major factor in the support of an adequate circulation is the function of the heart.

Both the sympathetic and parasympathetic branches of the autonomic nervous system project efferent fibres to the heart, and the two tracts have opposing actions. Sympathetic stimulation increases heart rate, and contractions occur with added force. These effects are mediated by β-adrenergic receptors. The pattern of contractile (inotropic) and frequency (chronotropic) response depends on the duration and intensity of stimulation. Thus Liard and his colleagues (1976) observed an immediate increase in blood pressure, cardiac output and heart rate on stellate ganglion stimulation of conscious dogs. Yet when the procedure was continued for seven days, cardiac output did not remain elevated, but peripheral resistance rose to sustain the hypertension. In the same way, noradrenaline infusion augments cardiac performance acutely, while peripheral resistance slowly increases with long-term transfusion (Moss *et al*, 1966).

Contrasting responses follow vagal stimulation, since the heart rate is slowed. The tonic activity and interactions between the cardiac sympathetic and parasympathetic fibres differ between species (Levy, 1977). Animals such as the squirrel monkey have high resting sympathetic tone, while the vagus dominates in dog and man. Thus in humans, strong vagal stimulation generally overrides sympathetic inputs; furthermore, the "intrinsic heart rate", assessed after complete autonomic blockade, is higher than the normal resting frequency, reflecting tonic inhibition by the vagus. Such species differences are significant, as they affect the responsiveness of autonomic pathways during psychosocial stimulation.

Feedback processes and the cardiovascular system

The regulatory factors outlined in the last sections are functionally linked by a series of feedback loops, designed to maintain stable arterial pressure. Each loop has its own time course and sensitivity, operating maximally over a different range of pressure. Circulatory function is corrected through the efferent pathways already described, while the feedback mechanisms are activated by receptors responsive to particular types of cardiovascular disturbance (Coleridge and Coleridge, 1980).

The most rapid response to changes in pressure is countered by the baroreceptor reflex. The baroreceptors are found in the walls of the carotid sinuses, aortic arch, and other pulsatile regions of the system. They are sensitive to stretch, and are also influenced by local ionic balance (Kezdi, 1977). They are excited at normal levels of arterial pressure, responding to the distortion of the vessel wall induced by the fluid bulk. Since flow is pulsatile, the output from the receptors is phasic, as may be seen in Fig. 2.1. The afferent activity from the baroreceptors is thus closely associated with the instantaneous state of the circulation, and larger deviations in pressure lead to recruitment of more units. Information from the units is integrated with the efferent

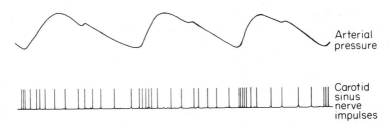

Fig. 2.1. Schematic outline of the relationship between carotid baroreceptor discharge and variations in systemic arterial pressure.

arm of the reflex in the central nervous system; the resultant feedback loop acts to sustain pressure at a uniform level. Thus an increase in arterial pressure is compensated by bradycardia, and a reduction of vasoconstrictor tone.

The baroreflex is a rapidly acting, short-term feedback loop, and serves to counter immediate fluctuations in pressure. Although destruction of the brainstem regions responsible for baroreflex action leads to fulminating hypertension in some animals, deafferentation of the reflex generally has little lasting effect on pressure level (Reis *et al.*, 1977). Cowley *et al.* (1973) showed that denervation in the dog led to a great increase in the variability of pressure, without altering mean values; the cardiovascular system became more responsive, since short-term fluctuations were poorly buffered.

Receptors that are sensitive to the chemical constituents of the blood are also present at several sites. Reflexes mediated by the chemoreceptors, and by central ischaemia, are particularly important at low levels of arterial pressure and during hypoxia, when oxygen supply is deficient. In addition, elements that respond to mechanical stimulation have been found in the atria and ventricles of the heart. Their role has yet to be fully explored; however, they too direct afferent impulses to the higher integrating centres. When variations in pressure are sustained, these neural reflexes are reinforced by other feedback loops. The renin- angiotensin system is stimulated by pressure reduction, while vascular and volume regulation mechanisms may also be mobilised. Thus in a condition of prolonged pressure imbalance such as essential hypertension, each control pathway may be involved at a different stage.

Since so many elements are concerned in regulation, the manner in which they interlock becomes crucial. Integration is effected in the central nervous system, and it is there that psychological state and behaviour may have an impact on circulatory control.

Central integration of regulatory mechanisms

The traditional accounts of central cardiovascular integration conceive of a series of vasomotor or cardiovascular centres in the brainstem. Each might be identified by the type of response (e.g. pressor or depressor) elicited through local stimulation or lesion, and regulation could then be explained in terms of the balance between different centres.

However, it has become apparent that such a picture is incomplete (Korner, 1971; Hilton, 1975). Although cardiovascular reactions can be separated experimentally with selective stimulation, in practice the system is complexly integrated. It may be misleading to delineate a "centre" for increases in arterial pressure (itself a multidetermined variable), or one for controlling heart rate. Despite the important role of the brainstem in regulation, circulatory control can be demonstrated after its destruction. Thus the chronically isolated spinal cord can sustain arterial pressure, while lesions in the brainstem "pressor centre" do not abolish the ability of the organism to support an adequate blood supply (Koizumi and Brooks, 1972).

It is more fruitful to consider cardiovascular activity as integrated longitudinally by the central nervous system into more general patterns of adjustment (Hilton and Spyer, 1980). Vegetative reactions are not isolated, but are essential correlates of the organism's behavioural output. The medullary zones may not be independent centres, rather regions through which biologically significant tracts pass. This neural traffic between brainstem and higher regions is two way, and involves both ascending and descending transmission.

The organisation of the baroreceptor reflex illustrates the extent to which concepts of brainstem control centres have to be modified. The primary neurons from the receptors terminate on the nucleus of the tractus solitarius (NTS). The NTS exerts a negative, inhibitory influence on the regions modulating vasomotor tone; it also connects with vagal nuclei, thereby affecting parasympathetic output (Palkovits and Zorborszky, 1977). Stimulation of the NTS causes frequency dependent hypotension and bradycardia, presumably by depressing sympathetic discharge while augmenting vagal tone (DeJong *et al.*, 1977b). Conversely, interruption of NTS output will inactivate the baroreflex, leading to chronic pressure lability.

However, there is abundant evidence that interventions higher in the brain can modify baroreceptor activity. Hilton (1963) examined the baroreflex while stimulating cats in the anterior hypothalamus. Following 10 s. of current, the reflex was completely suppressed, due to central inhibition rather than alterations in receptor threshold. A number of experiments were carried out by Gebber and Snyder (1970) to determine the mechanism of this inhibition. They concluded that the reflex was overridden both by increased sympathetic output and by attenuation of vagal activity. In contrast, stimulation at the level of the amygdala heightened vagal tone, and enhanced the bradycardia (Gebber and Klevans, 1972). The nearby septal region appeared to modulate amygdaloid activation. Thus limbic and hypothalamic factors interact dynamically in the production of the cardiovascular response. Similar work is now in progress on elaborating the role of higher brain structures in other basic reflexes, such as those associated with the chemoreceptors (Zanchetti, 1976).

It is significant that the hypothalamus is involved in cardiovascular regulation, since the importance of the region in the integration of behaviour, neuroendocrine and vegetative reactions has long been known. Hypothalamic stimulation provokes catecholamine secretion,

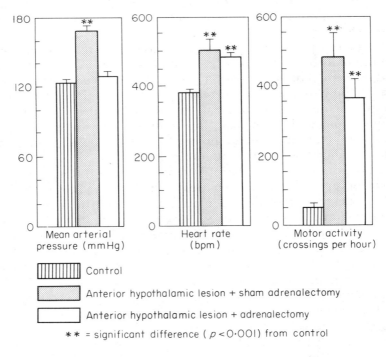

Fig. 2.2. Effects of bilateral denervation of the adrenal glands on changes in arterial pressure, heart rate, and motor activity produced by anterior hypothalamic lesions. Means $\pm$ S.E. are plotted. (Reis *et al.*, 1976.)

and selective release of adrenaline and noradrenaline has been elicited with electrodes located at the appropriate sites (Folkow and Von Euler, 1954). It is even possible to distinguish the neural and adrenomedullary components of sympathetic excitation at this level (Reis *et al.*, 1976). Fig. 2.2 summarises results from an experiment in which rats with bilateral lesions in the anterior hypothalamus developed hypertension, accompanied by motor agitation and tachycardia. The pressure rise, and not the other components of the response, was abolished by adrenal denervation or removal. Similarly, stimulation of the anterior hypothalamus evoked pressor reactions after 6-OHDA treatment; in both cases, the pressure elevation may have been due to the vaso-constrictor influence of circulating catecholamines, mediated via α-adrenergic receptors.

The central nervous system not only affects haemodynamics through modulating peripheral vasomotor tone and cardiac innervation, but by altering kidney function. Brainstem stimulation facilitates renin release, as well as inducing renal vasoconstriction. The interrelation between these responses was examined in a series of experiments that are illustrated in Fig. 2.3 (Richardson *et al.*, 1974). When the kidney was denervated (Study A), stimulation of the brainstem failed to alter either renal blood flow or renin release, indicating the neural origin of the reactions. However, after α-adrenergic blockade of the intact kidney (Study B), renin increased on stimulation, despite the abolition of vasoconstriction. On the other hand, β blockade (Study C) inhibited renin without affecting blood flow. Hence the two components of the renal response are transmitted through α- and β-receptor pathways, both of which originate centrally. Furthermore, it appears that much of the vasomotor effect of angiotensin is mediated centrally. Infusions of angiotensin in the dog have direct effects on the brainstem control regions, promoting sympathetic vasoconstriction (Ferrario *et al.*, 1972). Hypothalamic stimulation can alter renin output as well (Zanchetti *et al.*, 1977).

The responses to hypothalamic interventions have behavioural as well as neuroendocrine and vascular components. One of the first integrated behavioural–vegetative action patterns to be examined in detail was the defence reaction (Bard, 1960). It may be elicited by stimulating the medial forebrain bundle in the lateral hypothalamus and midbrain of the cat. Behaviourally, the response includes alerting, head turning, piloerection, hissing and flattening of the ears. Con-committant increases in cardiac performance, visceral vasoconstriction and muscle vasodilatation are observed. The long-term consequences of activation were documented by Folkow and Rubinstein (1966);

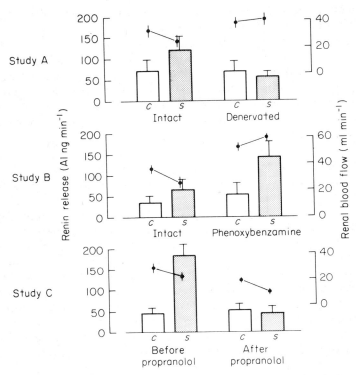

Fɪɢ. 2.3. Summary of experiments on the effects of brainstem stimulation on renin release (histograms) and renal bloodflow. In each case *c* = control values; *s* = response to stimulation. Study A (top) – denervated kidney; Study B (middle) – α-adrenergic blockade of intact kidney; Study C (bottom) – β-adrenergic blockade of intact kidney. (Zanchetti *et al.*, 1977.)

although the electric current levels were so low that no behaviour modifications were observable, repeated stimulation in the lateral hypothalamus of rats resulted in the development of fixed hypertension.

Other integrated behavioural–circulatory patterns, such as those associated with sleep, diving, feeding, orienting and exercise, have been identified, although few have been examined in detail. The hypothalamus does not, however, modulate brainstem mechanisms and circulatory output in an unrestricted way, since it is subject to higher control. The limbic system, a rich source of responses, is closely associated with emotional behaviour; yet it can be argued that not only emotional, but cognitive factors are involved in cardiovascular pathology. Evidence for cerebral cortical influences on circulatory dynamics has been collected in both animals and man.

Cerebral cortical influences on circulatory control

Cortical functions are commonly explored experimentally with lesions and electrical stimulation. In the last decades of the nineteenth century, several laboratories reported that cerebral cortical stimulation might modify blood pressure and heart rate (Hoff *et al.*, 1963). These observations were doubted, and it was suggested that responses were due to spread of the current into subcortical regions. Yet Hoff and Green (1936) later carried out careful studies on etherised animals, and demonstrated a range of haemodynamic adjustments following interventions in the motor cortex. The responses that are observed under anaesthesia are now considered to be unrepresentative, since pathways may be differentially suppressed; nevertheless, the modifications after cortical stimulation have since been confirmed in alert animals. Delgado (1960) exploited chronic monkey preparations, producing changes of blood pressure or heart rate selectively, and even provoking ventricular extrasystoles. Both pressor and depressor responses were observed, together with renal vasoconstriction of a severity sufficient to precipitate ischaemia and tubule damage.

The elimination of artefactual changes in vasomotor tone continues to present methodological problems however. For example, Clarke *et al.* (1968) argued that stimulation of the motor cortex elicited vasodilatation in skeletal beds independently of striate muscle tone. When movements were blocked pharmacologically, or by section of the spinal nerves, regional blood flow was still modified by cortical stimulation. Yet after Hilton and colleagues (1979) had taken special precautions to avoid contaminating sources of cardiovascular response, they only observed skeletal vasodilation secondarily to muscle contraction. Nevertheless, it is probable that a wide range of haemodynamic adjustments can result from interventions in the neocortex. These effects are not simply consequences of generalised autonomic activation, since precisely differentiated adjustments may be elicited. Commonly the responses are more specific than those from lower structures, while the thresholds for stimulation are higher (Hoff *et al.*, 1963). The descending anatomical connections that translate such effects were explored by Wall and Davis (1951). Three distinct pathways from different cortical regions were identified. Stimulation of the somatomotor area provoked pressure changes through tracts that bypassed the hypothalamus, although responses were abolished after lesions of the pyramidal fibres. On the other hand, modifications elicited from the postorbital surface were mediated hypothalamically. A third pathway, descending from the anterior temporal cortex, was independent of both the hypothalamus and the pyramidal tract. Large, prolonged changes in pressure, often associated with respiratory responses, could be evoked through this temporopontine bundle. While the significance of these different mechanisms for normal regulation is not known, their existence reflects the complexity of neocortical influences on the circulation.

Cortical involvement in human cardiovascular reflexes

There have been occasional opportunities to study the cardiovascular responses to direct stimulation of the neocortex in man as well. Chapman *et al.* (1950) investigated patients undergoing lobotomy or cortical excisions, and provoked reactions analagous to those seen in lower animals. Thus pressor changes, with and without respiratory adjuncts, were elicited from frontal and temporal areas. Parallel results emerged from Goldstein's (1942) classic series of brain injured patients, where either generalised or specific modifications in haemodynamics were observed.

Such methods cannot be used in healthy humans; moreover, electrical stimulation may provoke atypical responses, as the levels of current will differ from those present during normal brain function. Yet it is not easy to show the selective influence of the cortex from intact organisms, since cardiovascular reactions are commonly components of integrated programmes of behaviour and vegetative adjustment.

However, some modifications of basic circulatory reflexes by cognitive activity have been demonstrated in man. For example, the sensitivity of the baroreflex alters during performance of mental arithmetic (Brooks *et al.*, 1978). Similarly, the degree of bradycardia elicited by breath holding under water (the diving reflex) may be attenuated by mental work. This was documented by the author, collaborating with Alvin Ross, during a study in which volunteers held their breath for 60 second trials (Ross and Steptoe, 1980). Breath holding was carried out in air, and during face immersion in 15°C water, and on half the trials mental arithmetic was performed at the same time. Essential results are plotted in Fig. 2.4. Although some heart rate changes were registered on breath holding in air, the bradycardia was larger under water, with the reduction in rate averaging 15·9 per cent. The degree of heart rate change was significantly lessened by arithmetic; in this condition, the mean decrease from baseline was 15·0 bpm, compared with 19·1 bpm without the task.

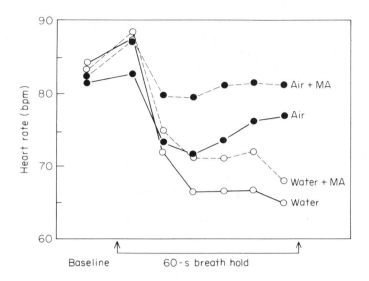

Fig. 2.4. Heart rate responses during breath holding with and without face immersion. Means for the 30-s baseline and each 10-s epoch of the 60-s breath holds are plotted. ●———●, Breath holding in air without mental arithmetic; ●-----●, breath holding in air with mental arithmetic; ○———○, breath holding in water without mental arithmetic; ○-----○, breath holding in water with mental arithmetic. (Ross and Steptoe, 1980.)

Since the physical and postural aspects of face immersion were identical during arithmetic and no arithmetic trials, it is unlikely that the divergence in heart rate was artefactual. Peripheral haemodynamic mechanisms, such as alterations in venous return and raised intrathoracic pressure, may be involved in the diving reflex. However, the bradycardia is thought to be primarily a product of neural reflexes, with stimulation of temperature sensitive receptors in the face provoking vagal inhibition of heart rate. The study therefore suggests that this "automatic" reflex can be modified by neocortical activity.

A further case in which the effects of central command were isolated was examined by Goodwin and associates (1972). Participants were asked to maintain constant isometric muscle contraction with the biceps, and an oscillatory vibrator was applied to the tendon. This stimulated the spindle endings, eliciting reflex tension in the muscle; consequently, a proportion of the contraction was supplied locally. Less central command was then required to maintain tension, so that the influence of cerebral control could be assessed. Fig. 2.5 summarises the cardiovascular and respiratory responses during one such study. The differences in rate and pressure modifications under stimulation and no stimulation conditions were due to variations in central command, and not to muscular effort *per se*.

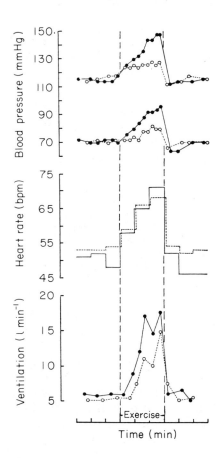

FIG. 2.5. Changes in systolic and diastolic pressure, heart rate and ventilation during two isometric contractions of the biceps (tension of 3·2 kg). ●———●, Normal contraction; ○-----○, contraction during vibration of primary afferents from the muscle spindles of the biceps. This induced reflex contraction, reducing the level of central command. (Goodwin *et al.*, 1972.)

A final technique that exploits direct neocortical influences on the cardiovascular system is biofeedback. Subjects are provided with stimulus displays that vary contingently with the fluctuations of a selected circulatory parameter. This information may then facilitate the voluntary control of increases and decreases in the activity. Several aspects of haemodynamics, from regional blood flow to blood pressure, have been modified with some success (Steptoe *et al.*, 1974; Steptoe, 1979a). The biofeedback literature also supports the contention that the cerebral cortex is involved in cardiovascular regulation in a variety of ways.

The mechanisms discussed thus far form the basis from which psychosocial and behavioural factors might disturb circulatory regulation. Their involvement in the development of high arterial pressure will be discussed further in Chapter 3. Yet there are a number of additional processes whereby neural and endocrine activity affect cardiovascular pathology. The three most important are the neural influences on cardiac electrical stability, the neuroendocrine influences on myocardial metabolism, and the endocrine influences on platelet aggregation and thrombotic mechanisms. Each of these will therefore be considered in turn.

Neural factors and the electrical stability of the heart

Cardiac pathology involves not only disturbances of the power of the heart to pump blood, but unstable rhythm and electrical failures. The role of arrhythmias and ventricular fibrillation in sudden cardiac death was discussed in Chapter 1. Electrical instabilities can emerge in the ischaemic heart from disorders of impulse initiation or conduction, and the autonomic nervous system makes important contributions to such effects.

Unlike working muscle fibres, cells in the sinoatrial node of the heart have the property of "automaticity", due to an instability of membrane potentials. After depolarisation, the membrane potential returns to baseline, but the cells do not remain quiescent until the next excitatory pulse. Instead, there is a slow depolarisation, as membrane potential moves towards the threshold for excitation. This means that in the absence of external restraints, pacemaker cells will fire spontaneously, and may cause general cardiac contraction. Automatic depolarisation is normally controlled by stimulation from the autonomic nervous system, imposing a firing rate. Nevertheless, if the excitability of the node is depressed, the likelihood of ectopic impulses eliciting general activation increases, particularly in the later stages of the refractory period, when membrane potentials are approaching the threshold for depolarisation.

Ectopic beats may also originate through defective propagation of excitation from the sinoatrial node, or from anomalies in conduction that enable an impulse which has already excited the myocardium to re-enter the ventricle. Such pathways are often blocked by increases in the dominant rhythm (Cranefield *et al.*, 1973).

The influence of autonomic cardiac efferents on electrical stability is well established. Surgical and pharmacological interruptions of sympathetic traffic protect against disorders of rhythm, while stimulation has the opposite effect (Verrier and Lown, 1978). Moreover, the release of noradrenaline enhances the automaticity or rate of spontaneous firing (Hoffman, 1977). Catecholamines are also prominent in the genesis of multiple re-entry circuits following infarction.

Stellate ganglion stimulation reduces the threshold for ventricular fibrillation, and sympathetic blockade is protective (Vassalle *et al.*, 1968; Harris *et al.*, 1951). Higher nervous influences also appear to be mediated by sympathetic fibres. These have been explored experimentally using the sequential R/T pulsing technique. During repolarisation, the imposition of a train of electrical pulses provokes rapid extrasystoles; the current required to produce the fourth response in such a series provides an index of vulnerability to fibrillation (Thompson and Lown, 1972). Verrier *et al.* (1975) used the method to examine the effects of hypothalamic interventions on stability. Stimulation was carried out in the posterior hypothalamic area of 34 dogs, and of these 40 per cent showed a reduction in fibrillation threshold. The response was abolished by β blockade. Experimental interventions that raise arterial pressure through peripheral vasoconstriction tend to increase the threshold for ventricular fibrillation; there appears to be a protective reflex reduction in cardiac sympathetic tone under these circumstances (Verrier *et al.*, 1974). Blatt *et al.* (1977) observed that the heightened vulnerability to fibrillation after coronary occlusion was likewise reversed by acute arterial pressure elevation. In this case, propranolol returned the heart to its fragile state, since the protective decrease in sympathetic tone was attenuated by blockade. Thus depression of cardiac sympathetic activity results in enhanced myocardial stability.

In direct opposition to sympathetic effects, vagal stimulation raises fibrillation threshold and thus bolsters the unstable heart (Abildskov and Vincent, 1977). But vagal influences evidently depend on the presence of activity in cardiac sympathetic pathways. Kolman *et al.*

(1975) found that in the absence of β-adrenergic sympathetic provocation, vagal stimulation had no effect on vulnerability. Yet with stellate ganglion stimulation or catecholamine infusion, vagal activity protected the myocardium. Hence in the dog, the parasympathetic operates through countering sympathetic nervous challenge to the heart.

In 1935, Nathanson reported a formidable experiment confirming some of these observations in man. Elderly patients were injected with adrenaline, and within a few minutes a number developed acute arrhythmias, with ectopic ventricular contractions. These responses were abolished by prior injection of acetyl-β-methylcholin, a cholinergic stimulant. Disturbances of rhythm are also characteristic of some forms of central nervous damage following strokes.

Additionally, sympathetic pathways may be involved in the generation of arrhythmias during myocardial ischaemia; the β-adrenergic receptors in the heart are stimulated reflexively, while adrenaline may reach high concentrations in the blood (Lown *et al.*, 1977). The pain associated with myocardial ischaemia may be translated through somatic afferents, causing further elevations in cardiac sympathetic tone (Maythan *et al.*, 1977). Whilst the application of β-blocking agents in the post-infarction period remains controversial, beneficial antiarrhythmic effects have been documented experimentally (Ross *et al.*, 1978). On the other hand, sinus bradycardia may also occur in acute myocardial infarction, possibly through vagal dominance. The frequency of ventricular fibrillation is low in such patients, and their prognosis is good, suggesting that the rhythm may be benign (Neufeld *et al.*, 1978).

Occasionally, ischaemic-like ECG changes may occur in the absence of identifiable occlusions or pathology, reflecting a hypersensitivity to circulating catecholamines (Taggart *et al.*, 1979). It is also interesting that many patients with ectopic activity show a reduction in premature ventricular contractions during sleep. The pattern is paradoxical, in that heart rate is generally lower in sleep, and slow rates tend to promote arrhythmias. Yet sympathetic cardiac tone is also diminished, and this appears to reduce the instability of the heart (Lown *et al.*, 1973b).

The data outlined in this section indicate that the autonomic nervous system makes significant contributions to ventricular stability, particularly when the heart is in a fragile state due to coronary stenosis. Since the autonomic pathways are sensitive to higher nervous stimulation, it is possible that psychological influences may be translated through such mechanisms. Consequently, the role of behaviour in the precipitation of fibrillation and sudden cardiac death will be considered in later chapters. However, the responses to cognitive and emotional stimuli may also be mediated by neuroendocrine tracts, as will be seen below.

Neuroendocrine reactions and myocardial pathology

Amongst the steroid hormones secreted by the adrenal cortex, the ones of greatest significance in cardiovascular pathology are the 17-hydroxy-corticosteroids (17-OHCS). These are classified into mineralocorticoids and glucocorticoids. The former include aldosterone, and are involved in the renal mechanisms regulating fluid volume and blood pressure, through their effects on sodium and potassium. On the other hand, the glucocorticoids, such as cortisol and corticosterone, are important in stimulating metabolism and the release of fuel supplies.

The synthesis and release of corticosteroids is controlled by adreno-corticotrophin (ACTH), secreted by the anterior pituitary. Since the pituitary is in turn stimulated by chemical agents of hypothalamic origin, steroid production is under the direct control of the brain. Furthermore, there is some autonomic involvement, as the adrenal cortex is innervated by the splanchnic nerve (Mikhail and Amin, 1969). This sympathetic pathway may act permissively in allowing ACTH to regulate steroidogenesis; sympathetic stimulation itself does not elicit the release of corticosteroids (Ciaranello *et al.*, 1976). The relationship mirrors control mechanisms in the adrenal medulla, where glucocorticoids are necessary but not sufficient for catecholamine secretion. Thus although the pituitary–adrenocortical and sympathatic–catecholamine axes are distinct, they are mutually dependent for some of their actions.

The activity of the adrenal cortex is governed by a series of feedback loops. Glucocorticoids inhibit ACTH release at a central level, while ACTH itself is involved in a negative feedback loop. Nevertheless, ACTH output is not entirely under autonomous control, but is powerfully influenced by other inputs to the median eminence of the hypothalamus. The role of neocortical and limbic processes has been widely documented with experimental interventions. Selective lesions in limbic structures such as the amygdala, septum and fornix appear to disturb the reactivity of ACTH to stimulating agents, while lesions in the frontal cortex affect glucocorticoid output (Murgas and Kvetnansky, 1973; Trulson, 1977). Electrical stimulation of diencephalic and mid-brain structures may also modify ACTH secretion (Slusher and Hyde, 1966). These factors are seen in the control of diurnal rhythms of circulating corticosteroids; plasma concentrations tend to be highest in the early morning, declining slowly over the day. The diurnal curve is not smooth, since cortisol is secreted in periodic bursts, punctuated by quiescent phases (Hellman *et al.*, 1970). Moreover, the circadian rhythm can be disrupted by limbic interventions (Ganong, 1974). These and other phenomena indicate that the control loops regulating pituitary–adrenocortical function can be overridden by central nervous impulses.

Both glucocorticoids and the catecholamines play important roles in the mobilisation and utilisation of stored fuels. They facilitate the release of free fatty acids (FFA) from triglycerides stored in adipose tissue (lypolysis), and similarly both support gluconeogenesis, or the production of glucose from carbohydrates. If these fuels are not consumed, they may contribute to the serum lipoprotein complement. Thus a substantial proportion of patients with excess cortisol have elevated serum triglycerides, while the hepatic production of very low density (VLD) lipoprotein is directly stimulated by cortisol. The effects of catecholamines on serum FFA can be inhibited by propranolol, suggesting a β-adrenergic mechanism. These circulating neuroendocrine agents are therefore implicated in long-term atherosclerotic processes, particularly when mobilised energy supplies are not utilised.

Furthermore, corticosteroids and catecholamines have direct and potentially damaging effects on the myocardium. Selye and his followers carried out experimental studies of the myocardial damage provoked by administration of corticosteroids and electrolytes (Selye and Bajusz, 1959; Selye, 1976). Rats were treated with the steroid fluorocortisol, and electrolytes such as sodium acetate. They rapidly developed massive cardiac necroses, and the effects were reproduced by replacing electrolytes with noradrenaline. The role of this steroid mechanism in the development of human cardiac disorders remains elusive however.

The responses to catecholamines are more firmly established. While sustained noradrenaline infusion can lead to degeneration and necrosis of cardiac tissue, the doses required may be outside the normal physiological range (Schenk and Moss, 1966). More important may be the fact that even small amounts of noradrenaline raise the oxygen demand of the myocardium, by stimulating local metabolism. If the oxygen supply cannot rise, because of coronary stenosis, ischaemia may develop. Thus sympathetic cardiac stimulation and circulating catecholamines may increase cardiac work in the absence of complementary improvements in coronary perfusion. There is some evidence that β-adrenergic blockade can reduce the size of experimental infarcts, attenuating regional contractile dysfunctions (Ross *et al.*, 1978). Moreover, a trial of sympathetic receptor blockade in victims of subarachnoid haemorrhage, showed that myocardial lesions were confined to the placebo group (Neil-Dwyer *et al.*, 1978). This aminergic mechanism is again dependent on the adrenal cortex, since corticosteroids appear to inhibit the neuronal uptake of noradrenaline, leading to accumulation in extracellular spaces.

Additionally, FFA are significant in myocardial ischaemia and infarction (Oliver, 1978). Both experimental and clinical studies indicate that high plasma FFA concentrations increase myocardial irritability. Vetter *et al.* (1974) carried out investigations from a mobile coronary care unit immediately following infarction. Catecholamine concentrations were high at the earliest sampling times, preceding the peak in FFA by a short period. Plasma cortisol was also raised, together with growth hormone. The mechanism of this FFA effect is not clear, but there may be an uncoupling of oxidative phosphorylation; it is significant that antilypolytic treatment in post-infarction patients can reduce the incidence of ventricular arrhythmia and tachycardia (Rowe *et al.*, 1975).

Platelet aggregation, thrombus formation and catecholamines

Catecholamines have an impact on still another aspect of cardiovascular pathology, since they are involved in blood coagulation and platelat aggregation. One   of the first responses to vascular injury is the formation of a temporary haemostatic plug from platelets. This process pathology, since they are involved in blood coagulation and platelet aggregation. One of the first responses to vascular injury is the fornormal endothelial cells, but to an exposed sub-endothelial basement membrane. Following aggregation, the temporary plug is converted into a fibrin clot, itself a product of a complex series of reactions. The importance of platelets in the formation of arterial thrombi is now well recognised, particularly when lesions or arterial damage have led to the exposure of the basement membrane (Born, 1977; Sherry, 1977). Dietary fats, especially the long-chain saturated fatty acids, and high arterial pressure, facilitate platelet aggregation (Hornstra and Haddema, 1977).

The sympathetic–catecholamine axis is concerned at several stages. Adrenaline and noradrenaline enhance both adhesion and aggregation of platelets. Fig. 2.6 shows the induction of platelet aggregation by

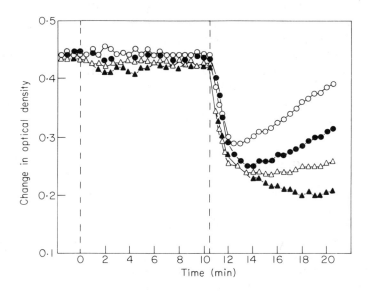

FIG. 2.6. Platelet aggregation induced by ATP, and potentiated by adrenaline. Aggregation assessed by changes in optical density. O———O, Saline control. Adrenaline concentrations range from $2 \cdot 5 \times 10^{-8}$ M ($\bullet$———$\bullet$) to $2 \cdot 6 \times 10^{-6}$ M ($\blacktriangle$———$\blacktriangle$). Adrenaline was added to plasma containing 290 000 platelets mm^{-3} at time 0, and ATP was added at 10·5 minutes. (Ardlie *et al.*, 1966.)

the nucleotide ATP (Ardlie *et al.*, 1966). The stimulating effect of adrenaline is plotted, and similar responses were recorded for other catecholamines. The stickiness of platelets may be increased secondarily by catecholamines, through the action of FFA.

Adrenaline is also associated with fibrin formation and the later stages of the clotting mechanism. Infusion raises the concentration of Factor VIII, and shortens whole blood clotting time. These actions can be abolished by propranolol, indicating a β-adrenergic mechanism (Britton *et al.*, 1974). Gunn and Hampton (1967) demonstrated that Factor VIII concentration was augmented after electrical stimulation of the hypothalamus or reticular formation, and reduced by limbic stimulation. In man, coagulation of the ventrolateral thalamic nucleus elevated concentrations of Factor VIII in the blood, although other insults to the central nervous system, such as electroshock, had no effect (Manucci *et al.*, 1971). Adrenocortical processes may also modify Factor VIII, and thereby influence fibrin activation. The adrenergic stimulation of this clotting factor is inhibited after adrenal-ectomy, while clotting time is shortened by ACTH in a dose-dependent fashion (Landaburu and Castellano, 1973).

Neuroendocrine responses are therefore implicated in both platelet and fibrin stages of coagulation, and may be concerned in the formation of arterial and venous thrombi. If psychological factors are associated with pathological disturbances of haemostasis, they could be mediated by these mechanisms.

Summary and conclusions

A number of the basic physiological mechanisms which mediate behavioural effects on the cardiovascular system have been discussed in this chapter. The regions of the brainstem that have a primary role in haemodynamic regulation do not operate autonomously, or inde-pendently of higher cortical nervous structures. Rather, circulatory control is integrated longitudinally in the brain, with patterns of response varying in complexity at different levels.

The components of any animal's response to environmental stimuli include skeletal muscular actions and circulatory adjustments. But these are not separately organised entities; rather, they reflect one closely meshed programme of action. The modifications in haemo-dynamics effected through autonomic nervous pathways are best understood with reference to the overall behaviour of the organism.

The brain also plays a major role in the release of catecholamines and corticosteroids, and may override peripheral regulatory mechanisms under appropriate conditions. These agents have powerful effects on haemodynamics, the mobilisation of stored fuels, and blood clotting processes. Their influence may either be adaptive, in preparing the organism to face threats from the environment, or harmful.

Several additional mechanisms through which the autonomic nervous system and humoral agents promote cardiovascular disturb-ance have been discussed. The electrical stability of the heart is modified by activity in the sympathetic and vagal cardiac fibres, while myocardial integrity may be weakened by the metabolic effects of circulating hormones. Experimental physiological studies suggest that neocortical interventions can influence these pathways—but it is for the behavioural scientist to determine the conditions under which psychological factors are significant for pathology.

3
Essential Hypertension and the Autonomic Nervous System

High arterial pressure holds a special place amongst disturbances of cardiovascular function. Although it is often benign in itself, hypertension is implicated in atherogenesis, and in the development of a number of non-sclerotic lesions. Furthermore, it can become malignant, leading directly to fibrinoid necrosis of the small arteries and arterioles. High blood pressure may be secondary to conditions such as pyelonephritis, phaeochromocytoma and coarctation of the aorta, but the majority of cases are not associated with specific diseases, and are classified as essential or primary. It has become increasingly clear, however, that essential hypertensives vary a great deal; thus a significant proportion are characterised by low plasma renin activity (PRA), while a "hyperkinetic" circulation is frequent in the early stages of the disorder (Birkenhager and Schalekamp, 1976). These differences are relevant to the role of neurogenic factors, and will therefore be discussed below. More detailed accounts of central nervous involvement in hypertension are available elsewhere (De Jong *et al.*, 1977a; Julius and Esler, 1976a).

High blood pressure is ubiquitous in industrialised nations, and the prevalence amongst middle-aged European men has been estimated as high as 15–30 per cent (Richard, 1976). A major screening programme in the USA indicated that the frequency of diastolic pressures above 90 mmHg was some 20 per cent in white males under 30, rising to 35 per cent in older men (Stamler *et al.*, 1976). These figures actually underestimate the problem, since cardiovascular morbidity varies continuously with pressure level, and does not depend on arbitrary categorisation of the distribution (see Fig. 1.1). Smaller and smaller elevations in arterial pressure are being considered appropriate targets for intervention (Perry and Smith, 1978).

It was argued in Chapter 1 that high arterial pressure is a relative phenomenon, and that no absolute cutoff between normal and hypertensive groups can be made. Blood pressure is a dynamic rather than fixed parameter, and levels vary considerably over the day. This was documented when Riess *et al.* (1967) provided 50 mild essential hypertensives with portable sphygmomanometers, and recordings were taken throughout everyday activities. The average clinic readings of 171/99 mmHg contrasted with mean portable levels of 144/90 mmHg; average values varied over the day between 169/105 mmHg and 123/74 mmHg. Studies with continuous 24-hour intra-arterial recordings have confirmed this pattern (Bevan *et al.*, 1969). Pressures are markedly reduced during sleep, and show wide fluctuations in the day-time. There is little evidence that people with very high pressures display less variability than healthier groups (Tarazi *et al.*, 1976; Pickering and Sleight, 1977).

Furthermore, the classification of a reading as high depends on the age of the individual, since arterial pressures tend to rise as people grow older. Fig. 3.1 is derived from Miall and Oldham's (1963) cross-sectional survey of pressure levels from a sample living in South Wales. The flattening or downturn of the curves in older groups may

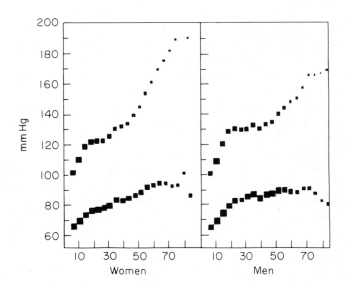

FIG. 3.1. Mean systolic and diastolic pressures in two Welsh populations, categorised by age and sex. The area of each square is inversely proportional to the standard error of the mean. (Miall and Oldham, 1963.)

have been due to greater survival amongst those with lower pressures; however, the pattern has been confirmed in longitudinal investigations (Harris, 1967).

Yet these trends are not universal. Many people show very little rise in arterial pressure with age, and some populations fail to conform with the expected distributions. Fig. 3.2 summarises data from cross-sectional observations of four groups; for convenience, only the systolic pressures of men have been plotted. The populations vary in race, environment and culture, but in each case pressures do not change with age. The same phenomenon has been recorded from samples in Russia, Japan and Kenya (Henry and Cassel, 1969). Such groups are not protected genetically from pressure increase, since under different environmental conditions the conventional pattern is followed. Thus the lowland relatives of the Chilean group plotted in Fig. 3.2 start at the same modest pressure in youth, but typically exhibit marked rises with age (Cruz-Coke *et al.*, 1973).

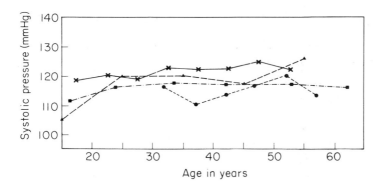

FIG. 3.2. Distributions of systolic blood pressure amongst males in selected populations, showing the stability of pressure level over age. ▲------▲, Highland Chileans (Cruz-Coke *et al.*, 1973); ■—·—·—■, Najafgarh of India (Padmauati *et al.*, 1959); ×——×, US Aviators (Oberman *et al.*, 1976); ●-----●, Navajo Indians, USA (Fulmer and Roberts, 1973).

An age-related increase in arterial pressure is not inevitable, but may be a consequence of exposure to particular environmental factors. In considering the role of psychology and behaviour, it is important to clarify the extent to which hypertension can be accounted for by constitutional or physical risks.

Factors associated with essential hypertension

Several factors predispose individuals to develop sustained hypertension, but they do not apply in all cases. The evidence for genetic involvement is considerable, and need not be recounted in detail (Pickering, 1968, p. 236 et seq.). Both racial and familial differences are related to heredity, and transmission is thought to be polygenic. It has been estimated that genetic linkage accounts for 36–67 per cent of the variance in arterial pressure; whatever the proportion, it is clear that the environment must make a substantial contribution.

The presence of high pressure early in life, even if it is only temporary, is another major risk. Levy and his colleagues (1944) studied the medical records of over 22 000 army officers, and identified variables that predicted subsequent fixed hypertension. They defined transient hypertension as a moderately high reading on a particular occasion (systolic over 150 mmHg, or diastolic over 90 mmHg) that was not maintained at later examinations. Men manifesting transient high levels in early adulthood were some three and a half times more likely to develop sustained high pressure than others (Levy et al., 1945). When the pressor episodes were also characterised by tachycardia, the ratio rose to 7·5/1·0 (Fig. 3.3). The pattern has also been observed in the health records of students; both systolic and diastolic levels were directly related to later incidence of hypertension, in a continuous association that did not depend solely on the occurrence of very high readings (Paffenberger et al., 1968; Thomas and Greenstreet, 1973).

It should be emphasised that stable hypertension is not an inevitable consequence of early pressor episodes. As with other vulnerability factors, the risk is relative. Fejfar and Widimsky (1962) followed up 54 juvenile hypertensives over five years; of these, only 35 per cent showed definite progression, while pressure returned towards age-expected norms in 40 per cent. A substantial proportion of patients with diagnosed mild hypertension regress towards the population mean on follow-up (Miall and Brennan, 1979). At the same time, many children and young adults who show somewhat elevated blood pressure, tend to remain above their contemporaries in later years (Julius and Schork, 1971).

Two other factors associated with the development of high arterial pressure are the amount of salt in the diet, and body weight. Clinically, it has been observed that severe salt deprivation will lead to reductions in pressure, and mechanisms based on experimental hypertension have been proposed. Dahl (1961) demonstrated that feeding rats with

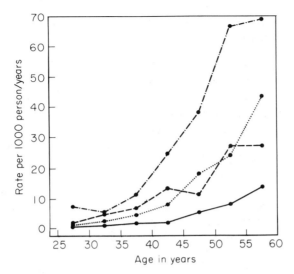

Fig. 3.3. Annual incidence of development of sustained hypertension at different ages, according to the presence or absence of transient tachycardia or hypertension. ●——●, No transient tachycardia or hypertension; ●———●, transient tachycardia only; ●·····●, transient hypertension only; ●—·—·—·—●, transient tachycardia and hypertension. (Levy *et al.*, 1945.) (Copyright © 1945, American Medical Association.)

large amounts of salt led to pressure increase, and that an hereditary sensitivity to salt could be produced through selective breeding. High salt intake may provoke elevations in arterial pressure by raising extracellular fluid, and thereby disturbing volume regulation mechanisms (Fries, 1976).

The general significance of salt intake for essential hypertension can however be over emphasised. Dahl and Love (1957) argued that dietary salt in different populations correlated with average pressure levels, but this is not always the case. The Buddhist farmers of Thiland for example, have an average salt intake of 20 g per diem, yet have uniformly low pressures that do not rise with age. Dietary salt intake is not consistently associated with pressure variations within populations either. Miall (1959) categorised a Welsh sample according to reported salt use, and found no systematic differences in pressure between light and heavy users. Similarly in the Framingham study, 24-hour sodium excretion rates were poorly correlated with the pressure distribution of males (Dawber *et al.*, 1967). Moreover, the physiological mechanisms affected by salt are not always disturbed in hypertension. Plasma and extracellular fluid volumes are within the normal range, or may even be reduced (Birkenhager and Schalekamp, 1976; Chau *et al.*, 1978). Page (1976) has argued that salt is more important in the very young rather than in adults, although the evidence for such a pattern is not strong (Török, 1979). Essential hypertensives may, however, vary in their ability to handle salt metabolically (Kawasaki *et al.*, 1978). Another possibility is that the sodium–potassium balance, and not the sodium level *per se*, is the crucial factor.

Body weight is also associated with blood pressure, and correlations have been reported in both longitudinal and cross-sectional surveys. Much of the power of this association may be due to the extremes of the distribution, since hypertension is almost invariable in the very obese. Thus in Framingham, body weight was considered to account for only 10 per cent of the variance in pressure, and was not therefore a principle factor (Kannel and Dawber, 1973). Some authorities have claimed that reductions in weight may lead to decreases in arterial pressure, even when there is no concomitant fall in salt intake, but the effect is controversial (Reisen *et al.*, 1978).

Weight tends to increase with age in industrialised societies, and may contribute to the rise in pressure. Yet firm correlations between pressure and weight increases are not always found (Page *et al.*, 1974). For example, when women in Warsaw were divided into underweight, normal and overweight subgroups, pressure increased with age in all three categories (Alexandrow, 1967). Weight may therefore operate independently of age-related changes; excessive adiposity at an early age is, however, a strong predictor of hypertension (Miller and Shekelle, 1976).

The association of arterial pressure with both weight and salt emphasises the importance of eating behaviour in essential hypertension. Both factors may best be managed through behavioural interventions, and the psychologist can contribute usefully to such programmes. Salt and weight are also significant in the changes of pressure that occur on migration and material development in primitive cultures (Ostfeld and D'Atri, 1977); they are thus relevant to the discussion of psychosocial change and migration in Chapter 8.

In summary, both constitutional and environmental factors are involved in the genesis of high arterial pressure. Yet much of the variation in pressure level remains unexplained. Higher nervous influences may be important as well; but in order to understand their contribution, the haemodynamic mechanisms underlying disturbances in arterial pressure must be described.

The haemodynamics of essential hypertension

Our understanding of the circulatory balance in essential hypertension has been greatly expanded by detailed investigations of patients at different stages in the development of the disorder. Pickering (1968) summarised early work on small groups of well established hypertensives, and concluded that high pressure was sutained by an elevated vascular resistance in most tissues of the body. It is now apparent however that the physiological mechanisms maintaining hypertension vary with the severity and duration of the condition.

Bello *et al.* (1967) divided patients into severe, medium and mild hypertensives. Those in the severe group, who showed signs of cardiac, renal and retinal disease, had pressures associated with abnormally high peripheral resistance. But amongst mild hypertensives, the common pattern was of high cardiac output, and a peripheral resistance within the normal range; thus the increased arterial pressure was due to cardiac rather than resistive mechanisms. A similar haemodynamic state was observed in borderline hypertensives by Julius and Conway (1968), while Lund-Johansen (1967) found that only a small proportion of early essential hypertensives had elevated vascular resistance. Frohlich and associates (1970) categorised over 100 hypertensive patients into four degrees of severity according to the variability of pressures, and the presence of secondary symptoms. Cardiac index was significantly higher in the group with moderate hypertension, and declined with the severity of the dysfunction. Thus in the most serious cases, cardiac index was actually below normal, while the total peripheral resistance was correspondingly increased.

The haemodynamic pattern in which cardiac output is elevated, while resistance is in the normal range, is known as the hyperkinetic state. It is most common amongst borderline hypertensives — those who show occasional readings above 150/90 mmHg, or who have persistent pressures between 150/90 mmHg and 160/100 mmHg (Julius and Esler, 1975). These patients were formerly considered to have "labile" hypertension, but the distinction is now discredited; it was based on a dichotomous view of hypertension, in which pressures fluctuating above and below an arbitrary criterion (such as 150/95 mmHg) assumed special significance. Continuous pressure recordings have not confirmed that variability is greater when the average level is only moderately elevated (Pickering and Sleight, 1977). Even well-established hypertensives may show the hyperkinetic pattern, with considerable systolic lability and high cardiac output; conversely, young or borderline patients show variations in haemodynamics as complex as those at later stages (Tarazi *et al.*, 1976; Fouad *et al.*, 1978).

Since arterial pressure is maintained by the balance between cardiac output and peripheral resistance, it is probable that even in hyperkinetic conditions, the resistance mechanisms are disturbed. The raised cardiac output "ought" to be compensated by low vascular resistance, but this is not the case. Julius *et al.* (1971) found the peripheral resistance of borderline hypertensives was no different from normal, despite the elevated cardiac index; yet when plotted at comparable levels of cardiac index, the resistance of hypertensives was higher. Additionally, responses to stimuli which normally result in reductions of resistance are impaired. For example, the decrease in vascular resistance during exercise is small, as is the response to volume expansion (Julius *et al.*, 1971; Safar *et al.*, 1973). The hyperkinetic pattern should not therefore be considered purely as a defect in cardiac activity, but as one involving a breakdown between output and resistance.

Although hyperkinetic disturbances may occur amongst patients with sustained high blood pressure, there is controversy over its significance in borderline hypertensives. In some series, hyperkinetic subjects evidently have benign prospects, but the state may also be a precursor of high resistance patterns (Julius *et al.*, 1979). This is implied in the cross-sectional data, where high cardiac indices are more prevalent at moderate pressure levels. It has also been confirmed in longitudinal surveys. Eich and co-workers (1966) followed up patients who initially showed transiently elevated pressures. After 5 years, the raised cardiac outputs were replaced by high total peripheral resistance, and the latter maintained the increased arterial pressure. A high cardiac index was originally recorded in a cohort of untreated young hypertensives in France (Weiss *et al.*, 1978). On 4-year follow-up average systolic and mean arterial pressures were both significantly greater. Cardiac index had, however, fallen within normal limits, while total peripheral resistance had risen. Similarly, Lund-Johansen (1977) retested untreated hypertensives after 10 years. Even though the average arterial pressure had not changed, the peripheral resistance was elevated at the expense of cardiac output. The switch seems to be gradual, and there is no sharp dichotomy between people with high cardiac index and high vascular resistance (Safar *et al.*, 1973).

The crossover between cardiac and vascular processes in hypertension has also been documented experimentally during prolonged stellate ganglion stimulation in dogs (Liard *et al.*, 1976). Arterial pressure rose immediately, together with cardiac output. But when stimulation continued for 7 days, peripheral resistance increased while cardiac output normalised.

These data have important implications for understanding the development of essential hypertension. The rise in pressure seems to be initiated by cardiac rather than resistive mechanisms. This is consistent with evidence that alterations in peripheral resistance do not themselves provoke permanent adjustments in arterial pressure. For example, when all four limbs are removed, the total peripheral resistance may be 160 per cent above normal, yet pressure does not increase (Guyton, 1978). Conversely, disorders such as beriberi and Paget's disease lead to reductions in resistance without changing blood pressure. Students of circulatory dynamics have argued against taking the pattern of fixed hypertension as primary:

> There still remains widespread belief that by far most instances of hypertension result from some primary factor that increases the total peripheral resistance. This is very unfortunate, because this belief has led to virtually all research workers in the field of hypertension to search endlessly for the factor or factors that cause the primary increase in total peripheral resistance, while relatively little effort has been expended in looking for the causes of primary elevation of cardiac output.
>
> Guyton *et al.* (1976), p. 73

One haemodynamic mechanism that could lead to the hyperkinetic pattern is an abnormal venous pressure in the cardiopulmonary (central) circulation. This would increase the preload on the myocardium, causing elevations in cardiac output. Since plasma volume is not expanded, high central venous pressure might be due to re-redistribution of blood in favour of the pulmonary capacitance bed. A number of studies examining the relationship between cardiopulmonary blood volume and cardiac index have been carried out in recent years. After careful evaluation of these, Birkenhager and Schalekamp (1976) concluded that increased central blood volume was not generally a cause of the high cardiac index. However, the relevance of this factor may vary with the renin status of patients, becoming more important in those with low PRA (see p. 52).

An alternative explanation of the hyperkinetic pattern is that there is a disturbance of autonomic nervous regulation. This possibility will be discussed in the next section, along with other evidence for elevated sympathetic neural tone in essential hypertension.

Sympathetic nervous activity in hypertension

Sympathetic nervous hyperactivity is involved in a number of experimental hypertensions. If rats with one kidney removed are injected with the synthetic mineralocorticoid deoxycorticosterone (DOCA), they will develop high blood pressure, provided they are given saline

to drink (DOCA-Salt hypertension). Radioactively labelled noradrenaline was injected into these animals by De Champlain *et al.*
(1968). An increase in transmitter turnover was recorded, and this
was dependent on the degree of pressure elevation. When salt was removed from the diet, pressure returned to normal, as did noradrenaline
metabolism. Some genetic influences on high arterial pressure may
also be mediated autonomically; for example, the pressue rise typical
of the Okamoto strain of spontaneously hypertensive rats can be
blocked by neonatal sympathetectomy (Provoost *et al.*, 1977). Yet it
cannot be inferred from these data that autonomic pathways are
disturbed in human hypertension — more direct evidence is required
(Ferrario and Page, 1978).

Many inconsistencies have emerged from the study of catecholamines and sympathetic tone in essential hypertension. These have
been due in part to the grouping of patients with different haemodynamic dysfunctions. A distinction should therefore be drawn between sympathetic nervous involvement in established hypertension,
and in the borderline and hyperkinetic types.

The evidence for autonomic overactivity in hyperkinetic groups is
strong. The sympathetic and vagal inputs to the heart were blocked
pharmacologically by Julius and co-workers (1975), and the responses
are plotted in Fig. 3.4. Both components of cardiac output were ele-

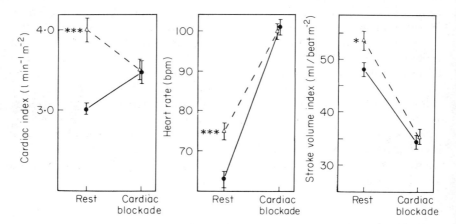

FIG. 3.4. Cardiac index and its components, heart rate and stroke volume, at rest and
after complete cardiac blockade with atropine and propranolol. $\triangle$ ---- $\triangle$, 25 young
hypertensives with elevated cardiac output; ●——●, 28 control normotensives.
Bars represent standard errors of the mean. Significance levels: $*p < 0.05$; $***p < 0.001$.
(Julius *et al.*, 1975.)

vated at rest, and together accounted for the raised blood pressure. The heightened myocardial performance was not due to intrinsic disturbances of contractility, nor to increased central blood volume, but to traffic in the autonomic pathways. The sympathetic mechanism has been confirmed with measurements of systolic time intervals, and consistent negative correlations have been recorded between pre-ejection period and plasma catecholamines (Wikstrand *et al.*, 1976; Cousineau *et al.*, 1978).

The cardiac sympathetic tone may be disturbed even before pressure levels are unduly elevated, since moderately raised pressure in children is associated with tachycardia and a hyperkinetic circulation (Török, 1979). A survey of 13–23-year-olds identified individuals with casual pressures of more than 140/90 mmHg (Hofman *et al.*, 1979). On reassessment 2–4 years later, pressures had returned to the age-expected range in a proportion. However, even after secondary hypertensives had been excluded, some subjects remained with pressures averaging 139/76 mmHg. The plasma noradrenaline of this group was significantly higher than that of age-matched controls, and was closely correlated with the levels of systolic pressure.

Other investigations suggest that autonomic reactivity, rather than resting tone, is disturbed. Chobanian *et al.* (1978) found no differences in plasma catecholamines at rest, between mild hypertensives and matched controls. However, the responses to 70° tilt and cold pressor challenges were exaggerated in the patients. The response to tilt may be so great in some cases as to provoke orthostatic hypertension (Safar *et al.*, 1973). The changes in pressure correlate with noradrenaline excretion rates (Esler and Nestel, 1973a).

Some aspects of autonomic involvement in hyperkinetic patterns are not well understood. Effects vary with the renin status of patients, as will be seen in the next section. The myocardial adjustments could be sustained by sympathetic hyperactivity alone, but there may also be disturbances of vagal input. Some investigators have found β blockade normalises the cardiac state, while others have reported that parasympathetic pathways must also be inhibited (Julius *et al.*, 1975; Tarazi *et al.*, 1976). Nevertheless, there is a strong possibility that higher cortical inputs play a role in the production of the exaggerated sympathetic tone.

The contribution of sympathetic tracts to established hypertension is more ambiguous. One way of evaluating this effect is to study the responses to total sympathectomy. However, the operation has never been subjected to a controlled trial; it was commonly found that pressure fell after surgery, but gradually rose again in all but a small proportion of patients (Pickering, 1968). The abolition of innervation was rarely complete in this operation, which has long been abandoned. Furthermore, denervated organs become supersensitive to circulating catecholamines, and this may have diminished the response (Sleight, 1975).

The success of β blockers as antihypertensive agents is prima facie evidence for sympathetic involvement. Yet the mechanism of action is not clear; although these drugs reduce myocardial contractility and heart rate, the change in cardiac output may not be responsible for the hypotensive effect. A fall in output occurs in both responders and non-responders, and a high initial cardiac output does not guarantee effective action (Ulrych *et al.*, 1968; Birkenhager and Schalekamp, 1976). However, it is interesting that the cardioselective β blocker atenolol reduces blood pressure and heart rate only during the day, according to 24-h monitoring records (Millar-Craig *et al.*, 1979). Sympathetic nervous activity may be diminished at night, and the implication for psychological theories is obvious (see also p. 198).

Chronic changes of sympathetic tone have been investigated by measuring plasma catecholamine concentrations in hypertensives. De Quattro and Chan (1972) found significant resting differences between hypertensives and normotensive controls, and greater responses to standing in the former as well. This suggested elevations in both the tonic output and reactivity of the sympathetic–adrenomedullary system. Unfortunately, age-matched controls have been omitted from many studies, and the hypertensive patients are frequently older. Plasma catecholamine levels are generally found to rise with age (Axelrod, 1976). Lake and associates (1977) showed that the plasma noradrenaline concentrations of young normotensives and older hypertensives fell on the same age-dependent regression line; furthermore, when age-matched normal controls were used, no differences in plasma noradrenaline were observed by this group (Lake *et al.*, 1976).

Another factor confounded in this research has been the effect of anxiety and unfamiliarity on catecholamines. Many patients find the sampling of blood distressing, while physicians and laboratory staff take it in their stride. Yet scientists, technicians and clinical personnel are commonly used as the controls against which patients are compared (e.g. Franco-Morselli *et al.*, 1977). Such individuals are clearly inappropriate for the purpose.

One investigation that avoided both these problems assessed catecholamines from healthy men applying for vasectomies (De Quattro *et al.*, 1975). Three groups with the same average age were formed. Group 1 were normotensive (mean 125/70 mmHg), group 2 had high systolic pressure (mean 149/74 mmHg), while both systolic and diastolic were elevated in group 3 (153/95 mmHg). Total plasma catecholamines were excessive in the two hypertensive groups, averaging 66 per cent and 60 per cent respectively above controls.

The results of plasma catecholamine studies have thus been somewhat inconsistent, and a clearer picture will emerge when careful allowance is made for confounding factors, and with the refinement of methods for evaluating sympathetic tone. Moreover, many of the variations may be genuine, since essential hypertensives are not an homogenous group. In particular, sympathetic disturbances appear to be related to the plasma renin status of patients.

Renal function, PRA, and sympathetic tone

The kidney is of such importance to cardiovascular regulation that it is almost inevitably involved in all sustained haemodynamic disturbances. Yet although renal dysfunctions are characteristic of malignant hypertension and primary aldosteronism, it has been difficult to identify abnormalities in essential hypertension. Nevertheless, disturbances of the renin–angiotensin system are implicated. The plasma renin status of patients is not fixed, but may alter as essential hypertension progresses; and these variations interlock with the autonomic disturbances discussed in the last section.

The number of essential hypertensives with PRA above or below normal is difficult to estimate reliably. Low PRA is found in some 20–30 per cent, but the proportion increases with age (Guthrie *et al.*, 1978). High PRA is more common in younger people with borderline hypertension, where the proportion may reach 30 per cent (Esler *et al.*, 1977). PRA is inversely related both to the diastolic level, and to the total peripheral resistance in hypertension (Thomas *et al.*, 1976). It is therefore probable that as pressure rises, PRA is suppressed. However, these trends are complicated by the fact that high PRA may also be recorded in the late or malignant stages of the disorder — in such cases, the renin status is generally a product of kidney damage.

There is a good deal of evidence that the high PRA found in young and borderline patients is due to sympathetic nervous stimulation. Levels of plasma and urinary catecholamines are elevated in this subgroup, while traffic in the cardiac sympathetic fibres is intensified (Chobanian *et al.*, 1978). β blockade has greater effects on the heart rate and cardiac index of high PRA patients compared with others, with total autonomic blockade normalising arterial pressure as well

(Esler *et al.*, 1977). The response to β blockers as therapeutic agents may also be greater in these patients (Conway 1978). The alternative hypothesis, that high blood pressure is a product of stimulation by angiotensin rather than automatic hyperactivity, has been tested by infusing angiotensin II blocking agents (De Quattro *et al.*, 1977); in patients with high PRA and high plasma noradrenaline, the depressor effect was very modest, suggesting a primary autonomic dysfunction.

The pattern in low renin hypertension is rather different. Both tonic levels of catecholamines, and sympathetic reactivity are below normal (Esler and Nestel, 1973b; Chobanian *et al.*, 1978). Adrenergic discharge to the kidney may therefore be suppressed, so that renin is not strongly stimulated. Low PRA is also characteristic of primary aldosteronism, and it has been suggested that mineralocorticoids play a part in this subgroup of essential hypertensives as well (Biglieri, 1978). It may be significant that there is a high incidence of adrenal abnormalities amongst low PRA patients (Guthrie *et al.*, 1978). Nevertheless, the data are inconclusive, since over-secretion of mineralocorticoids is not common in essential hypertensives. Julius and Esler (1976b) proposed that blood is distributed disproportionately to the cardiopulmonary circulation in low renin hypertension, so that stimulation of the cardiac mechanoreceptors reflexly inhibits autonomic discharge to the kidney. This is consistent with the observation that the ratio of central to total blood volume is disturbed in some hypertensives (Simon *et al.*, 1977).

These data on renal function help to explain why assessments of sympathetic activity have been inconsistent. The mechanisms underlying the hypertension may vary according to the stage of development. In early phases, PRA is stimulated as one component of neurogenic (β-adrenergic) hyperactivity. Subsequently, renin is suppressed as an adaptive response, since reduced PRA inhibits angiotensin and aldosterone feedback loops, promoting decreases in arterial pressure through lowering fluid volume. However, this adjustment is evidently unsuccessful, as raised pressure may be maintained. Finally, in the late stages of the disorder, PRA begins to rise once more.

The degree of autonomic or renal disturbance will therefore vary between different patients. Some individuals show no progression, with fixed hypertensive mechanisms. Yet the fact that high arterial pressure can persist in the face of low PRA and reduced adrenergic tone is important; it suggests that non-neural factors come to play a major part in the maintenance of the condition. This is reflected in Weiss's (1978) follow-up study of haemodynamics in young hypertensives. On the first examination, heart rate and cardiac index were reliably correlated, while cardiac index and blood volume were unrelated. But at follow-up 4 years later, the pattern had reversed. There was a growing dependence on the mechanical properties of the circulation, and autonomic activity diminished in importance. In some hypertensives, elevated pressure is unaffected by complete autonomic blockade (Korner, 1976). Two of the processes that may take over the task of sustaining high blood pressure are discussed in the following sections.

Baroreflex activity in essential hypertension

The baroreceptor reflex acts to counter fluctuations in arterial pressure by modifying autonomic vasomotor and cardiac tone. However, it has been known for many years that the carotid baroreceptors adapt to prolonged increases in pressure. McCubbin *et al.* (1956) demonstrated that after a few days of experimentally induced renal hypertension, the frequency of discharge from the receptors was reduced. The system "resets" to modulate cardiovascular activity around a new, high pressure level. The pattern is illustrated in Fig. 3.5, where activity in baroreceptor fibres was recorded directly in normal and hypertensive dogs (Pickering and Sleight, 1977). In both cases, output rose with increased sinus pressure, but there were important differences. The threshold for firing was higher in the hypertensive, while the sensitivity to pressure change was depressed; furthermore, the maximal firing frequency was lower. The latter effect may be due to limits in the distensibility of the carotid sinus, rather than to receptor saturation. The ability of the reflex to compensate for fluctuations is thus reduced at high levels of arterial pressure.

A similar pattern has been observed in man. Direct recordings of efferent sympathetic activity are possible using microneurographic techniques (Wallin *et al.*, 1973). Signals are not precisely quantifiable, as they depend on electrode placement and the number of units engaged; nevertheless, variations in discharge can be detected. These indicate that vasoconstrictor tone is inhibited by the baroreceptor reflex at a higher arterial pressure in hypertensives than controls. Assessments of reflex sensitivity may be made indirectly with the phenylephrine pressure-interval method. Gribbin and colleagues (1971) showed that the sensitivity of the baroreflex varied inversely with age and pressure level. Thus in patients with high blood pressure, the reflex buffered fluctuations only poorly. This pattern has been con-

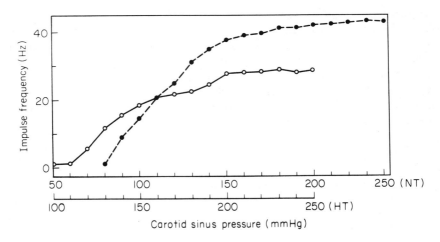

FIG. 3.5. Impulse frequency from baroreceptor fibres at different carotid sinus pressures in the normotensive (●----●) and hypertensive (○———○) dog. The axes are arranged so that resting mean arterial pressures in unanaesthetised animals (100 mm for the normotensive, and 150 mm for the hypertensive) are aligned. (Pickering and Sleight, 1977.)

firmed by others using more direct measures of reflex sensitivity (Mancia *et al.*, 1978).

The effects of carotid endarterectomy are also relevant, since the receptors are neurally isolated by this procedure. Over an 11-year period, Wade (1970) found that 38 per cent of patients developed hypertension, while many others showed poor reflex control and considerable pressure variability.

The mechanism by which the reflex resets is complex, since both central and peripheral factors may be involved. The influence of higher centres was discussed in Chapter 2, and these may also have a role in hypertension. Simon *et al.* (1977) used a gradual atropinisation procedure to determine the dose at which the reflex was abolished at different pressure levels. Amongst normotensives, the threshold fell as pressure increased; but this pattern was not observed in hypertensives, indicating a vagal dysfunction. Important peripheral factors include atheroma of the carotid sinus. Pathological changes make the wall stiffer and more resistant to stretch, and hence the impact of alterations in pressure on the receptors is deadened (Sleight, 1975).

In the early stages of hypertension, the reflex opposes pressure increases for short periods, before it is reset. Subsequently, modifications of baroreceptor activity help to maintain high arterial pressure, since after resetting they counter any reductions of level. However, a primary role of baroreceptor sensitivity in the initiation of essential hypertension is unlikely. An intriguing aspect of this mechanism is that stimulation of the carotid baroreceptors inhibits afferent tracts to the cerebral cortex, and reduces discharge from pyramidal cells (Coleridge *et al.*, 1976). It is possible that the reflex thus modulates the intensity of sensory inputs to the higher centres, and is functionally involved in central processing.

Structural changes in the vasculature

Folkow has championed the hypothesis that structural changes are responsible for the increased systemic resistance characteristic of sustained hypertension (Folkow *et al.*, 1970; Folkow and Neil, 1971). The high resistance is not due simply to elevated vasomotor tone, since even under conditions of complete vascular relaxation, forearm blood flow is low in hypertensives. A mechanism, based on medial hypertrophy of resistance vessel walls, has been proposed, leading to a raised wall/internal lumen ratio. The process is seen as a form of "structural autoregulation", where increases in intrinsic resistance protect the capillary beds at a local level from high pressure. This may result in a chronically high vascular resistance amongst hypertensives, even in the absence of elevated smooth muscle tone. Furthermore, although a vasoconstrictor influence may produce the same shortening of muscle fibres as in normotension, it will provoke exaggerated increases in resistance, as the vessel lumen is squeezed by the wall mass (Folkow, 1976). Hence both the high peripheral resistance, and the heightened response to vasoactive agents, may be accounted for by the physical properties of the vessels themselves.

There is much support for this theory. Folkow *et al.* (1970) infused noradrenaline into the large hind limb vessels of Okamoto strain hypertensive rats. The threshold for constriction was identical with that of normal controls, but the subsequent response curve was steeper. However, it is possible that vascular hypersensitivity to vasoconstrictors is also present, decreasing the response threshold in some cases. Lais and Brody (1975) found that the catecholamine threshold was reduced by some 60 per cent in hypertensive rates; sensitivity changes have been shown to precede hypertension in DOCA-Salt and spontaneously hypertensive rats, and must therefore come before wall thickening (Bohr and Berecek, 1976). Experimentally, selected vascular beds can be protected from the effects of hypertension by chronic obstruction, and this should prevent structural alterations of the type suggested by Folkow. Yet when this is done, sensitivity to catecholamines still rises. Moreover, a circulating agent may modulate sensitivity. Bloom *et al.* (1976) potentiated the response of an arterial preparation to nor-adrenaline, by adding plasma from hypertensives to the medium. A corpus of evidence thus suggests that vascular sensitivity can be in-creased in hypertension, contributing to the effects described in the structural theory.

These mechanical processes may underlie the heightened peripheral resistance of hypertensives. The vascular hypertrophy is thought to be a response to changes in pressure load, rather than a primary cause. Increases in vascular reactivity imply that "normal" levels of catecho-lamines or sympathetic tone may produce exaggerated changes in resistance.

Summary and conclusions

Many studies of behavioural and psychological factors in essential hypertension have been confounded by variations in the disorder. Different mechanisms sustain the elevated arterial pressure at dif-ferent stages, and only some of these are likely to be affected by higher cortical activity.

The pathways most accessible to psychological influence are the autonomic tracts. It is important to distinguish alterations in reactivity from differences in chronic sympathetic outflow. A heightened sym-pathetic tone is strongly implicated in the hyperkinetic syndrome, and in borderline hypertensives with high renin status. Cardiac output is likely to be elevated, although disturbances of resistance may also be present.

Once arterial pressure has been raised through cardiac mechanisms, other factors help maintain the new level. These include renal pro-cesses, alterations in baroreceptor control and structural vascular adjustments. Variations in salt intake, weight and hereditary con-stitution, may add to the vulnerability of these systems. Under such circumstances, the role of autonomic overactivity will diminish, al-though heightened reactivity may persist. It is not clear whether the progression to higher pressure is confined to subgroups of patients exhibiting particular patterns of autonomic and renal dysfunction, or whether there are general trends.

An implication of these observations is that the search for cognitive and behavioural influences is best focused on early or borderline hypertension, since autonomic dysfunction is more prominent at this stage. Furthermore, in view of the complexity of mechanisms, it is not sufficient to examine gross circulatory variables such as heart rate and arterial pressure; more detailed investigations may be required, if hypotheses concerning psychosocial factors are to be refined.

Section 2

4
Experimental Investigations of Psychological Influences on the Cardiovascular System

Environmental inputs can conveniently be segregated into those that cause tissue damage, such as radiant heat or toxins, and behavioural stimuli. The fact that the latter frequently evoke cardiovascular reactions scarcely requires documentation; such effects are inevitable, considering the manner in which the activity of an animal is integrated with metabolic and circulatory adjustments. However, the demonstration of psychological influences is only the first step. The additional aim is to evaluate the significance of these factors in pathological conditions. It is therefore necessary to go beyond straightforward description, to the analysis and integration of experimental results.

The interpretation of laboratory data involves extrapolation beyond the immediate experimental context. Certain assumptions are made about the stability and generality of the phenomena observed. The present chapter is concerned with a number of problems in the interpretation of experimental data on animals and man; evidence is cited here only by way of illustration, and detailed evaluation will be delayed until Chapters 5 and 6.

Measurement artefact

It is customary to preface any discussion of behavioural research on cardiovascular and neuroendocrine systems with warnings about measurement. Unfortunately, a cautious attitude is only too justified, since the techniques used in monitoring can influence recordings quite considerably. The reactivity of the circulatory system is a mixed blessing. On the one hand, this responsiveness provides opportunities for psychological research, since the connections between cognitive or emotional factors and cardiovascular function are rich. On the other hand, reactivity makes standardisation of measurement a major problem. The participant's familiarity with the setting or equipment, the obtrusiveness of recording methods, and the significance of the occasion may all contribute. They affect not only the level of function, but changes over time. Such influences can distort fine-grained analysis of circulatory adjustments, and their modulation by behaviour.

These factors all come into play during arterial blood pressure measurement from humans (Steptoe, 1980a). Continuous intra-arterial monitoring may not be as disturbing as is often assumed, but it is nevertheless inconvenient in many experimental settings, and also involves some risk (Beamer and Shapiro, 1973). However, conventional sphygmanometric recordings show wide variation both within and between occasions (Armitage and Rose, 1966). This is due to natural fluctuations, inaccuracies in measurement systems, and also to re-cording conditions.

Familiarity has a powerful influence. Dunne (1969) found that pres-sures measured during the first visit to the clinic were invariably higher than those taken on subsequent occasions. The amount of time required for adaptation was examined by Benson and his associates (1971). Before carrying out a behavioural study of hypertensives, they waited for blood pressure to reach a stable level, and patients therefore at-tended the laboratory repeatedly until pressure readings no longer fell between visits. Up to 16 sessions were needed before stabilisation was achieved. The emphasis that Smirk (1957) has placed on "basal blood pressure" is a further reflection of this effect.

Yet arterial pressure does not simply fall progressively as recordings are repeated; readings are also modified by the importance attached to the occasion. The idea that pressure and pulse rate are lower when taken by a nurse as opposed to the more prestigious doctor has circu-lated anecdotally for many years, and has been systematically confirm-ed. Thus Surwit *et al.* (1978) showed that the pressures recorded during the physician's examination that preceded a treatment study of hyper-tensives were a great deal higher than values found in the case notes. The readings on this occasion also exceeded the levels measured in the first visit to the laboratory—a striking observation, since introducing patients to the unfamiliar setting and equipment might have been expected to provoke pressor responses.

When recordings are taken outside clinical settings, the discrepancies between arterial pressures in different situations are even more marked. Fig. 4.1 illustrates the "physician effect" on pressures re-corded with a portable cuff system; the levels were a great deal higher than others monitored during the day (Werdegar *et al.*, 1967). Other

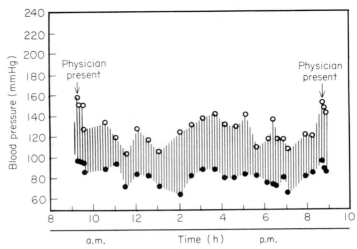

Fig. 4.1. Portable blood pressure recordings from one patient, showing variations over the day, and responses to visits to the physician. (Werdegar *et al.*, 1967.)

investigators have found little correlation between pressures assessed in the clinic and those taken elsewhere (Fouad *et al.*, 1978).

An added problem in experimental studies is that repeated measurement with a cuff may itself distort variations over time. The arm becomes sensitive after frequent occlusion, adding an extra dimension to the impositions on the participant. Thus sphygmanometrically monitored blood pressure does not always fall gradually even in normotensive subjects sitting quietly in the laboratory (Steptoe, 1977a).

These combined influences imply that pressure reactions are not necessarily the products of the experimental stimuli imposed by the investigator. Failure to control for tonic fluctuations and the order of experimental manipulations compromise the interpretation of studies. Nor is this pattern exclusive to blood pressure, since the measurement of neuroendocrine parameters raises similar difficulties. In order to avoid the disturbance of repeated blood sampling, many resort to the assessment of substances such as catecholamines in the urine. Concentrations are higher than in the blood, while collection is less hazardous. Yet unfortunately, levels in the urine are not consistently related to secretions from the adrenal medulla or sympathetic terminals. Only some 6 per cent of catecholamines appear in unchanged form in the urine, due to prior catabolism and incomplete clearance by the kidney (Axelrod, 1965). Urinary concentrations are also affected by renal blood flow; since decreases in flow occur in precisely those circumstances in which the adrenal medulla is stimulated, catecholamine output may be seriously misrepresented.

Furthermore, catecholamines are highly sensitive to novelty (Frankenhaeuser, 1975). Thus the use of laboratory staff as controls for patients is clearly unjustified. Nor can experiments in which conditions are manipulated progressively be easily interpreted (e.g. Frankenhaeuser and Rissler, 1970); the confounding of novelty and repetition of measurement with independent experimental variables makes it difficult to identify responsible causes. The recording of adrenocortical responses is also subject to methodological problems (see Smith, 1973).

These measurement artefacts do not only occur in human studies, although they have received little attention in animal research. Bühler and co-workers (1978) identified situational influences on plasma catecholamine levels in a variety of species. Basal recordings from dogs, cats and rats were made through chronically indwelling catheters, long after these had been inserted. Plasma adrenaline and noradrenaline concentrations were well below values reported in most other studies, and showed little variability. Yet gentle handling of rats for 30 seconds prior to sampling was sufficient to increase adrenaline concentrations tenfold, while noradrenaline rose by 300 per cent. Brief restraint, a technique still employed during measurement, produced adrenaline levels 20 times above basal, while catecholamine concentrations from decapitated animals were vastly inflated.

Thus measurement technique can distort the effects of experimental manipulations in animals as well as man. A case in point may be Shapiro and Horn's (1955) attempt to assess the blood pressure response of cats to anxiety–conflict procedures. Blood pressures were taken by restraining cats on their backs and puncturing the femoral artery. Even after repeated experience, the animals continued to struggle, and failed to adapt to the board. Arterial pressures recorded during light anaesthesia were only inconsistently related to values from conscious animals.

Metabolic demands and cardiovascular responses

One of the fundamental tenets of psychosomatic theory is that psychological factors such as emotional condition or environmental stimulation may have deleterious effects on physical state. However, all behaviours put motor demands on the organism, and these in turn have cardiovascular concomitants. It is therefore important to determine whether responses in noxious conditions are simply adjuncts of motor output. A related question is whether the circulatory adjustments under aversive stimulation are qualitatively different from those produced during other behaviours such as exercise or eating. These problems have generally been neglected in behavioural research, although they are central to the study of interactions between psychological factors and the cardiovascular system.

In many cases, motor responses are found to have a powerful impact on haemodynamic reactions. For example, squirrel monkeys were trained to press a key in order to avoid electric shocks, programmed to occur in the presence of a visual stimulus (Kelleher *et al.*, 1976). If the key was pressed a predetermined number of times (Fixed Ratio schedule), the light was extinguished and no shock was given. These conditions elicited high levels of lever pressing, together with phasic increases in heart rate and arterial pressure. The pressor responses varied with the number of key presses required on the schedule, so that greater changes were produced at higher Fixed Ratios. Hence cardiovascular reactions did not depend simply on the aversiveness of stimulation, but on motor requirements.

Furthermore, it was found that circulatory responses were similar when food was substituted for electric shock; although key presses then led to the presentation of food pellets rather than shock avoidance, the phasic changes in heart rate and blood pressure persisted. Likewise, classical conditioning for rewards and punishment in the rhesus monkey both elicited cardiovascular adjustments (Randall *et al.*, 1976). A low tone was regularly followed after one minute by food, while a high tone preceded electric shock. In each case, heart rate, blood pressure and ventricular contractility rose during the anticipation period.

One parameter that may distinguish cardiovascular reactions in negative and positive conditions is the size of responses. Adjustments are generally larger in threatening settings. Fig. 4.2 summarises the cardiac responses to classical aversive conditioning in the monkey; normal animals were compared with those subjected to total surgical denervation of the heart (Randall *et al.*, 1976). In the latter, the acute pressor responses were eliminated, reflecting mediation by neural pathways. Yet in their place, low-level long-latency reactions were observed. These may have been due to the delayed effects of circulating catecholamines, secreted during shock anticipation. No secondary reaction of this type was found on food trials, suggesting that the physical activation was less pronounced in appetitive conditions.

However, if circulatory responses to perturbing stimuli are merely

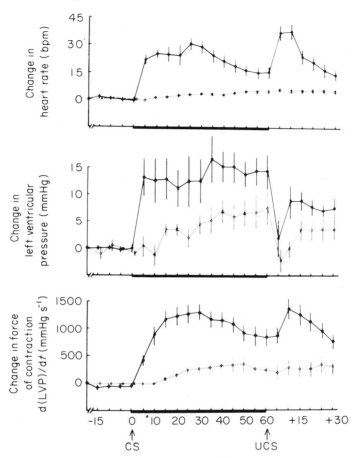

Fig. 4.2. Cardiac responses to classical aversive conditioning in 10 normal (solid line) and 5 monkeys with denervated hearts (dotted line). Mean changes ±s.e. from average resting values in the 30 s prior to CS. (Randall *et al.*, 1976.)

larger, it might be predicted that comparable changes would emerge during exercise. This is not always the case, since detailed haemo-dynamic studies suggest qualitative differences in reactions. Thus Vatner (1978) monitored mesenteric and renal blood flow telemetri-cally from unrestrained baboons. Pressor responses were recorded during moderate exercise, but there was no reduction of flow in these visceral beds. In contrast, the emotional excitement generated by tantalising animals, provoked decreases in flow of more than 80 per cent; resistance in the renal and mesenteric vessels rose some ten times.

The cardiovascular modifications in aversive conditions may be disproportionately large for the metabolic demands put on the system. Langer *et al.* (1979) measured oxygen extraction from the blood by sampling arterial-mixed venous oxygen $(A-VO_2)$ difference in dogs. Running exercise produced work-dependent increases in cardiac output, heart rate and $A-VO_2$. The correlations between these parameters were significant, indicating that the cardiac response was associated with fuel demand. But during sessions of shock avoidance, the correlations between cardiac output and $A-VO_2$ difference fell to low or non-significant levels. The oxygen extraction was less than would be expected for the level of cardiac output. There was an excessive rise in cardiac activity that was not warranted by metabolic requirements.

In experimental research on man, the motor components of laboratory tasks have tended to be ignored. For example, verbal mental arithmetic is frequently used as a "psychological stressor"; yet this test involves articulatory responses, and interference with normal breathing, both of which may affect cardiovascular function. Other forms of stimulation, such as disturbing or unpleasant films, require no response apart from passive observation. Variations in motor output may thus make important contributions to the pattern of cardiovascular adjustment.

This is not to say that reactions in man are solely functions of motor activity. Some investigators have held behavioural responses constant while varying mental task difficulty, and have recorded different degrees of tachycardia (Kahneman *et al.*, 1969). Haemodynamic adjustments may again be disproportionate to motor demands. Gliner *et al.* (1979) monitored heart rate and cardiac stoke volume from volunteers before an important public speech, and then during physical exercise on a bicycle. Exercise was regulated so that heart rate increased to the degree measured under the psychological stress; the average cardiac index was then found to be identical under the two conditions, despite the fact that the metabolic demands during anticipatory threat were much lower.

Another method of testing the link between cardiac activity and physical demand is by recording heart rate and oxygen uptake at different levels of treadmill exercise (Blix *et al.*, 1974). A curve relating the two variables can then be plotted, and the heart rate expected for various degrees of oxygen consumption during other activities may then be estimated. When helicopter and aircraft pilots were subsequently monitored while performing takeoffs and landings, their heart rates were well in excess of those predicted from the oxygen uptake curve; these tachycardias or "additional heart rates" were disproportionate to metabolic requirement.

Data from humans and laboratory animals indicate that the cardiovascular responses in noxious conditions are not products of motor activity alone. Nevertheless, it cannot be assumed that all reactions are due to psychological factors (such as mental work or emotional arousal). Attention must be paid to this aspect of experimental conditions if the true origins and organisation of cardiovascular adjustments are to be identified.

Acute and chronic cardiovascular reactions

Experimental studies of animals and man are generally brief in comparison with the time scale of pathological processes. Two strategies are therefore commonly used in the design and interpretation of laboratory findings.

a. When working with animals, it is common to hasten or telescope pathological changes by applying acute, very severe stimulation. This method is regularly employed in pathophysiological research; the Goldblatt preparation for renal hypertension, the feeding of animals with very high cholesterol diets, and DOCA–salt hypertension all utilise the technique. Similarly in behavioural laboratories, animals are exposed to intense traumatic conditions in an effort to provoke tissue damage that might otherwise only develop after years. It is assumed that the mechanisms mobilised during acute or severe interventions are similar to those that mediate chronic, lower level stimulation. If this assumption is at fault, much physiological as well as psychological research on the circulation may be of little direct value.

b. Strategy (a) cannot be applied to man, so an alternative argument is proposed. It is suggested that the small size and reversibility of circulatory responses is due to the brief duration of experiments. If stimulation were to be continued or repeated, reactions such as hypersecretion of glucocorticoids, vasoconstriction or increases in blood pressure, might become sustained. The assumption here is that short-term responses parallel long-term pathology.

The difficulty with all such inferences from acute observations is that the circulation is both flexible and adaptive. Many interventions, even of a gross nature, can be accommodated homeostatically. Consequently, it cannot simply be taken for granted that reactions seen in the short

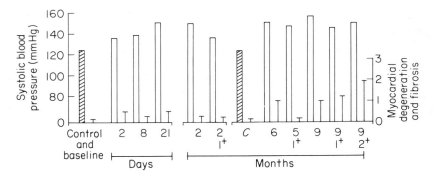

Fɪɢ. 4.3. Cardiovascular pathology in male mice following varying durations of psychosocial stimulation in population cages. The histograms indicate average systolic pressures, while the bars represent degree of myocardial necrosis. The time scale refers to the length of time spent in the population cages. C = control values from animals kept in isolation. 2+1, 5+1, 9+1 and 9+2 represent groups returned to isolation for one- or two-month periods following psychosocial stimulation. (Henry *et al.*, 1975.)

term will necessarily progress to pathological conclusions; the hypothesis must be substantiated by documentation of long-term change.

Chronic disturbances have been recorded for some experimental preparations. Henry and his colleagues (1975) have studied male mice raised in isolation and then put into large colonies for varying periods of social stimulation. These mice are hyperaggressive, and living in the colony therefore involves repeated confrontation and the inhibition of territorial behaviour. Considerable cardiovascular pathology is observed in these animals, as can be seen in Fig. 4.3. Generally, the responses are transient in the short term, but irreversible damage may develop after prolonged stimulation. In primates such as the squirrel monkey, a high incidence of coronary atherosclerosis has been elicited after animals performed a shock avoidance task daily for more than two years (Lang, 1967). A variety of experimental hypertensions have also been produced in monkeys, and these will be discussed in Chapter 5.

On the other hand, there is evidence that cardiovascular and neuroendocrine responses may habituate after repeated exposure to behavioural stimuli. Leenen and Shapiro (1974) measured the plasma renin activity (PRA) of rats subjected to regular, inescapable electric shocks. Although rapid increases in PRA were generated within a few minutes, longer experience of 8 to 24 hours with shock was associated with a return to control levels. Likewise, the habituation or adaptation of adrenocortical hypersecretion during long-term stimulation has been documented in both rodents and primates (Brady, 1965; Mikulaj *et al.*, 1976).

The relationship between short- and long-term responses in man will receive special consideration in Chapter 7. There are, however, three factors that may contribute to the variations in response duration. Firstly, some neural and endocrine pathways may only react acutely, and be incapable of long-term disturbance in response to behavioural stimuli. This possibility can only be resolved empirically, although much evidence may already be marshalled against it. Secondly, there may be differences between species in the duration and salience of reactions; and in the third place, the response pattern may vary with the type of stimulation imposed. These last two explanations will be considered separately.

Reactivity in different species

There are marked variations in the cardiovascular reactivity of animals to behavioural stimuli. Fig. 4.3 illustrated the responses of mice placed in socially competitive colonies. They contrast with the effects of keeping rats in overcrowded conditions for several months; despite the selection of animals from strains susceptible to hypertension, high arterial pressure did not develop at a rate exceeding that of control siblings (Dahl *et al.*, 1968). Thus crowding and competition for food are not necessarily powerful provoking agents in themselves.

Some important differences are also observed amongst primates. The squirrel monkey is highly vulnerable, and readily develops hypertension and cardiac pathology in shock avoidance studies (Corley *et al.*, 1977). Yet baboons maintained in similar experiments for up to 12 months do not show these changes (Brady, 1965). Rhesus monkeys may be intermediate, for although high arterial pressure does emerge, few signs of vascular or cardiac necrosis are manifest even after prolonged periods (Forsyth, 1969).

Differences may be related to the organisation of cardiac innervation. The contributions of sympathetic and vagal inputs to the heart can be assessed by pharmacological blockade of both pathways. The resulting "intrinsic" heart rate is higher than the resting level in man, indicating that chronic vagal inhibition is normally present. This pattern underlies the difficulty in demonstrating sympathetic nervous influences on human heart rate. Over a series of experiments, Obrist and his colleagues studied phasic heart rate changes during anticipation of electric shock. Responses were predominantly modulated by the vagus, and sympathetic reactions were observed only on threat of extremely severe stimulation (Obrist, 1976; Obrist *et al.*, 1974).

The squirrel monkey, however, has an intrinsic rate somewhat below resting levels (Herd *et al.*, 1974). Thus the sensitivity of this species to behavioural stimulation may be a consequence of high cardiac sympathetic tone, and the significance of responses for human pathology must be qualified. The dog and rhesus may be more comparable with man in terms of cardiac innervation patterns. In the case of coronary vascular distribution, however, the primate has been recommended as the most appropriate model (Bruyneel and Opie, 1974). The anatomy of the coronary arteries and collaterals, together with the form of infarcts, makes the primate preferable to the dog in myocardial infarction research.

Experimental and natural stimuli

A variety of stimuli, ranging from immobilisation to electric shock, are used in psychological studies of animals. The primary concern may not be with these stimuli themselves, but with the behavioural contingencies under which they are imposed. Thus electric shock may signalled or unsignalled, or presented at regular or irregular intervals. However, experimental studies generally employ forms of stimulation that are not naturally encountered by animals. Psychophysiological investigations of humans may also involve relatively artificial threats or taxing mental puzzles. It is therefore important to rule out the possibility that experimental stimuli provoke artificial cardiovascular responses.

Fortunately, advances in measurement technology have permitted natural forms of stimulation to be explored in detail, and parallels with experimental stimuli have been established. For example, the circulatory activation and redistribution of blood flow that occurs when cats are exposed to threats such as a barking dog, are mediated sympathetically (Mancia *et al.*, 1974). As in the responses to laboratory stimuli, both autonomic vascular innervation and the adrenal medulla are involved. This was confirmed by monitoring renal blood flow in cats with unilaterally denervated kidneys. Fig. 4.4 illustrates the distinct effects of neural vasoconstriction and catecholamine release on renal flow in this preparation. In the left-hand panel, the modest vasoconstriction in response to immobile confrontation with another cat is restricted to the innervated kidney. But under the more severe threat of supportive fighting with a dog (right-hand panel), vaso-

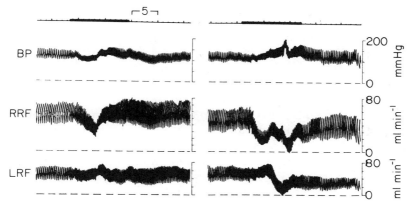

FIG. 4.4. Arterial blood pressure and renal blood flow in the cat during immobile confrontation (left) and supportive fighting (right). RRF, blood flow to the innervated right kidney; LRF, blood flow to the denervated left kidney. (Mancia *et al.*, 1974.)

constriction is observed in the denervated organ as well. This suggests that in the more taxing condition, adrenal medullary catecholamines bolster neurally mediated vasoconstriction.

In primates, Zbrozyna (1976) reported substantial pressor responses, together with reductions in renal flow, when animals were frightened by snakes. Corticosteroid output is also sensitive to natural stimuli, and secretion in both rodents and primates depends on the position of the individual in the dominance hierarchy (Chamove and Bowman, 1978; Christian, 1971).

Responses to non-painful behavioural stimulation in humans cover the gamut of mechanisms discussed in Chapters 2 and 3, from endocrine responses and changes in blood coagulability, right through to flow redistributions and pressor responses. Yet although parallels may be drawn between different types of stimuli, the conditions under which they are imposed remain crucial. It will be argued in subsequent chapters that the presentation of stimuli, and the cognitive or behavioural responses that are mobilised to cope with them, are vital factors in determining cardiovascular reactions.

The concept of stress

Some of the work discussed in subsequent chapters might pass under the general rubric of stress. Although Selye's original work was concerned primarily with the pituitary–adrenocortical system, the applications of the term have extended greatly. Psychological stress is an umbrella covering almost every way in which the environment, emotion, behaviour or personality might affect the organism's physical well-being. Yet this very ubiquity is itself a handicap; the expression has become an excuse for careless thinking, and can deter more exact investigation.

It will become apparent in later sections that the general concept of stress has little explanatory value in the analysis of cardiovascular disorders. However, it is relevant here to mention some semantic and theoretical shortcomings (see Steptoe, 1980b). There are a number of terminological ambiguities in the definition of stress. Selye (1976) has used the term to describe the "non-specific response of the body to any demand", yet also refers to people being "under stress", implying that stress is a stimulus rather than a reaction. When commentators describe the stress of urban life, does this label identifiable responses, is it a characteristic of external conditions, or perhaps an inference about the apparent noxiousness of stimuli impinging on the individual? The expression has also been defined as the interaction or transaction between person and environment (Lazarus and Cohen, 1977).

The introduction of "psychological stressor" to describe stimuli has done little to clarify ambiguities, since stressors cannot be specified by their physical characteristics, only by their consequences. For example, electric shock is an archetypal experimental stressor; yet it will be seen that the cardiovascular responses to shock depend not simply on qualities such as duration and intensity, but on predictability, prior experience, behavioural response requirement, pattern of presentation, cognitive appraisal, the availability of coping strategies and other factors. Under the circumstances, labelling shock as a stressor conveys very slight information.

These are not merely semantic quibbles, since they introduce a vagueness into the discussion of stress that can inhibit serious analysis. Stress may be used as a glib explanation of phenomena that are not understood, discouraging the search for other causes of disturbance. For in the absence of *a priori* definitions, arguments based on stress are frequently irrefutable; almost any difference in circulatory response between groups may be "understood" in these terms. For instance, it has been suggested that church attenders are protected from stress, since they have access to social supports, group cohesion, and coping strategies backed by religious tenets (Kaplan, 1976). On the other hand, the religious may be under more stress than others; the bases of faith are increasingly challenged by cultural demands, while contradictions between the requirements of a religious life and the means of survival or achievement in contemporary materialist society widen.

The term stress is too fluid to provide an adequate theoretical framework.

A further problem is that unwarranted generalisations are made about stress responses. Stress is used to describe reactions in the cognitive, emotional, behavioural, neuroendocrine and physical domains, but it cannot be assumed that reactions are congruent. There is abundant evidence that phenomena in these different categories are not closely correlated. Psychological stress, however defined, is not consistently associated with disturbed biological function, and does not always lead to the same alterations in overt behaviour. Conversely, extreme physical stress, provoked for example by haemorrhage or cold, can be produced in anaesthetised preparations, where the behavioural or mental parameters are completely unaffected. Even within the cardiovascular and neuroendocrine fields, no generalised reactions are seen to all imposed stressors. This problem has been explored in detail by Mason in his discussions of non-specificity (Mason, 1972, 1975; Mason *et al.*, 1976).

It is evident that allusion to stress in the present narrative would only cause confusion. The expression will therefore be avoided as far as possible. Some reference is made to behavioural stressors, but this is in the limited context of particular studies, where the phrase is an acceptable shorthand for describing the experimental contingencies applied to an organism.

Summary and conclusions

Several assumptions and inferences governing experimental approaches to psychological influences on the circulation have been outlined. These place limitations on the conclusions that may be drawn from such investigations.

Recordings of cardiovascular and neuroendocrine variables are affected by measurement conditions, including the techniques employed, the subject's prior experience, and the significance of the circumstances in which monitoring takes place. If these factors are not appreciated and controlled, data may be uninterpretable.

Behavioural studies involve physical as well as psychological demands on the organism. Cardiovascular reactions cannot necessarily be interpreted in terms of emotional or mental disturbance, but may be concommittants of motor activity.

Acute cardiovascular and neuroendocrine responses do not all endure in the long term, and some may therefore be of little significance in chronic disease aetiology. There are variations between species in the form of reactions, and not all respond in the same way as humans. Although in many cases, circulatory changes in experiments parallel responses to natural threats, the conditions under which the stimulation is imposed may be crucial. The experimental approach has an important role in identifying the dimensions of environmental influence that are involved in cardiovascular disorders. However, the demonstration of a circulatory response to a particular form of stimulation does not mean that the pathway is necessarily of any relevance to pathological conditions.

The experimental literature covers a wide variety of phenomena, with different species, stimuli and physiological variables exploited. Much may be learned from negative results — about the circumstances that do not provoke reactions — as well as from the positive.

5
Neuroendocrine and Cardiovascular Reaction Patterns in Animals

Haemodynamic reactions during psychological stimulation

Animals typically respond to painful or threatening stimulation by preparing for confrontation or flight. The precise form of behaviour varies between species, but may include displays such as arching the back, piloerection and baring the teeth. These actions are accompanied by acute mobilisation of the cardiovascular system. The haemodynamic components of the response were identified by Cannon (1915), and involve increases in the force and rate of cardiac contraction, together with preferential diversion of blood to skeletal muscle at the expense of visceral beds. The alteration in arterial pressure is variable, depending on the balance between skeletal vasodilatation and constriction in other tissues. These responses are mediated in the short term by increased traffic in the sympathetic nervous pathways, augmented by catecholamine secretions from the adrenal medulla; in addition, vagal tone to the heart may be withdrawn. The entire response pattern mirrors the defence reaction elicited with hypothalamic stimulation (see Chapter 2).

Haemodynamic adjustments are not themselves dangerous or pathological, but are inevitable consequences of the integration between behavioural output and its vegetative concomitants. Nevertheless, the responses to threat share a number of significant features. Firstly, some components are mobilized in response to motor activities, while others are prepared in anticipation of physical work. Thus sympathetic cardiac tone may increase before any action is taken, together with peripheral vasoconstriction; on the other hand, much of the vasodilatation in skeletal beds is a consequence of local metabolic factors evoked by muscular work itself, and is not a direct result of neural outflow (Adams *et al.*, 1969). Secondly, acute haemodynamic

73

adjustments are provoked under conditions where prolonged exercise and muscular work are not required. Cardiovascular mobilisation may therefore occur when flight or fight are inappropriate behavioural responses.

Most important for the study of circulatory dysfunction is the observation that reaction patterns are not the same under all aversive or potentially noxious conditions. This variation provides a key for exploring those elements of environmental stimulation and behavioural demand that are involved in promoting high blood pressure. Circumstances in which large modifications are recorded may be compared with those that provoke little haemodynamic response. Unfortunately, most behavioural scientists are intent on maximising blood pressure change, and do not exploit negative results. Nevertheless, it is clear that the production of substantial pressor responses depends not simply on the intensity of stimulation, since reactions are modulated by a network of associated factors. The animal's experience may be complex, as in the mouse colonies briefly described in Chapter 4 (p. 66), or relatively simple; it is easier to consider responses in less complicated conditions in the first instance.

Dahl and associates (1968) studied the effects of two forms of behavioural stimulation on blood pressure in rats bred for their susceptibility to hypertension, and fed a diet including salt. In one group, animals were administered unavoidable electric shocks at random intervals in sessions that spanned more than four months. A second group was given unavoidable shocks paired in the first place with a warning signal (a classical conditioning format), but later occurring independently of the tone or light. In neither instance did experimental animals develop higher blood pressure than control siblings.

Even if differences in pressor response had been observed under these circumstances, they could not have been attributed solely to psychological disturbance. Electric shock is painful, and may provoke direct tissue reactions independently of the higher nervous system. The most appropriate way of evaluating behavioural or emotional effects is to subject different groups to identical physical threat or deprivation, while varying psychological contingencies (Steptoe, 1980b).

This was done in a further study of rats from a pressor-sensitive strain (Friedman and Dahl, 1975). They were divided into the five groups outlined in Table 5.1. Groups 1 and 2 were both trained to press a lever, and food was delivered according to an intermittent (Variable Interval) schedule of reinforcement. In addition, lever presses by Group 1 periodically resulted in electric shock administration (Variable Ratio schedule); thus Group 1 was in a state of conflict,

TABLE 5.1
Experimental groups in Friedman and Dahl's (1975) study

Group	Treatment
1. Conflict	Food and electric shock delivered on lever presses
2. Yoked shock	Food on lever press, shocks yoked to Group 1
3. Yoked food	No shock, food yoked to Group 1 or 2
4. Yoked food and shock	No lever press, food and shock yoked to Group 1
5. Control	Ad lib food, no shock

since both food and shock were dependent on behavioural responses. The remaining groups were "yoked" to Group 1, controlling for the various aspects of physical distress. For example, Group 2 received an identical pattern of shocks to Group 1, while Group 3 was given the same number of food pellets without experiencing any shock. These yoked control procedures removed the element of conflict, while matching the physical dimensions of Group 1.

The results of this study are complex, since blood pressure was elevated above control levels in all four experimental groups at some point. However, the greatest and most consistent pressor response was recorded in the conflict condition (Group 1). In contrast, the group yoked for shock (Group 2) showed no sustained pressure rise. Using a strain of rats bred for susceptibility to borderline hypertension, Lawler *et al.* (1980) also found conflict to be a potent elicitor of high blood pressure.

These studies suggest that the cardiovascular response varies according to the relationship between noxious stimulation and the organism's behaviour. When shock was imposed independently of behaviour, increased pressure was not provoked even in genetically susceptible rats. Similar response dimensions are relevant to the pressor reactions of primates.

Behaviourally induced hypertension in primates

When monkeys are subjected to sequences of electric shock over which they have no control, tonic increases in arterial pressure and heart rate are seldom found; this has been documented even when schedules of shock were continued for several sessions (Forsyth, 1968; Benson *et al.*,

1970). On the other hand, haemodynamic adjustments are prominent when the administration of shock depends on the animal's behaviour. Characteristically, the investigations of behavioural hypertension amongst primates have employed variations on the shock avoidance strategy.

Thus Forsyth (1969) equipped adolescent rhesus monkeys with implanted arterial catheters, and monitored them systematically for more than a year. After periods of adaptation and the assessment of basal pressure, experimental animals performed on Sidman avoidance schedules for extended daily sessions. Under these conditions, the animal receives an electric shock at a predefined interval following the last lever press, unless a further response is made. Each lever press resets the timer, so that by responding regularly, the monkey avoids shock for much of the time. Four monkeys were trained on schedules with a 20-second delay between response and shock, compared with controls that were given shock without being able to avoid it. Over the first three months, blood pressures did not rise, but gradual increases were subsequently observed in three of the four monkeys. By the seventh month, systolic pressure averaged 28 mmHg and diastolic 19 mmHg above pretraining levels. Diurnal variations of cardiovascular function

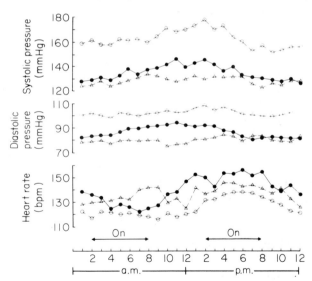

FIG. 5.1. Mean levels of arterial pressure and heart rate throughout the diurnal cycle for one monkey. ●———●, Baseline period ($N = 12$ per hour); Δ - - - - Δ, after 3 months avoidance conditioning ($N = 30\,\mathrm{h}^{-1}$); ○- - - -○, after 8 months avoidance conditioning ($N = 30\,\mathrm{h}^{-1}$). (Forsyth, 1969.)

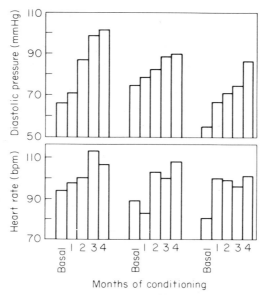

Fig. 5.2. Average heart rate and diastolic blood pressure for each of three baboons during "conditioning off" (rest) periods at different stages of blood pressure conditioning. Values for the pre-experimental baseline, and the first four months of conditioning are shown. (Harris and Brady, 1977.)

in one of these animals at different stages of the experiment are illustrated in Fig. 5.1; while the contour of fluctuation remained stable, the pressures were maintained at considerably higher levels by the eighth month. The fourth shock avoidance monkey showed little pressor response, but instead a marked tachycardia emerged—this may reflect individual variability, even in these precisely controlled environmental conditions.

Similar patterns of cardiovascular response have been observed in the squirrel monkey, where behavioural hypertension may be rapidly induced (Benson *et al.*, 1969). The baboon however behaves differently. Findley and his colleagues (1971) programmed the entire lives of two baboons, allowing specified periods for eating and sleeping, together with two 6-hour avoidance sessions in each day. Throughout the ten-month investigation, haemodynamic reactions were consistently elicited, with higher levels of blood pressure and heart rate during shock avoidance than while eating or sleeping. But the pattern was stable, with no trend towards greater responses after long exposure, and no maintenance of hypertension outside avoidance phases.

A second strategy is to condition pressor responses directly, by making shock avoidance depend on pressure level itself, so that the animal learns to maintain hypertension. Harris and Brady (1977) made both food availability and shock avoidance contingent on the level of diastolic pressure produced by a series of baboons. The criterion pressure was gradually raised, so that higher and higher levels were needed in order to avoid shock and receive food. Under these conditions, systolic and diastolic pressures were elevated throughout the 12 hour sessions, even though only one or two shocks were actually administered. Moreover, the haemodynamic adjustments were eventually established outside conditioning sessions, over the rest of the day. Fig. 5.2 summarises diastolic pressure and heart rate averaged over rest periods in consecutive months of training. Despite the absence of any shocks or response requirements during these phases, pressure progressively increased. These changes were reversible on removing the baboons from the conditioning programme in the early months, but later the high pressure became fixed.

Studies of this type have been carried out on only a few animals, and even between these there is much variation. The investigations are expensive, unpleasant, and take a long time to complete; nevertheless, the data indicate that stable levels of high arterial pressure may be produced with challenging environmental contingencies. In some cases, the parallel with human hypertension may extend to the underlying patterns of haemodynamic adjustment. Forsyth (1971) reported a switch-over from cardiac output to peripheral resistance mechanisms as shock avoidance was continued for an extended session. Monkeys performed Sidman avoidance for 72 hours, and were periodically injected with radioactively labelled microspheres. These were dispersed to tissues in proportions that reflected the distribution of cardiac output at different stages of the study. Consequently, a picture of the changes in blood flow over time could be built up, as shown in Fig. 5.3.

Hypertension was sustained throughout the experiment, but the mechanism underlying the response altered progressively. In the early stages, the pressor reaction was underpinned by a high cardiac output, while total peripheral resistance did not alter. As the experiment proceeded, however, resistance rose at the expense of cardiac output, and eventually accounted for the raised blood pressure entirely. Furthermore, the distribution of blood in the early phases of avoidance reflected typical cardiosympathetic activation, with vasodilatation in the coronary and skeletal beds, and reduced flow to the skin and viscera. Later in the study, flow to voluntary muscle diminished, and this may have been responsible for the net rise in peripheral resistance.

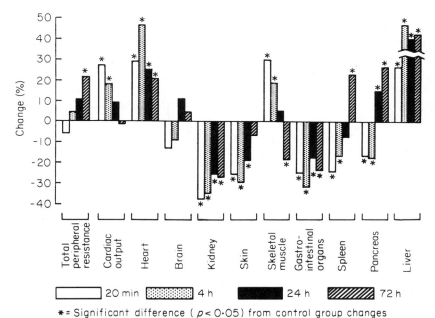

Fig. 5.3. Modifications in total peripheral resistance, cardiac output, and regional distribution of blood during 72 hours of continuous Sidman avoidance (from Forsyth, 1971).

These results illustrate in microcosm the haemodynamic progress of some human hypertensives, and mirror the responses to stellate ganglion stimulation described in Chapter 3 (p. 46).

Forsyth's study again demanded alert responding from the animal in order to avert shock. Unfortunately, it cannot be concluded that behaviourally induced hypertension occurs only when noxious stimulation is dependent on the animal's actions. Durable hypertension has been documented in rodents under conditions of passive distress, when aversive events were not contingent on behaviour. Buckley (1977) for example, subjected albino rats to four hourly sessions of severe sensory stimulation three times a week. Large cages containing 20 rats were vibrated on an Eberbach shaker at 140 cycles min^{-1}, during exposure to high-intensity noise and flashing lights. Under these conditions, arterial pressure rose over several weeks to levels above those of unstressed animals. In a rather different experimental environment, Marwood and Lockett (1977) kept pairs of rats in a soundproofed room for prolonged intervals. Pressures were raised in comparison with controls housed under normal laboratory conditions, and eventually stabilised at a high level. The pressor response was reversible on removing rats from the silent environment, but only if transfer occurred within five weeks; after longer exposure, the hypertension became permanently established.

The discrepancies between outcomes in rodent and primate experiments may be species dependent. Alternatively, patterns of response may be subtly different, varying with the mechanisms of cardiovascular activation. Careful analysis of different experimental paradigms suggests that the circulatory adjustment elicited during active (behaviour-dependent) threat is more closely associated with cardiac sympathetic and catecholamine pathways than the responses in passive conditions.

Behaviour-dependent stimulation and the mechanisms of cardiovascular activation

The patterns of cardiovascular adaptation that underlie pressor responses in different circumstances are best explored within single experimental settings, instead of attempting to generalise across studies. Much attention has been focused on the reactions of dogs trained in shock avoidance (Anderson and Brady, 1973). Modifications in cardiovascular function are observed both in anticipation and during avoidance sessions, but the patterns of circulatory activation are different in the two cases. Avoidance training itself provokes large, immediate and durable increases in systolic and diastolic pressure, together with tachycardia. Yet in the period preceding avoidance, pressure rises gradually without elevations in heart rate.

The two response configurations were examined with detailed haemodynamic monitoring by Anderson and Tosheff (1973). Their results are summarised in Fig. 5.4. In the preavoidance period, high arterial pressure was maintained by resistive factors, whilst cardiac output increased abruptly at the start of avoidance. Lawler *et al.* (1975) found that myocardial contractility rose when behavioural responses were initiated, and the β-adrenergic cardiac activation has been confirmed with direct intracardiac recordings (Galosy *et al.*, 1979). Moreover, propranolol has no effect on the preavoidance pattern, while reliably attenuating the tachycardia in avoidance itself (Anderson and Brady, 1976).

These studies of dogs clearly show the manner in which cardiac sympathetic tracts are relatively undisturbed by passive anticipatory distress, but are strongly stimulated during alert behavioural per-

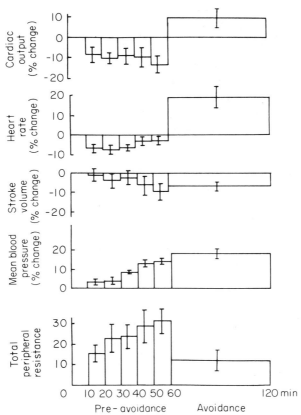

Fɪɢ. 5.4. Cardiovascular function (averaged across 20 sessions for 4 dogs) during successive 10-minute intervals of the pre-avoidance hour and for the 60-minute avoidance session (Anderson and Tosheff, 1973).

formance. Similar β-adrenergic effects are recorded in other settings. For example, Blair and associates (1976) measured high levels of PRA in baboons both during and immediately after avoidance sessions. The reactions were not directly correlated either with shock administration or lever presses. The tachycardia displayed by baboons during shock avoidance sessions is reduced by propranolol, while pressor responses are attenuated with combined α and β blockade (Harris *et al.*, 1977).

When cardiovascular arousal does occur in response to stimuli that are not contingent on the organism's behaviour, high levels of cardiac sympathetic tone do not persist. Initial reactions may be mediated β adrenergically, but their importance to the overall circulatory adaptation rapidly diminishes. This is seen during classical (**Pavlovian**) aversive conditioning. When dogs were exposed to a tone followed after 7 seconds by shock, conditioned responses to the tone included elevations in heart rate and cardiac contractility (Obrist *et al.*, 1972). However, contractility changes disappeared after the first trials; the tachycardia, which persisted, was not abolished by β blockade, suggesting a vagal mechanism. Dykman and Gantt (1960) showed that tonic arterial pressure did not alter even when classical conditioning was continued for more than a year — in striking contrast to the chronic responses in avoidance experiments. It appears that under passive aversive conditions, heart rate is predominantly regulated by vagal tone, rather than β-adrenergic mechanisms (Galosy and Gaebelein, 1977). In the rabbit, the cardiovascular response during classical conditioning does not include increases in heart rate and blood pressure at all; rather, a vagally mediated bradycardia is induced (Sampson *et al.*, 1974).

A low sympathetic output is characteristic of other responses during passive noxious stimulation. Hallbäck and Folkow (1974) exposed spontaneously hypertensive rats to intense auditory, visual and vibratory stimulation for a single session. Under resting conditions, β blockade elicited greater bradycardia from these animals than from normal control rats, suggesting high tonic traffic in the sympathetic pathways. Yet even against such a background, the reactions to environmental stimulation were not attenuated with propranolol — rather, vagal blockade with atropine was necessary to reduce the cardiac response. Sustained hypertensive reactions may also be independent of sympathetic activity. Thus during the development of high arterial pressure in the sound-proofed environment described on page 79, plasma catecholamines actually fell below control levels.

There appears to be considerable support for the hypothesis that β-adrenergic sympathetic responses, and even catecholamine mobilisation, are prominent only when psychological threats are contingent on the organism's behaviour. During passive stimulation, haemodynamic reactions may occur, but they are not likely to be sustained by these pathways. In view of the importance placed on sympathetic nervous activation in the early stages of human hypertension (see Chapter 3), these distinctions have important implications for evaluating the contribution of behaviour and environmental factors.

Nevertheless, these conclusions must be qualified in several respects:

a. *Duration of responses.* The initial reactions to noxious conditions tend to include sympathetic and catecholamine mobilisation, regardless of the precise contingencies (see p. 00); the distinctions discussed here emerge only after chronic stimulation. Thus β-adrenergically mediated changes in cardiac contractility and PRA have been recorded during classical aversive conditioning, and can be extended by spacing experimental trials widely (Randall *et al.*, 1976; Schramm *et al.*, 1975). Significant alterations in other functions, such as platelet aggregation, may also be elicited with acute, severe, uncontrollable stimuli (Haft and Fani, 1973).

Yet these reactions are not persistent. In the case of PRA for example, the time course of responses over extended periods of inescapable shock was explored by Leenen and Shapiro (1974). Although reliable increases were measured during the first hour, PRA responses diminished as the experiment continued, and had returned to baseline by the eighth hour. The early rise in PRA was suppressed by propranolol, confirming the β-adrenergic mechanism. Parallel effects have been recorded over a longer time scale in rhesus monkeys restrained chronically in primate chairs (Perlow *et al.*, 1979). Excretion of adrenergic metabolites was significantly greater in the first few days than after three weeks of restraint.

One reason why the pattern of neuroendocrine activation alters when animals are helplessly exposed to unpleasant conditions is that behaviour may change. In the early stages, the animal attempts to struggle and escape, thus mimicking the alert actions seen during avoidance conditioning. As these efforts to master the environment cease, β-adrenergic mechanisms no longer exert a powerful influence. This illustrates a second hazard in generalising about cardiovascular reactions under disturbing conditions.

b. *Eliciting conditions and behavioural responses.* The distinctions drawn between haemodynamic reactions under active and passive (or contingent and non-contingent) noxious conditions are facets of the animal's behaviour, not of the stimulation *per se*. Thus although some experimental operations are programmed independently of voluntary actions, the animal may not perceive the situation in the same way. For example, very large increases in plasma catecholamines are recorded from rats immobilised for 150-minute epochs, and these responses may persist for several sessions (Kvetnansky and Mikulaj, 1970). Yet while this is a passive stressor, in that the rat is released after the same period irrespective of behaviour, the organism may engage in attempts at active coping. It will struggle to escape, and be rewarded for its efforts after 150 minutes. Consequently, the patterns of cardiovascular arousal parallel those generated by response-contingent stimulation. Struggling and other motor responses are typical in immobilisation, and may promote adrenomedullary secretions (Shapiro and Horn, 1955; Kvetnansky *et al.*, 1979). Indeed, there is some doubt whether immobilisation can be considered purely as an emotional or behavioural stressor at all (Feldman *et al.*, 1970). When the hypothalamus is isolated surgically from the rest of the brain, immobilisation continues to elicit ACTH responses, despite the absence of higher neural inputs. Thus central integration is not a prerequisite of neuroendocrine reactions to immobilisation.

Similarly, responses may differ when animals are alone or in groups during aversive stimulation. If rats are shocked in pairs they fight, and the pattern of cardiovascular and adrenocortical reactions is not the same as in solitary animals (Conner *et al.*, 1971; Williams *et al.*, 1979). When stimulation is apparently dependent on another animal, active reprisal becomes a possibility, and the context of passive helplessness is transformed. Thus experiments such as those described by Buckley (1977), in which groups of rats were stressed simultaneously, are difficult to interpret.

The need to consider the animal's precise behaviour, and not simply the operational conditions of the experiment, is amply documented by investigators of the mouse colonies described in Chapter 4 (Henry, 1976; Henry and Stephens, 1977). Blood pressure and PRA rise as soon as the mice are introduced into the colony, and there are large increases in turnover of catecholamine synthesising enzymes during the first few weeks (Vander *et al.*, 1978). Confrontations and aggressive interactions are common in this period. However, after several months, the activity of these enzymes falls back towards control values; the change reflects alterations in the social conditions, as the ageing males tend to fight less, and the pattern of psychosocial stimulation is modified.

c. *Interactions between neural pathways and other factors.* A further caveat is that the autonomic tracts do not determine the haemodynamic reactions to behavioural stimulation in isolation. Even when noxious events are dependent on behaviour, circulatory adjustments are not due entirely to neurogenic activation. Thus although β blockade reduces the tachycardia of dogs and primates performing shock avoidance, it does not necessarily have a depressor effect (Anderson and Brady, 1976; Herd *et al.*, 1974). Combinations of α and β inhibitors may not eliminate blood pressure reactions entirely (Harris *et al.*, 1977). Nor does the sympathetic nervous system respond in an unified manner (Williams *et al.*, 1979).

These observations suggest that non-neural factors also contribute to the pathological responses, and may act in concert with autonomic traffic. Some interactions of this kind have been identified. Forsyth and associates (1971) chronically infused angiotensin at low concentrations into rhesus monkeys. At the dosages employed, the agent evoked little cardiovascular response. However, when the monkeys also began shock avoidance conditioning, large increases in blood pressure were produced. The pressor reactions were greater than those measured during shock avoidance alone. Likewise, Shapiro and Melhado (1957) found that the hypertensive responses to long-term electric shock schedules developed more rapidly in rats made vulnerable by kidney damage. Reactions to some forms of environmental stimulation may also be exaggerated amongst rats with a genetic susceptibility for hypertension (Hallbäck and Folkow, 1974; Friedman and Iwai, 1976).

While recognising these limitations, it can be inferred that the cardiovascular reactions provoked when animals are passively exposed to noxious stimulation generally differ in mechanism and durability from those induced under active conditions. As far as the pathogenesis of essential hypertension is concerned, the β-adrenergically mediated responses to contingent stimulation are most significant. However, when reactions in the pituitary–adrenocortical axis are considered, settings of passive helplessness may be more important.

Responses of the pituitary–adrenocortical system

The adrenal cortex has been subject to an immense amount of behavioural research, since Selye (1976a) identified its central role in the General Adaptation Syndrome. The data were thoroughly reviewed by Mason (1968), and need not be elaborated here. Reactions occur during restraint, crowding and other forms of stimulation in most common laboratory species.

Nevertheless, the system is not equally responsive to all forms of behavioural distress; the type rather than intensity of stimulation is crucial in modulating corticosteroid release.

Moreover, the circumstances provoking maximal haemodynamic and sympathetic nervous adjustments do not favour adrenocortical secretions. Brady (1965) imposed repeated 72-hour sessions of Sidman avoidance on rhesus monkeys — such conditions elicit sustained pressor responses, as were described on p. 76). Yet despite an increase in corticosteroid excretion over the first months, the reactions diminished, so that few changes were observed later in training. Similarly, Feldman and Brown (1976) monitored plasma cortisol from chronically indwelling cannulae in monkeys learning shock avoidance. Concentration was elevated when the animals were first acclimatised to restraining primate chairs, and later at the beginning of the avoidance programme. Yet in each case, high cortisol levels did not persist, and there was complete adaptation to the stressor. The pattern is reflected in the rat, where corticosterone output is only slightly raised after avoidance behaviour has been well learned (Coover *et al.*, 1973).

A further analysis of the contingencies articulating adrenocortical responses was furnished by Hanson and his collaborators (1976). Rhesus monkeys were administered high-intensity noise under two conditions. Group 1 could press a lever after each 13-minute noise segment, and the stimulation was terminated. A second group had no control, and were yoked for noise duration to Group 1. Perceived control over the noise was associated with lower levels of plasma cortisol than no control; thus although the length of noise was identical in the two groups, the monkeys who made behavioural responses to stop the stimulation showed diminished adrenocortical output. In the second phase of the experiment, Group 1 lost control over noise, and their cortisol concentrations promptly rose to equal those of Group 2.

These results suggest that activation of the pituitary–adrenocortical axis is promoted when animals are passively or helplessly exposed to aversive environments. Other evidence is consistent with this generalisation. For example, corticosterone was monitored in the experiment described on p. 83, where PRA showed rapid adaptation to inescapable shock; despite this attenuation of sympathetic nervous responses, high steroid concentrations were maintained throughout (Leenen and Shapiro, 1974). A comparison in rats of shock avoidance and yoked shock controls revealed that adrenocortical secretions were greater in the latter (Corum and Thurmond, 1977). Primates too react with high corticosteroid output during inescapable threat. Thus Sidman *et al.* (1962) imposed non-contingent "free" shock on animals which were already working on avoidance schedules; 17-OHCS rose to concentrations above those generated even with the most demanding avoidance. These reactions may also occur when no shock is actually administered, as in the conditioned suppression paradigm (Mason *et al.*, 1957). The pattern contrasts strikingly with sympathetic–cardiovascular arousal, where responses are enhanced by escape or avoidance.

Additional hypotheses have been put forward about reactions during passive exposure to noxious stimulation. Weiss (1970) compared the corticosteroid responses to predictable and unpredictable shocks, administered through electrodes attached to the tails of rats. Each shock was preceded by a 10-second tone in the predictable condition, while no tones were sounded in the unpredictable case. Fig. 5.5 summarises the reactions measured at two stages of the experiment; although steroid levels fell over the extended session, concentrations remained higher when shocks were unpredictable. This result parallels the behavioural preference animals display for signalled stressors, and identical effects may be seen in other aspects of physiopathology (Furedy and Biederman, 1976). For instance, Miller *et al.* (1978) assessed the myocardial uptake of a radioactively labelled drug (TC-99m-MDP) in rats given either signalled or unsignalled footshock; uptake was higher in the unpredictable condition. Procedural variations in such experiments may be significant however, since these differences between predictable and unpredictable stimulation have not been observed universally (Hennessey *et al.*, 1977).

Corticosteroid output not only varies with the predictability of environmental events, but the degree of uncertainty may also be important (Levine *et al.*, 1972). It is interesting to note in this respect

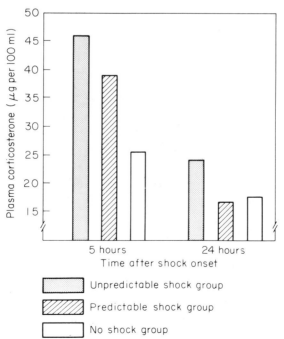

Fig. 5.5. Mean levels of plasma corticosterone for groups of rats ($N = 10$ per group), sacrificed at different stages of the shock experiment (Weiss, 1970).

that the adrenal cortex responds very strongly to novelty; in many studies, the largest changes occur on transfer of animals from their living quarters to experimental cages, even before the imposition of any aversive stimuli.

Similar dimensions may also modulate adrenocortical secretions under natural conditions. When animals are dominant and are able to regulate and control aggressive interactions with others, corticosteroid levels remain low. But subordinates that are relatively helpless in social confrontations produce high concentrations. Sassenrath (1970) found that dominant rhesus monkeys showed smaller corticosteroid responses to ACTH injections than subordinates, and the same pattern has been monitored in rodents (Christian, 1971). Thus the higher the social rank of an individual, the smaller the adrenocortical response. Dominance positions can be manipulated experimentally by introducing animals from established groups into new hierarchies (Chamove and Bowman, 1978). Rhesus monkeys with the same rank from different groups were placed together in new social systems, where ranking had to be redetermined. In the experimental groups, plasma corticosteroid levels rose with decreasing rank. The differences were greater in monkeys which had enjoyed a high rank in their original

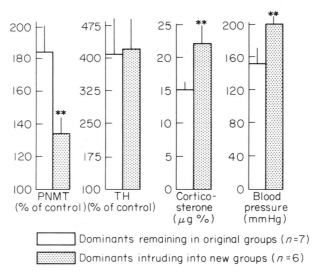

Fig. 5.6. Physiological responses of dominant mice transferred to new population cages. PNMT, enzyme controlling adrenaline production; TH, rate-limiting enzyme for noradrenaline synthesis; ** = significant difference between groups. (Henry and Stephens, 1977.)

group; previously dominant animals which could sustain only subordinate positions in the new hierarchies were the most reactive.

An intriguing pattern has also been recorded amongst mice (Henry *et al.*, 1974). Dominant animals from the colonies described earlier have high rates of catecholamine turnover, and cope aggressively with challenge. However, when these mice are transferred to new population cages, they become subordinated as intruders. The neuroendocrine correlates are plotted in Fig. 5.6. Enzyme activity in the adrenal medulla falls dramatically as the individual looses control over social interactions. Simultaneously the corticosteroid secretions associated with passive subordination increase. Blood pressure may also rise under these circumstances, through the action of mineralocorticoids.

Adrenocortical responses may be sufficiently intense to precipitate permanent damage, such as that seen by Von Holst in his studies of tree shrews (1972a). Adult males were put into cages with experienced fighters, who rapidly subjugated them. The animals were then physically separated, while remaining in visual contact through a screen, and fights were repeated only occasionally in order to maintain the dominance pattern. The defeated animals lay still for most of the daily activity phase, and died within some 20 days. Behaviourally, these tree shrews were submissive and passive, rapidly ceasing to threaten the fighter's position. Death was not due to wounds, but to renal damage following chronic overproduction of corticosteroids. Although some sympathetic nervous activation may have reduced renal blood flow, the pattern of development of uraemia indicated that steroids were the primary cause of renal insufficiency. It is interesting that glucocorticoid levels fell at the start of the study, and only rose after a few days (Von Holst, 1972b); in the early stages, the tree shrews may have attempted aggressive challenge, only taking a passive, helpless position after repeated defeats.

The conditions that provoke maximal adrenocortical and sympathatic–catecholamine activation thus appear to differ. Secretions of corticosteroids are facilitated when the organism is the helpless recipient of aversive stimulation; and even when threat is dependent on behaviour, the level of glucocorticoid output depends critically on feedback of response effectiveness (Sidman *et al.*, 1962). The circumstances favourable to pituitary–adrenocortical activity include both laboratory conditions of inescapable stress, and subordinate positions in social confrontations.

Nevertheless, despite these differences, the pituitary–adrenal and sympathetic pathways are not independent, and the interactions between the two may have severe pathological consequences.

Behaviour and interactions between neurohumoral systems

Autonomic and neuroendocrine mechanisms are interdependent, so the circumstances in which behavioural stimuli elicit generalised activation may present the greatest threats to cardiovascular integrity. The potentially lethal combination of high noradrenaline and corticosteroid levels in the myocardium has been noted in Chapter 2; it is possible that severe emotional and behavioural threats may provoke this pattern of secretion. Raab and his associates (1961) showed that rats injected with fluorocortisol manifest few cardiac lesions, despite high levels of circulating mineralocorticoids. Likewise, immobilisation produced little effect, but the two treatments in combination had severe consequences for myocardial pathology. Cardiac necrosis was attenuated by adrenergic antagonists, suggesting that the behavioural stimulation was translated through sympathetic tracts.

It may be inferred from the data already presented that conditions which promote chronic hyperactivity in both the adrenal cortex and medulla will be comparatively rare. However, a series of experiments by Cairncross and Bassett (1975) suggest cardiovascular damage may ensue even when neuroendocrine reactions are submaximal. Rats were subjected to a series of shock avoidance trials for several days; this procedure elicited moderate corticosteroid responses. But when the atria and ventricles were removed and assayed fluorimetrically, the endogenous catecholamine levels in the myocardium were found to be reduced. The corticosteroid concentration may have been sufficient to inhibit neuronal uptake of noradrenaline, a possibility that was confirmed with radioactive labelling techniques. The interaction may have led to the presence of dangerously high levels of catecholamines in the extracellular spaces of the heart.

The neuroendocrine responses induced during behavioural stimulation may also interact with other factors such as fat in the diet. Cairncross and Bassett (1975) fed rats with diets that were either high or low in saturated fats; both groups were then exposed to irregular inescapable signalled footshock for 70 days. On autopsy, mild oedema of the intima and media of arterioles, and congestion of the large venules, was recorded in the two conditions. Additionally, the saturated fat group showed infarct-like lesions, with cardiac fibrosis and leucocyte infiltration. The response to noxious stimulation was thus more severe in the animals with high proportions of saturated fat in their diets.

The reverse phenomenon, with aversive conditioning modifying the impact of dietary variables, has also been examined (Rothfeld *et al.*,

1973). Rats were maintained on a high lipid diet, but half of the group experienced unpredictable shocks and loud tones. Radioactively labelled cholesterol was injected at various intervals, so that its deposition in different tissues could be measured. Even after two days, more cholesterol had been laid down in the aortic walls of stressed animals. By day 8, levels were higher in the liver and serum as well. Serum cholesterol has similarly been modulated by shock avoidance in rats fed with high lipid diets (Uhley and Friedman, 1959); in this case, differences in blood clotting time, and ratings of coronary atherosclerosis were also documented.

Atherosclerosis, and disturbances of cardiac metabolism, have rarely been observed in the absence of diets rich in saturated fats (Lang, 1967). It is not clear whether the degrees of neuroendocrine secretion elicited by behavioural threats are adequate to produce such pathology in isolation, without dietary predisposition. Nevertheless, psychological factors have a critical impact on other aspects of cardiac functioning, as may be seen in the next section.

Behavioural stimulation and electrical disturbance of the heart

It was argued in Chapter 2 that the electrical stability of the heart, and its vulnerability to fibrillation, were adversely influenced by cardiac sympathetic inputs. Conversely, stimulation of the vagus may provide protection against ventricular fibrillation.

Since these electrical disturbances of the heart may be elicited by acute increases in cardiac sympathetic tone, they may be displayed during the initial experience of many forms of psychological threat (see p. 82). Thus changes in fibrillation threshold have been recorded from dogs, both during shock avoidance and classical aversive conditioning. The threshold for repetitive ventricular extrasystoles was determined during Sidman avoidance by Matta and associates (1976). The electrical current required to induce extrasystoles fell 49·5 per cent below control levels in 10 dogs, and the effect could be abolished by β-adrenergic blockade. Another index of ventricular fragility is the effective refractory period (ERP); a reduction in ERP reflects increased danger of fibrillation. Data from a study in which the ERP was recorded during shock avoidance are plotted in Fig. 5.7. ERP was reduced throughout the session early in training, but not in later periods. Thus under these circumstances, the danger to myocardial

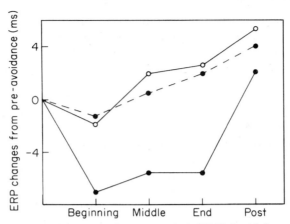

FIG. 5.7. Changes in the effective refractory period (ERP) for 10 dogs at four stages of the 90-minute conditioning session. ●——●, Day 1; ○——○, day 3; ●----●, day 5. (From Lawler *et al.*, 1976.)

stability may be severe, although comparatively brief (Lawler *et al.*, 1976).

Dramatic changes in fibrillation threshold have also been observed during classical conditioning to intense shocks. Lown *et al.* (1973) placed dogs in Pavlovian slings, and gave them single 5-joule transthoracic shocks on three successive days. When the animals were placed in the apparatus on Days 4 and 5, no shocks were administered, but the threshold for repetitive extrasystoles fell to one third of control, while heart rate increased to high levels. In a supplementary study, morphine was shown to attenuate this vulnerability (De Silva *et al.*, 1978). Morphine elevates vagal tone, and its effect on fibrillation threshold was countered with atropine.

These modifications have been provoked from healthy animals, yet cardiac responses may be even more severe in ischaemic preparations. Corbalan and co-workers (1974) for example, used the Pavlovian sling, having first induced experimental infarctions by temporary coronary occlusion. Post-infarction, premature ventricular contractions were monitored as dogs were put in the sling, and these disturbances of rhythm persisted for the next three sessions. A similar strategy has been used in the rhesus monkey, and in at least one case, the conditioned response was so severe that it precipitated a further infarction (Randall and Hasson, 1977; Randall *et al.*, 1979). In some species, pathological reactions may occur in the absence of artificially induced ischaemia. Pigs are particularly susceptible—a single session of restraint and inescapable shock is enough to bring on T-wave inversion, sinus bradycardia, subendocardial haemorrhage and even sudden death (Johansson *et al.*, 1974). The lesions in this case are similar to those produced with catecholamine injection or temporary coronary occlusion.

These data indicate that β-adrenergically mediated myocardial instability may occur under many conditions of acute psychological disturbance in animals. However, there is a further form of cardiac vulnerability that has also engaged the interest of behavioural scientists. It has been suggested that intense bradycardia, mediated to vagal overstimulation, will lead to sudden death in some cases (Hellerstein and Turrell, 1964). Such effects may be characteristic of conditions in which animals helplessly endure environmental threat.

Behavioural influences on vagal tone have been documented in several species. Newton (1967) reported a "psychogenic vagotonia" in beagle dogs as they oriented to unexpected stimuli. Heart rate slowed, and there were cases of atrio-ventricular block. The reactions were relieved by atropine, confirming their functional origin in vagal overstimulation. Similarly, a strain of pointer dogs has been bred that is characterised by a high incidence of atrio-ventricular block (Newton *et al.*, 1970). These animals also show a slow resting heart rate, suggesting strong tonic vagal output. Behaviourally, the dogs are not agitated and hyperactive, but nervous and withdrawn; they react to stimuli with exaggerated freezing and other passive behaviours. Many other breeds of dog show transient bradycardia when they are petted by humans, and the responses can be classically conditioned (Gantt *et al.*, 1966).

More dramatic reductions in heart rate have been registered in rats during shock avoidance studies by Brener and his colleagues (1977). When rats were reinforced for lowering heart rate, some animals responded rapidly with bradycardias of more than 100 bpm, and profound disturbances of rhythm were observed. In a subsequent experiment, avoidance of shock was contingent on increasing either heart rate or ambulation in a running wheel (Brener *et al.*, 1980). Several rats failed to learn the response, and were consequently exposed to high densities of shock; they also exhibited disruptions of the close linkage between heart rate and oxygen consumption, reflecting suprametabolic autonomic stimulation of the heart. Both sympathetic and vagal innervations appeared to contribute.

Vagal overstimulation has also been invoked as an explanation of the swimming deaths first described in detail by Richter (1957). Wild rats were made to swim in glass jars from which there was no escape. Tachycardia was recorded from the animals early in the swim, but attempts to struggle and escape did not persist. The rats developed marked bradycardia, fell to the bottom of the jar, and died within a few minutes. Richter considered that the animals "gave up" in the face of inescapable noxious conditions. More recently, the phenomenon was reproduced in laboratory rats (Binik *et al.*, 1977). While some animals showed stable heart rates and steady swimming for several hours, others rapidly became uncoordinated, frequently sank, soon stopped moving and dropped to the bottom. This behaviour, which was associated with a slow heart rate, did not appear to be due to exhaustion, since it occurred within minutes.

These swimming studies may parallel electric shock experiments, showing vagal hyperstimulation in states of learned helplessness. However, there are alternative explanations for the pattern of swimming deaths, suggesting they are simply due to drowning (Hughes and Lynch, 1978). The bradycardias may reflect the diving explorations of animals trying to escape (Hughes *et al.*, 1978). Various manipulations that modify the likelihood of death, such as cutting the vibrissae, may make it more difficult for rats to swim efficiently. Moreover, when animals are pretreated in ways thought to induce helplessness the probability of death is not increased (Binik *et al.*, 1979). At present, therefore, inferences about human cardiac pathology cannot reliably be drawn from these observations of swimming deaths in animals.

The complex pattern of behavioural influence on cardiac pathology is amply documented in the series of studies emerging from Corley's laboratory (1975; 1977; 1979). The experimental design used by these investigators involves comparisons between squirrel monkeys performing shock avoidance and animals yoked for shock but unable to avoid it. Corley *et al.* (1975) stressed monkeys for 8-hour sessions, and found pathological changes in both groups of animals — the patterns of damage were, however, different in the two cases. Greater myocardial necrosis was found in avoidance monkeys, suggesting responses to catecholamine accumulation, such as those described on p. 90. The helpless group remained healthy for long periods, until acute bradycardia suddenly developed, leading rapidly to death.

Later studies employed more intense 24-hour continuous sessions, followed by sacrifice. Under these circumstances, the sympathetic – catecholamine pathology was accentuated; thus avoidance animals displayed marked myofibrillar degeneration, while yoked monkeys showed few signs of damage. The necrosis was eliminated by propranolol, confirming the importance of β-adrenergic cardiac receptors (Corley *et al.*, 1979). In contrast, cases of cardiac arrest and death persisted in groups pretreated either with propranolol or vagotomy, suggesting that both autonomic pathways are involved in the response.

It seems, therefore, that permanent cardiac damage may result from contingent or non-contingent stimulation, but that the form of lesions varies in the two cases.

Summary and conclusions

The arguments presented in this chapter have ranged across several areas. For although cardiovascular and neuroendocrine adjustments occur in response to all manner of behavioural stimuli, certain distinctions can be made. The conditions that favour chronic activity in different pathways are distinct.

During the early or acute stages of aversive stimulation and psychological threat, large undifferentiated reactions tend to be observed. These include pressor responses, haemodynamic redistribution and adrenocortical hypersecretion. The electrical stability of the heart is particularly vulnerable at this stage; however, ventricular fibrillation rarely occurs in the absence of predisposing ischaemia.

With chronic exposure, differences between pathways emerge. The activation of cardiac sympathetic tracts is most prominent when stimulation is dependent on the organism's responses. In most investigations, the animal has been able to escape or avoid shock with appropriate actions. However, the ability to modify stimuli may not be crucial; rather it is the potential mastery of the environment that is important. The autonomic and neuroendocrine reactions may lead to sustained hypertension, increases in PRA, and signs of catecholamine hypersecretion. Platelet aggregation and thrombus formation have not been extensively studied in this context, so it is not clear whether these processes are also stimulated under such conditions.

Enduring modifications of adrenocortical activity occur in rather different settings. They are prominent when the animal is subject to inescapable unmodifiable stimuli which are administered irrespective of behavioural responses. Reactions are also large when appropriate behaviours have yet to be acquired, or are unavailable. When paired with predisposing factors such as high fat diet, the deleterious effects of neuroendocrine hyper-stimulation are extended.

Bradycardia and increases in vagal tone may also be characteristic of passive exposure to stressors. However, the significance of the pattern with respect to cardiovascular pathology is not clear.

The contrasts between environmental conditions have been exaggerated here, in order to try and identify the underlying dimensions of behavioural stimulation. The distinctions are not rigid, and there is considerable interaction between pathways. The impact on any organ system depends on the mutual interplay of neural and endocrine inputs. Combined activity is also important; pathological damage to the myocardium, for example, may require noradrenaline release in the presence of adequate levels of corticosteroids.

The nature of the behavioural stimulation depends not only on the conditions imposed, but on the way they are appraised by the organism. Thus the availability of an active coping response, even if it is irrelevant to the source of stimulation, may do much to modify reactions. Careful consideration must therefore be given to the animal's history, and to the cues present in the immediate environmental context.

There has been no mention in this chapter about the involvement of neuroendocrine responses in learned behaviours. This area has generated much research, and various reviews are available (De Wied, 1974; Van Toller and Tarpy, 1974). The results are broadly consistent with the arguments presented here, since adrenocortical secretions are associated with passive behaviours, while catecholamines are more prominent during the acquisition of active avoidance. Such work is not central to the present arguments however, since it has been concerned with the role of neurohumors in behaviour, rather than the physiological reactions *per se*. Similarly, the large strides made towards understanding the relations between central neurotransmitters and behaviour have not been considered (Scmitt and Worden, 1979). I have also avoided speculation about the central nervous structures governing these different response patterns; however, Henry and Stephens (1977) have put forward an integrated scheme, in which adrenomedullary and sympathetic activity is linked to the amygdala, while corticosteroid release is prompted by conditions of conservation and withdrawal, modulated via the hippocampus. Such hypotheses go beyond the cardiovascular realm, and may have implications for pathological responses in other organ systems (see Steptoe, 1980b).

6
Short-term Responses in Man

The haemodynamic adjustments that occur in response to harassing stimulation can readily be elicited in acute experimental settings. Typically, there are increases in both systolic and diastolic pressure, accompanied by tachycardia (Brod *et al.*, 1959). Regional blood flow follows a pattern which parallels in part the preparation for muscular work. Thus forearm blood flow is augmented during performance of mental tasks, due to preferential distribution into muscle beds (Mathews and Lader, 1971). There is some evidence that the lowering of vascular resistance in skeletal muscle is cholinergically mediated, although β-adrenergic vasodilator mechanisms also contribute (Holmberg *et al.*, 1965; Berdina *et al.*, 1972). Blood flow to the skin and viscera tends to fall in compensation (Ludbrook *et al.*, 1975). But since these differential tissue responses are variable, total peripheral resistance does not show consistent alterations; consequently, the pressor reaction is largely maintained by raised cardiac output. The extra demands on the myocardium are met by increases in coronary flow (Adsett *et al.*, 1952). These cardiovascular adjustments may be accompanied by heightened plasma noradrenaline, confirming that sympathetic auto-nomic pathways are mobilised (Baumann *et al.*, 1973).

Even amongst healthy volunteers, there are wide fluctuations in the size and duration of responses. Such differences may be associated with constitutional predispositions to vascular hyper-reactivity. However, they will also reflect familiarity with tasks, perceived threat, and other subtle aspects of the experimental setting. Cardiovascular reactions are measured under a range of conditions, from taxing mental tests, through psychomotor tasks to interviews of a personal nature. Subjects examined in the laboratory do not have uniform skills or experience of such challenges, and differ in their expectations about experiments. Thus the variations in response are not surprising.

It is possible that the size of modifications alters as a function of stimulation intensity. Those people who are exposed to severe, taxing conditions may show greater neuroendocrine and haemodynamic adjustments than individuals in more benign settings. There is some evidence for a relationship between cardiovascular activation and psychological or behavioural load. Ettema and Zielhaus (1971) employed a task in which participants had to press one of two pedals, tracking high and low tones sounded in random order. As the rate of signal presentation increased from 20 to 50 per minute, progressive rises in blood pressure, heart rate and breathing rate were noted. Such an experimental design unfortunately confounds information processing with physical response rate, so the contribution of the former cannot be distinguished. Danev *et al.* (1972) administered an arithmetic test under two conditions. Subjects were either self-paced and worked at their own rate, or a time limit was imposed. Although the duration of the two runs was similar, heart rates were significantly lower during self-paced performance. Yet other factors may again have influenced the outcome. Participants may have moved around more under time pressure, or breathed in a different manner; without measuring these parameters, the effects of intensity or emotional involvement alone cannot be evaluated.

The association between arousal and catecholamine excretion has also been explored. Two possible relationships can be considered; a monotonic increase of catecholamine output with emotion or stimulus intensity, or a U-shaped curve. Evidence for the latter was provided by Frankenhaeuser *et al.* (1971), when testing volunteers in three settings. In the first, they carried out a prolonged vigilance task with low levels of sensory stimulation. Secondly, they performed complex psychomotor tests, and finally read magazines or listened to the radio — this last condition was designed to provide an intermediate level of stimulation. Catecholamine excretion was lowest under intermediate stimulation, and highest with the complex tasks. However, since varying degrees of alertness and behavioural response were required in the different conditions, the pattern may reflect a simple linear increase of output with experimental demands.

Some support for this explanation emerges from other studies by the Swedish group. Thus Frankenhaeuser and Johansson (1976) compared two sets of subjects performing the Stroop test, in which there is a conflict between the name of a colour, and the shade in which it is printed. In one case, an additional stimulus interference (double conflict) was introduced, making the test even more taxing. Both groups later carried out a mental arithmetic task, and catecholamines were compared with excretion rates on control days. The results are sum-marised in Fig. 6.1. Unfortunately, the effects were somewhat con-founded by variations in excretion on the control day. Nevertheless, adrenaline levels were not only higher during the double conflict Stroop test, but were maintained by this group in the subsequent arithmetic task. Noradrenaline output did not distinguish conditions.

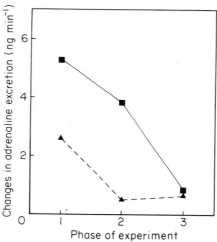

Fig. 6.1. Mean changes in adrenaline excretion assessed against values obtained during control session. Phase 1, colour/word conflict task (Stroop); Phase 2, mental arithmetic task; Phase 3, period of inactivity. ▲----▲, Subjects in the single con-flict condition (Phase 1); ■——■, subjects in the double conflict condition (Phase 1). (Frankenhaeuser and Johansson, 1976.)

On the other hand, close associations between stimulus intensity and catecholamine excretion have failed to emerge in many other cases (Frankenhaeuser, 1975; Frankenhaeuser and Lundberg, 1977). More-over, catecholamines are not linearly correlated with effort, since only at the highest work loads do levels rise above baseline (Frankenhaeuser *et al.*, 1969). It would seem therefore that cardiovascular activation and sympathetic–catecholamine arousal in the laboratory are not simple functions of the intensity of behavioural stimulation or emotional threat. Although adrenaline excretion often rises above basal levels, it does not link systematically with the strength of environmental challenge, except in the conditions discussed below. Rather, these physiological responses are sensitive to the patterns of demand, as appears to be the case in animals.

Modulation of responses by behavioural demands

It was argued in Chapter 5 that the pattern of cardiovascular activation depends on the behavioural contingencies implicit in the setting. Conditions in which the subject cannot avoid, modify or influence stimulus administration are conveniently categorised as passive, in contrast with circumstances where the individual's actions critically modulate aversive events.

The different patterns of haemodynamic adjustment have been elegantly dissected by Obrist and his co-workers (1978). Groups of healthy volunteers were subjected to three conditions: the cold pressor test (hand immersion in iced water), an explicit pornographic movie, and a shock avoidance reaction time (RT) task. The first two were passive forms of stimulation, demanding no specific behavioural responses. On the other hand, the speed of reactions in the RT test determined the occurrence of shock: with fast responses shock was avoided. Fig. 6.2 illustrates the range of modifications in cardiovascular activity. Systolic pressure and heart rate rose in all conditions, but the increase was most prominent in the RT test. Similarly, the index of cardiac contractility (carotid dp/dt) responded markedly only with the active task. Conversely, diastolic pressure changes fractionated in the reverse pattern, with greater alterations in the two passive conditions. The probable explanation is that the mechanism underlying the pressor response varied with experimental demands. During the passive stressors, the simultaneous rises in systolic and diastolic together with the

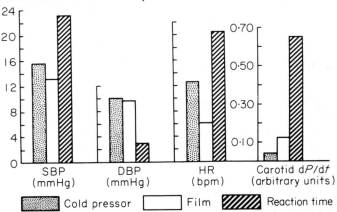

FIG. 6.2. Mean changes in systolic (SBP) and diastolic blood pressure (DBP), heart rate (HR) and carotid dP/dt during the initial 2 minutes of the pornographic film and reaction time task, and the 90 s of the cold pressor test. Changes from initial baseline. (From Obrist *et al.*, 1978.)

lack of contractility change, suggests that vasoconstrictor adjustments sustained reactions. In the active case, the augmentation of systolic, heart rate and contractility measures, associated with very modest diastolic pressure changes, implicate strong cardiac sympathetic (β-adrenergic) influence.

This possibility was tested in a further group, who participated in the experiment under β blockade. The results are plotted in Fig. 6.3, and comparison with Fig. 6.2 reveals a number of important differences. The cardiac (rate and contractility) modifications were attenuated in all cases by blockade, although the reductions were significantly larger in the RT task. Systolic pressure responses were also damped to the greatest extent in the RT test, reflecting the prominent β-adrenergic involvement in the active condition. Blockade had no effect on diastolic pressure except during RT performance, when the rise was exaggerated.

The propranolol intervention confirms that sympathetic influences on the heart are more salient in active avoidance than in passive con-

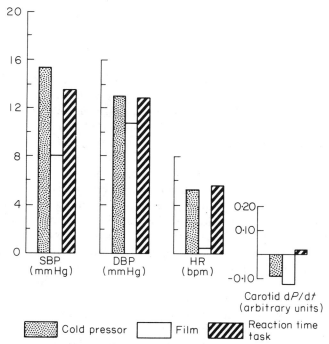

FIG. 6.3. Mean changes in systolic (SBP) and diastolic blood pressure (DBP), heart rate (HR) and carotid dP/dt during cold pressor, film, and reaction time task. Subjects were studied under β-adrenergic blockade with propranolol. (From Obrist *et al.*, 1978.)

ditions. The actual reaction times were uninfluenced by β blockade, so no performance decrement could be identified. Moreover, cardiovascular adjustments were not consistently related to measures of movement or activity. The β-adrenergically mediated hyperkinetic response may therefore have resulted from making shock contingent on behavioural efficiency.

Of course, an alternative explanation is that the distress is simply more severe when individuals are trying to avoid shock, compared with the pain of a cold pressor or the excitement of a pornographic film. However, Light and Obrist (1980) exploited the experimental paradigm further by assessing cardiovascular responses in the RT avoidance condition, and in a group yoked for shock but unable to avoid. The avoidance group was again characterised by greater cardiac sympathatic arousal, even though the number and intensity of electric shocks was identical in the two cases.

Other investigators too have shown that cardiac sympathetic traffic is not augmented during passive exposure to noxious stimuli. Gliner *et al.* (1977) monitored cardiac parameters such as stroke index during classical conditioning trials, in which a tone was regularly followed by electric shock. On occasions when the shock was omitted, a conditioned response emerged; it consisted of bradycardia without any change in stroke index. Vagal innervation appeared to dominate, without sympathetically mediated alterations in contractile state. Similarly, no changes in arterial pressure or heart rate were recorded during procedures such as skin venipuncture or mild burning of the skin (Gittleman *et a.*, 1968). Von Eiff and Piekarski (1977) reported that the systolic pressure responses to intense but inescapable noise were small and short-lived, being unaffected by the pattern of presentation (either continuous, periodic or irregular).

During passive experience of some threatening events, dissociations between haemodynamic adjustments and catecholamine release may also be observed. When volunteers watched violent movies, heart rate actually decreased in Carruthers and Taggart's study (1973). The response was largely unaffected by β blockade, confirming the dominance of the vagus under these conditions. Yet at the same time, small increases in plasma adrenaline were recorded. This pattern also emerged during dental procedures (Taggart *et al.*, 1976). Likewise in a series of stress experiments devised by Sapira and Shapiro (1966), subjects were the helpless recipients of painful or disturbing stimulation. In these cases too, cardiovascular and catecholamine responses were not consistently associated. More recently, Engel *et al.* (1980) observed significant correlations between plasma adrenaline and heart rate reactions during mental arithmetic performance, but not in passive conditions such as the cold pressor and noise. A similar comparison was reported by LeBlanc and colleagues (1979). The increase in plasma adrenaline was greater with mental arithmetic than the cold pressor, and it was associated with heightened tachycardia. In contrast, the modifications of systolic pressure and noradrenaline were similar in the two cases.

It is possible therefore to argue that passive aversive conditions seldom evoke substantial, coordinated hyperkinetic cardiovascular reactions. However, the components of behaviour-dependent stimulation and active coping remain controversial, and should be delineated with more precision.

Coping, control and cardiovascular reactions

There are widespread beliefs in the benefits of control over the environment. The hypothesis that haemodynamic reactions are actually more severe when an individual is challenged to cope actively with threatening conditions, may consequently appear discrepant. A lack of control has been identified as a major component in the stress of urban life, bringing with it the damaging experiences of helplessness and hopelessness (Glass and Singer, 1972). The positive effects of instrumental control, or belief in control, on behavioural efficiency have been documented, while the sense of helplessness has been proposed as a factor in diverse pathologies (Seligman, 1975).

However, it is misleading to think that "stress responses" in the emotional, behavioural, cardiovascular and neuroendocrine domains will necessarily be congruent (see Steptoe, 1980a). Moreover, the concept of personal control is complex, since it is used to describe a variety of phenomena (Averill, 1973; Miller, 1979). For example, cognitive control refers to the technique of interpreting or appraising threatening events in ways that modify disturbance, even though the external environment is not affected. Thus Lazarus and Opton (1966) showed volunteers a film about safety on the shop floor, in which a number of horrifying accidents were simulated. When a particular cognitive strategy was imposed, so that participants were told to deny the reality of the film, or to intellectualise its content, psychophysiological reactions were attenuated.

Such cognitive strategies may be important, and have already contributed to understanding of pain, and to methods of preparation for distressing surgical procedures (Johnson, 1975; Langer *et al.*, 1975).

However, they are peripheral to the issue of instrumental control, where the individual's actions can affect the occurrence of noxious events physically. The cardiovascular concomitants of alert coping behaviour are not only elicited when subjects are working to avoid threats; similar forms of activation have been recorded during performance of mental arithmetic and difficult psychomotor tasks (Steptoe, 1978a). Cardiac sympathetic stimulation may be promoted either when the behaviour required is challenging and engaging, or when a relatively simple response, such as releasing a key in a RT study, is carried out under threat.

Obrist's (1978) experiments are again germane. These investigators were able to clarify the contingencies provoking cardiac sympathetic tone by manipulating the reaction time criterion for shock avoidance. One group was given an easy target of 400 ms, which was generally met. Subjects in the Impossible condition were required to respond at a rate faster than 200 ms, a very short criterion that was rarely fulfilled. A third set of volunteers performed the task under intermediate Hard conditions. They were told to respond as fast as possible, but were given no fixed criterion. The Hard and Impossible groups were informed that shock would be administered on only some trials, and the number of shocks was matched. Participants were also shown their response times after each trial.

Fig. 6.4 outlines the changes in systolic pressure and heart rate at different points during the 14-minute task. Initially, substantial responses were observed in all conditions, but gradually distinctions emerged between groups; cardiovascular arousal was maintained to a greater extent in the Hard condition, declining more rapidly in the other groups. The correlations between pressor responses and measures of movement were inconsistent, while average reaction times did not differ between conditions; hence, the haemodynamic patterns were not simply functions of differential motor activity levels.

Haemodynamic reactions were more persistent when partial control could be exerted over the source of stimulation, and when the outcome of actions was uncertain. Hyperkinetic adjustments were not dependent on successful control, since sustained alterations were not recorded in the Easy condition. On the other hand, the Impossible group experienced repeated failure, and were under frequent threat of shock, yet cardiovascular reactions declined progressively—thus when the required behaviour was not in the repertoire, cardiac responses were attenuated.

Sympathetic activation is therefore provoked by alert and involving response demands, and not merely by conditions in which threats are

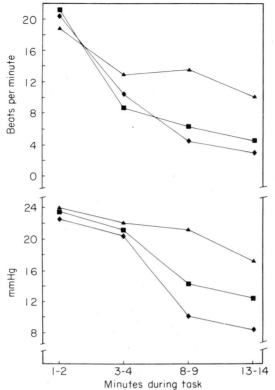

FIG. 6.4. Mean changes in systolic blood pressure (below) and heart rate (above), assessed as changes from the initial baseline, at four stages of the RT task. ◆——◆, Easy; ▲——▲, Hard; ■——■, Impossible. (From Obrist *et al.*, 1978.)

contingent on behaviour. Elliott (1969) reached similar conclusions about the availability of active coping responses, after a series of experiments on heart rate changes during cognitive and psychomotor tasks. This refinement suggests some of the reasons why the outcome of studies on instrumental control have been inconsistent. Two features are particularly important:

a. *The nature of the behavioural response.* When threatening stimuli can be controlled by trivial or simple actions, hyperkinetic cardiovascular responses may not be maintained. This was demonstrated by Hokanson *et al.* (1971), who administered Sidman shock avoidance to two groups of volunteers. One group was able to call a halt and take 60 s rest whenever it was wanted; the second group was yoked to the first for the number of time-outs, but had no control over their occurrence. The task and time-out periods were therefore identical in the two cases, the difference lying in the control exerted over the distribution of breaks. Large increases in systolic pressure (averaging over 25 mm) were recorded at the beginning of the test. But the levels in subjects with control were lower throughout the session. By the end, the systolic elevations above baseline were less than 10 mm in this condition, significantly below the 19 mm of the yoked subjects.

Certain aspects of Hokanson's methodology, including the manual measurements of blood pressure and the assignment of subjects to groups on the basis of pressure levels rather than reactivity, make the study difficult to interpret. Nevertheless, the basic pattern was confirmed by DeGood (1975). These experiments suggest that when control can be achieved through undemanding actions, pressor reactions may be attenuated. The point was explicitly tested by Manuck and associates (1978a), who varied the ease of avoidance by manipulating task difficulty.

Groups of normotensives performed a series of concept formation puzzles, presented either under easy or difficult conditions. Participants were also threatened with 115-dB "tone shocks"; for half the subjects, these were said to be random (no control), while for the remainder, tones were contingent on poor performance (control). Comparisons could therefore be made between control and no control, and between difficult and easy coping responses.

Table 6.1 summarises the average systolic and diastolic pressure reactions in the four conditions. No tones were actually administered, so unconditioned responses to noise did not account for changes. The greatest modifications were elicited from subjects with control, for whom the task was difficult. In the easy task condition, there was no reliable difference between control and no control groups. Diastolic

TABLE 6.1

Blood pressure reactions during task performance under threat of aversive noise
(Manuck *et al.*, 1978a)

Experimental groups (n=11 per group)	Average blood pressure changes from baseline (mmHg)	
	Systolic	Diastolic
Control — task difficult	23·4	7·7
No control — task difficult	12·1	3·9
Control — Task easy	9·4	3·6
No control — task easy	13·8	3·9

pressure changes did not diverge significantly. Thus systolic pressure reactions were potentiated by a demanding coping response with uncertain outcome. When aversive stimulation could be modified without straining personal resources, the systolic pressure adjustment was less marked.

b. *The intensity of the threat.* Another series of experiments, in which non-vascular parameters of sympathetic function were monitored, again apparently show the benefits of instrumental control. Geer *et al.* (1970) ran a two-part study, and measured skin conductance responses. In the first half, subjects were obliged to press a switch when picturds were presented, while being given 6-s shocks. During this period, the amplitude of skin conductance responses remained high. After 10 trials, two groups were treated differently. The perceived control group were told that fast reaction times would shorten shocks to 3 s. The no control group were simply informed that shocks would last 3 s, and not that their reaction times were relevant. Both groups in fact received 3-s shocks in part 2, but the skin conductance responses decreased significantly more in the perceived control condition. By making shock administration apparently dependent on performance, this index of sympathetic nervous arousal was damped.

The result runs counter to the arguments presented here, yet two factors raise serious doubts about its relevance to cardiovascular reactions. Firstly, the electrodermal response patterns were not replicated in a subsequent experiment using very similar procedures (Glass *et al.*, 1973). Secondly, the shocks employed were comparatively mild. The level was set at a value close to that previously labelled painful by each individual; thus participants were aware of what the shocks would feel like, and already had experience of them. But as Beecher (1966) has argued, the pain threshold is of little significance in evaluating the psychological threat of pain. Threshold levels of experimentally applied pain are insensitive to placebos and analgesics, since the affective components of the experience are largely absent (Sternbach, 1968). Moreover, mild shocks do not appear to provoke cardiac sympathetic arousal. Obrist *et al.* (1974) found that a current level 33 per cent above that judged as painful was required before hyperkinetic cardiac responses emerged. Even at intense levels, haemodynamic adjustments rapidly attenuate with shock experience (Light and Obrist, 1980).

There are alternatives to the actual administration of very intense shocks that have broadly similar effects. As has already been noted, these include taxing mental problems and the threat of shocks that are never given. For example, shock threat alone was used by Thackray and Pearson (1968). Volunteers were trained with a psychomotor task, and then divided into three groups: one acted as control while the other two were threatened with shock. The first group was told that shock depended on their task performance, and would be given when efficiency deteriorated. The second group was led to believe that random shocks would be administered in a non-contingent manner. Participants admitting to low and high fear of shock were subsequently distinguished, and heart rate changes during the test were monitored. The threat of contingent aversive stimulation resulted in a much greater tachycardia (averaging over 12 bpm) from high fear subjects, in comparison with those in the non-contingent condition (5·5 bpm). These differences were only apparent amongst people for whom the threat of shock constituted a frightening experience. The cardiovascular response is largely a product of anticipation, when the worrying but mysterious pain of shock is imminent. So when participants already have experience of shock, as in Geer's study, the autonomic responses are more fragile.

Thus hyperkinetic cardiovascular responses are augmented when coping involves alert actions with uncertain outcomes. If stimuli can be easily controlled, haemodynamic adjustments rapidly diminish. This distinction between active and passive conditions parallels the concept of "engagement", shown by Singer and her collaborators (1974) to modulate blood pressure reactions during personal interviews. There is also evidence that the output of catecholamines is governed by similar dimensions of coping.

Catecholamines, task requirements and emotion

During the 1950s, it was proposed that distinct patterns of adrenaline and noradrenaline excretion were associated with different emotions. Adrenaline was thought to predominate in fear or anxiety, while anger was accompanied by combined release (Ax, 1953; Funkenstein, 1956). The differentiation had implications for theories of emotion, and also provided a framework for psychosomatic thinking: an individual displaying particular emotions might be characterised by disorders prompted by the different catecholamines.

However, much of the corroborative evidence was indirect, based on inference from patterns of cardiovascular reactions. Although differential catecholamine excretion has been measured directly under some conditions, the effect is inconsistent (Elmadjian *et al.*, 1957;

Mendelson *et al.*, 1960). Variations in the amount of motor activity associated with emotional behaviours will confound recordings, and effort also makes important contributions (see p. 111). Thus using a chronically indwelling venous catheter and portable blood withdrawal pump, Dimsdale and Moss (1980) measured large adrenaline responses to public speaking, while noradrenaline was sensitive to physical exercise. The subjective intensity of different emotions remains difficult to monitor. It is also possible that the threshold for the appearance of noradrenaline in the urine is higher, so that the conditions provoking combined excretion may be more intense than those in which adrenaline only responds (Frankenhaeuser, 1975; Mason, 1975). Nevertheless, there may be certain groups, such as violent criminals, in whom the differential output of adrenaline and noradrenaline is of greater significance (Woodman *et al.*, 1978).

Catecholamine release is modulated not only by the intensity of disturbance, but by the behavioural response requirements. Active coping promotes adrenaline excretion, as may be seen in Fig. 6.1, and other experimental studies. Frequently, the catecholamine response is sufficiently intense to induce increases in FFA levels. Carlson *et al.* (1968) recruited three experimental groups; one acted as control, and the others had the task of sorting ball-bearings of different sizes, while being distracted by disturbing auditory and visual stimulation for a two-hour session. Noradrenaline excretion increased significantly in the experimental groups. Additionally nicotinic acid, a drug that inhibits the release of FFA by catecholamines, was injected into one set of volunteers. Fig. 6.5 illustrates the manner in which FFA were stimulated by catecholamines. Not only were correlations recorded between modifications in adrenaline and FFA levels, but FFA release was inhibited by nicotinic acid. Similarly, Peterfy and Pinter (1973) showed that FFA in the blood rose after hypnotic suggestions of intense emotion, but that the response was attenuated by β blockade.

These studies demonstrate the manner in which sympathetic–catecholamine reactions in actively demanding conditions may mobilise energy stores in adipose tissue. The fuel release is in excess of physical or metabolic requirements, since little motor activity is involved.

However, the association with active coping is not unique, since the adrenal medulla is also responsive to passive threat, or harrassment over which the individual has no control. Levi (1965) measured the urinary output of catecholamines while female secretaries viewed emotionally engaging movies. Unfortunately, the films were shown in a fixed order, so habituation of responses cannot be ruled out. Nevertheless, the first film, a neutral nature movie, was associated with decreases in excretion, in contrast with rises in catecholamine output during comedy and horror presentations. Changes in plasma catecholamines were likewise recorded by Carruthers and Taggart (1973) under similar circumstances.

Despite these effects, the significance of catecholamine responses to passive stressors is diminished by two factors. Firstly, as has already been noted, adrenomedullary output is not correlated with cardiovascular adjustments under such conditions (see p. 102). Secondly, the pathway is relatively insensitive to the parameters of stimulation; thus changes in the form or intensity of stimuli may not be followed by predictable alterations of catecholamine levels. For example, Frankenhaeuser and Lundberg (1977) had volunteers performing mental arithmetic during white noise interference. The noise was presented at 56-, 72·5- or 85-dB strength. Under these conditions, adrenaline excretion was elevated above control levels, but did not vary with noise intensity. On a second day, all participants were given 72·5-dB noise. This unexpected alteration in noise strength for those previously in the 56 and 85 dB conditions was not reflected in changing catecholamine output.

Even instrumental control over task-irrelevant aspects of noxious

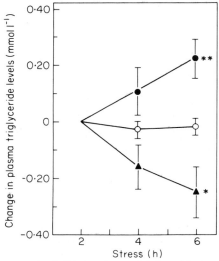

FIG. 6.5. Mean changes (± S.E.) in plasma triglyceride levels during and after experimental stress session. O——O, control; ●——●, stress alone; ▲——▲, stress + nicotinic acid. Significant differences from controls: *$p < 0.05$; **$p < 0.01$. (Carlson *et al.*, 1968.)

stimulation may not affect catecholamine responses. In a further experiment from the Stockholm group, 56-dB white noise was administered during mental arithmetic (Lundberg and Frankenhaeuser, 1978). Subsequently, half the participants were allowed to choose their own noise level, while the remainder were yoked for intensity. Yet this control over the stressor did not lead to reliable differences in catecholamine excretion, subjective discomfort ratings or task performance. Such results should be contrasted with Fig. 6.1, where modification of a salient component of task demands led to differential adrenaline excretion.

It is evident that although adrenaline and noradrenaline may be released during passive threat or stimulation, they are more sensitive to the requirements of alert coping. In this respect, the catecholamines reflect the patterns of sympathetically mediated cardiovascular response discussed earlier. There is no evidence that instrumental control over significant aspects of the stressor will attenuate reactions; the one study that showed such an effect confounded the control manipulation with habituation and the number of electric shocks administered (Frankenhaeuser and Rissler, 1970).

Within the context of active challenge to mental abilities, catecholamines may be further influenced by the degree of effort sustained by participants. In short-term laboratory settings, performance on the Stroop and other complex psychomotor tasks is positively correlated with adrenaline reactions (Johansson and Frankenhaeuser, 1973; Frankenhaeuser *et al.*, 1976). Levi (1972) studied the behaviour of soldiers in an intensive 72-hour experiment that simulated battle conditions. Sleep was prevented, and the time was divided into long periods of rifle shooting punctuated by brief rest intervals. Shooting accuracy correlated positively with adrenaline excretion, but negatively with noradrenaline.

Such associations may even reflect chronic styles of behaviour in different people. Bergman and Magnusson (1979) identified over- and under-achieving schoolchildren by cross-tabulating school performance with intelligence quotient. Catecholamine excretion was then evaluated in selected groups during a challenging mental arithmetic task, and a neutral movie. Amongst boys, both IQ and achievement were related to adrenaline excretion in the demand setting. Thus for a given IQ, achievement and adrenaline correlated positively, while at a fixed achievement level, adrenaline was negatively associated with IQ. Hence large adrenaline responses were characteristic of over-achievers. No differences emerged for noradrenaline, in the female students, or in the neutral setting.

It is therefore possible that adrenomedullary mobilisation is adaptive in the context of alert coping, having positive behavioural consequences in terms of performance efficiency. However, individuals who display the pattern chronically may be at greater risk for the pathologies associated with high circulating catecholamine levels.

Other neuroendocrine responses in the laboratory

Although neuroendocrine and biochemical agents outside the adreno-medullary axis have been studied in healthy subjects under laboratory conditions, the modifications elicited are generally very modest. For example, few normotensive volunteers increase PRA on exposure to laboratory tasks (Clamage *et al.*, 1977); experimental threats may be insufficiently intense to provoke substantial responses, since observations in real-life settings suggest that PRA is sensitive to emotional experience (see Chapter 7). Most of the evidence documenting associations between behavioural stimuli and serum cholesterol or blood clotting mechanisms has also been collected in field settings, although some laboratory studies have been performed (Peterson *et al.*, 1962; Palmblad *et al.*, 1977). The paucity of effects may again be due to the high threshold of response in these pathways, although recording methods are also less precise.

Even corticosteroids have proved relatively insensitive to laboratory manipulations, in striking contrast to the prevalence of reactions in everyday life (see Mason, 1968). The discrepancy may be due to the type of stimuli imposed in the laboratory. Data from animals, discussed in Chapter 5, indicate that corticosteroids respond under conditions of passive stress, and in man too adrenocortical function is heightened when individuals are helplessly exposed to threat (Bliss *et al.*, 1956). During active coping, reactions are attenuated. Thus Carlson *et al.* (1968) reported no change of corticosteroid output in volunteers performing the ball-bearing sort task described on page 109. Similarly, while adrenaline excretion increased during a self-paced reaction time test, cortisol output diminished (Lundberg, 1980). Raab (1968) used a combination of distracting non-contingent stimulation and a mental task to harass volunteer subjects. Cardiovascular adjustments were elicited, but mean plasma cortisol concentration did not rise, although the diurnal trend towards lower levels was delayed.

Another interesting parallel with the corticosteroid activity of animals is in the relationship with social dominance (see p. 88). Urinary concentration of 17-OHCS was monitored during an ethological study of young children, while social behaviours were closely categorised by observational techniques (Montagner *et al.*, 1978). Children characterised as leaders, who showed dominance without aggression, had lower levels of 17-OHCS throughout the day. In contrast, levels were high and fluctuating amongst children constantly employing aggressive tactics in trying to establish dominance. These patterns were seen in 2-3 year olds, and appeared consistent over 12 months, provided that the child's behaviour did not alter.

The significance of phasic cardiovascular responses

The reactions discussed thus far have involved tonic changes in haemodynamic and neuroendocrine function. However, a great deal of attention has also been directed at acute, phasic responses. This research is largely concerned with small heart rate adjustments that have little immediate relevance to pathology. Nevertheless, its relationship to dimensions of chronic stimulation and coping should be considered, since tonic modifications presumably develop in part through the accumulation of brief fluctuations.

The most influential hypotheses about the behavioural significance of phasic heart rate responses have been promulgated by the Laceys (Lacey, 1967; Lacey and Lacey, 1978). They noted variations in cardiac reactions associated with different tasks, and suggested that the continuum from "intake" to "rejection" of sensory inputs was important. The heart rate changes were thought to have causal significance in modulating central attentional processes, possibly through baroreceptor afferent inhibition of higher cortical activity (Coleridge *et al.*, 1976). Thus attention to external stimuli is linked with bradycardia, while performance of mental computations (where externally directed attention might interfere) is facilitated by increases in heart rate.

The field has generated considerable controversy, since not all investigators have found a similar response fractionation (Carroll and Anastasiades, 1978). The reductions in cardiac activity with "external" tasks are evidently fragile (Elliott, 1974; Herrmann *et al.*, 1976). Furthermore, the motor response requirements in the different task conditions make a significant contribution (Dahl and Spence, 1971).

However, the patterns of acute cardiac response appear to parallel on a small scale the differences seen under tonic stimulation. Thus pressor reactions and tachycardia are more pronounced with active cognitive tasks than on passive exposure to environmental stimuli

(Williams *et al.*, 1975; Herrmann *et al.*, 1976). Moreover, cardiac responses are larger and less dependent on somatomotor activity when alert behaviour is required. Obrist *et al.* (1974) conducted a pertinent study in which subjects made a small manual response to a tone presented 7 s after a preparatory signal. Subsequent electric shock was contingent on slow reaction times, while rapid responses were rewarded with money. The experiment was carried out under normal conditions and also during β-adrenergic blockade.

Fig. 6.6 summarises the modifications in heart rate and the carotid pulse index of myocardial contractility. Substantial phasic adjustments were produced before and after the behavioural response, but these were largely unaffected by pharmacological blockade. However, physiological arousal at the time of anticipated shock was lessened by propranolol. Thus cardiac sympathetic activation was not simply a function of alerting or the motor components of the behaviour, since

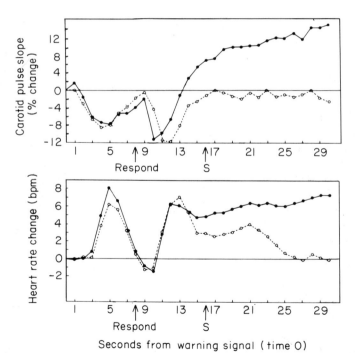

Seconds from warning signal (time O)

Fig. 6.6. Second-by-second changes in heart rate (below) and slope of the carotid pulse (above) from the warning signal (time 0) until after the shock is expected (S). ●——●, Intact; ○-----○, β-adrenergic blockade. (From Obrist *et al.*, 1974.)

the vagus dominated during performance of the response itself. Rather, sympathetic involvement was pronounced when the consequences of the action were unknown, and the outcome anticipated.

Hypertensive reactions and the prediction of dysfunction

The pattern of circulatory responses described in this chapter may be significant in the development of high blood pressure. Exposure to threatening environments that demand alert coping will result in β-adrenergically mediated haemodynamic adjustments. The mobilisation is in excess of metabolic demands, since it is adapted for vigorous physical exercise. Repeated or chronic stimulation may initiate the chain of pathological events, including modifications in vessel calibre, renal function and baroreceptor activity, that help to fix blood pressure at a new high level.

Three predictions can be drawn from this scheme. Firstly, hypertensive patients, in particular those at the early stages of dysfunction, will show exaggerated haemodynamic responses during behavioural stimulation. The hyperkinetic circulation that characterises some patients may itself reflect this reactivity. Secondly, responses to passive threats, which do not involve intense cardiac sympathetic stimulation, will not predict hypertension accurately. Thirdly, individuals who are at risk for cardiovascular disturbance may display heightened pressor responses when actively coping with laboratory tasks.

a. *Reactions in essential hypertensive patients.* There have been many comparisons between normotensives and hypertensives under laboratory conditions, and in general reactions are greater in the latter (Brod *et al.*, 1959). For example, Lorimer and collaborators (1971) found that blood pressure rose in both groups during a monotonous but taxing ball-sorting task. The average systolic pressure increase in patients was 27 mm, compared with 13 mm in controls.

However, the pattern of results is probably more complex. Resting pressure levels are of course elevated in essential hypertension, and although absolute changes are greater, it is not certain that reactions are proportionately exaggerated. Some investigators have found similar percentage changes, while others record disproportionate modifications from patients (Shapiro *et al.*, 1963; Holmberg *et al.*, 1965; Ulrych, 1969).

Many difficulties in interpreting studies of hypertensives undoubtedly result from grouping patients whose reactions differ in form as well as intensity. This was recognised by Brod *et al.* (1959) in their pioneer work, since not all of their hypertensive patients showed pressor responses that were sustained by cardiac output increases. Some individuals in both normal and hypertensive groups produced a fall in cardiac output together with a rise in total vascular resistance. Considerable variability was also seen in the redistribution of blood, since some people manifest little change in forearm flow. However, the renal vascular resistance rose consistently, and there was a tendency for this response to be greater amongst hypertensives. More recently, the catecholamine reactions to behavioural stimuli have been shown to vary with the renin status of hypertensives, being greatest in those with high PRA (Chobanian *et al.*, 1978).

Consistency may be enhanced by selecting homogenous groups of patients with borderline hypertension. Nestel (1969) compared such a series with normal subjects during the performance of complex visual puzzles. The pressor reactions of the borderline group were greater, both in absolute and percentage terms. Diastolic pressure for example rose an average of 25 mm (26 per cent) in patients, and 11 mm (15 per cent) in controls. Furthermore, these responses were associated with large elevations of urinary catecholamine concentration. The excretion of adrenaline increased some 120 per cent in patients, compared with 30 per cent in normotensives. The latter showed no noradrenaline response at all, while a 50 per cent rise was recorded in patients. The correlations between pressure response and catecholamine excretion were also significant. Similarly, Baumann *et al.* (1973) studied healthy subjects and young patients (aged 15 to 20) at the borderline stage. All performed mental arithmetic under time pressure. The arterial pressure response was significantly larger in the young patients, and levels also remained higher after the test, taking longer to return to baseline. Plasma FFA changes were more profound, although noradrenaline increments were of the same order in the two groups.

The data from hyperkinetic patients thus supports the present argument, although more evidence from well-defined groups is needed. People with high arterial pressure are not uniform in their reactions during psychophysiological experiments, and these variations may be significant in evaluating the physiopathology of different cases.

b. *Prognostic significance of passive coping responses.* The acute stressor that has perhaps been studied more than any other amongst essential hypertensives is the cold pressor. This is a passive threat over which the individual has no control, but must simply tolerate the pain.

There is some evidence that reactions are exaggerated, although effects are variable, being prominent only in sugbroups of the hypertensive population (Chobanian *et al.*, 1978). The pressure rises elicited are not closely associated with β-adrenergic mechanisms. Nicotero *et al.* (1968) measured reactions to the test in the normal state, and during β blockade. Pressor responses did not differ on the two occasions, indicating that cardiac sympathetic fibres do not make major contributions to the cardiovascular adjustments. This is reflected in the lack of correlation between adrenaline and pressure modifications during the cold pressor (Engel *et al.*, 1980; LeBlanc *et al.*, 1979).

Moreover, the cold pressor test is of little prognostic significance in essential hypertension. The arterial pressure changes are variable even within individuals, and patients do not necessarily display hyper-reactivity (Wolf *et al.*, 1948). Harlan and associates (1964) tested a group of 380 subjects with the cold pressor, and then repeated the assessment after 18 years. Large reactions at the first examination did not predict later elevations in tonic pressure level — the test was of no value in identifying people at risk.

These data suggest that cardiovascular reactions to a passive aversive test do not tap the mechanisms responsible for the initiation of essential hypertension. However, an alternative explanation is that reactive individuals may already be aroused in anticipation of the test, and hence show smaller magnitude changes. This possibility is supported by a study of adolescents in the highest 5 per cent of their age-related blood pressure distribution (Price *et al.*, 1979). Each child was matched with a normotensive control, and the cold pressor was administered. The high-pressure group did not produce exaggerated responses, but their anticipatory rise in heart rate and systolic blood pressure was greater. During the preparatory period, the cardiac sympathetic traffic may increase in such people.

c. *Hyper-reactivity during active coping.* These arguments suggest that responses to active demanding tasks that augment cardiac sympathetic tone may be more significant for future high blood pressure. Experiments have already been described in which borderline hypertensives produced heightened cardiovascular modifications under such conditions (e.g. Nestel, 1969); unfortunately, prospective surveys of the fate of normotensive hyper-reactors are not available.

Nevertheless, there is evidence that individuals who do respond during active coping with large circulatory adjustments, produce synchronous increases in heart rate and systolic pressure (Raab and Krywanek, 1965; Obrist and Light, 1979). A recent study carried

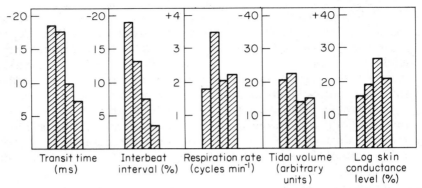

FIG. 6.7. Pattern of psychophysiological reactions during three mental task trials, plotted as changes from average baseline. Cohort divided into four subgroups ($n = 9$) on the basis of heart rate reactivity. (Steptoe and Ross, 1980a.)

out by the author with Alvin Ross, indicates that hyper-reactivity is not a function of general sympathetic nervous lability, but is localised in cardiovascular mechanisms (Steptoe and Ross, 1980a). 36 volunteers performed a series of demanding mental tasks, during which heart rate, pulse transit time, skin conductance and respiration rate were monitored; transit time is a measure of haemodynamic function that is responsive to changes in both arterial pressure and cardiac contractility (Newlin and Levenson, 1979; Steptoe, 1980a). Fig. 6.7. summarises responses to the tasks, with participants categorised on the basis of their heart rate changes. The whole sample was divided into quartiles, so that 9 subjects are represented in each group.

It is evident that heart rate increases were paralleled by modifications in transit time, suggesting a coordinated cardiovascular reaction, possible mediated β-adrenergically. However, this is not reflected in any differentiation of skin conductance level or respiratory change. There may therefore be a specific disorder of haemodynamic stability in the upper two quartiles that does not involve other autonomic disturbances.

The possibility of a selective dysfunction in cardiac responses is important, since it implies that people at risk for essential hypertension react idiosyncratically. This may explain why other groups who display hyperactivity in autonomic pathways, such as the chronically anxious, are not noted for a high incidence of cardiovascular disturbance. Such people may not show the selective hypersensitivity in cardiac sympathetic fibres that characterises individuals prone to essential hypertension.

Summary and conclusions

Experimental research into the behavioural aspects of cardiovascular reactivity in man is necessarily restricted. Many mechanisms, such as those involved in atherogenesis, thrombosis and sudden cardiac death, cannot easily be studied in the short-term on healthy individuals. The main focus has thus been on haemodynamic reactions, and on the cardiac sympathetic mechanisms that may be important in the aetiology of essential hypertension.

The evidence is consistent with work on non-human species, in that maximal activation occurs when the individual is alert and challenged, and when the threat of noxious events depends on behaviour. Such reactions are further promoted while the subject is uncertain about the outcome of actions. The inferences made by behavioural scientists about the benefits of instrumental control over threat have been too general; they do not apply to cardiovascular reactions, although control may attenuate hypersecretion in some neuroendocrine systems (Steptoe, 1980b). The alertness, uncertainty and involvement generated when noxious stimuli are contingent on performance, have a high cost in terms of cardiovascular integrity.

Similar dimensions of experience appear to be significant for catecholamine release. Thus although adrenaline and noradrenaline respond to passive stressors, more substantial effects are recorded during challenges to mental ability. In these circumstances, adrenaline output correlates with personal effort: when these efforts are successful, adrenaline is associated with performance efficiency, and thus fulfills an adaptive role. Other neuroendocrine and biochemical parameters have not been explored in such detail in the laboratory. Corticosteroid release may be selectively prompted in conditions of passive distress, and the pathway is suppressed during active challenge; this pattern too has much in common with effects in animals.

The extensive research into acute phasic cardiac and psychophysiological responses has not been discussed in detail. Much of it is concerned with issues that are tangential to the present context. Nevertheless, tachycardia and pressor reactions may be more prominent during performance of cognitive tasks than in conditions of passive sensory intake.

Psychophysiological laboratory studies may be valuable in identifying people at risk for essential hypertension. Exaggerated responses to mentally challenging tasks are seen in patients with diagnosed hypertension, particularly amongst borderline and hyperkinetic groups. Arterial pressure changes under passive conditions such as the cold pressor are of less significance prognostically. Normotensives who respond to demanding tasks with pronounced increases in heart rate and arterial pressure do not display generalised autonomic lability, but may have a specific predisposition towards cardiovascular dysfunction.

7
Long-term Influences on Cardiovascular Function

There are losses as well as gains in moving outside the laboratory into field surveys. It is rarely possible to define behaviours or environmental conditions precisely, since the challenges of everyday life are complex. Categorisation of stimuli or coping resources is therefore difficult. Additional variables that have little impact on acute investigations may confound naturalistic studies: diet, rhythmic fluctuations, smoking, exercise, and psychosocial pressures outside the investigator's control, may all contribute to the final pattern of cardiovascular or neuroendocrine response.

On the other hand, relatively artificial laboratory stimuli are replaced by environmental stressors with widespread currency. The limitations of time and experimental context do not apply, so that the range of reactions it is possible to explore is greatly expanded.

A major purpose of field surveys is to determine whether the responses monitored in the laboratory are reflected in natural settings. Chronic patterns of cardiovascular and neuroendocrine adjustment are rarely demonstrated experimentally in humans; it is possible that some of the mechanisms discussed in Chapter 6 are significant only in the short term, and that responses habituate. Field investigations therefore form a vital link between the healthy volunteer and the patient with cardiovascular disease.

It may be possible to extend the inferences drawn in Chapters 5 and 6 about the parameters of stimulation and coping, into observations of everyday life. Circulatory reactions to naturalistic stimuli may be modulated in patterns similar to those found in the laboratory; confirmation of this hypothesis would strengthen the case for considering such aspects in hypertension and ischaemic heart disease.

The persistence of reactions in different haemodynamic and endocrine pathways is variable. There is no support from field studies for the concept of an undifferentiated cardiovascular stress response, so the different mechanisms must be considered separately in the first instance. Two research strategies have been employed in the delineation of long-term response patterns (Steptoe, 1980b). In the first place, longitudinal surveys are performed; individuals are monitored in everyday life, or during periods of intense anguish, and associations are made between psychophysiological reactions and variations in emotional state or environmental demand. Such investigations are time-consuming and rare, while control groups are difficult to devise.

The economical alternative is cross-sectional rather than longitudinal, involving measurements during the routine behaviour of selected groups. If the setting is typical of the participants' normal experience, reactions monitored may reflect chronic patterns of adjustment. Much of the evidence discussed in this chapter was collected by such methods. The technique is valid, provided that the monitoring situation itself is undisturbing, and does not contaminate responses. In some cases, confusion has been caused by differences in measurement methodology. For example, Taggart *et al.* (1969) recorded large though variable increases in the heart rate while subjects were driving motor cars in urban traffic. Because of the equipment used, it was necessary for an experimenter to sit in the back seat throughout the journey. A later survey using portable apparatus permitted drivers to travel alone (Littler *et al.*, 1973); in this case, few fluctuations in arterial pressure were registered in healthy individuals or untreated hypertensives. Similarly, fewer ectopic beats or cardiac arrhythmias were seen in comparison with the earlier investigation. There is a strong possibility therefore, that the recording technique used by Taggart disturbed the responses to driving itself.

Blood pressure and heart rate

Medical research has frequently taken advantage of the tragic consequences of war and natural disaster, and this field is no exception. Life threatening conditions might be expected to provoke profound cardiovascular reactions, and this is confirmed by the increased frequency of high blood pressure during battle. Fig. 7.1 shows the distribution of diastolic pressures gathered by Graham (1945) from soldiers fighting in the Western Desert campaign of World War 2. They are compared with readings from similarly aged men in England (Cruz-Coke, 1960). Diastolic pressures over 100 mmHg were found in 26·9 per cent of soldiers, while 38 per cent had systolics of 160 mmHg or more. These

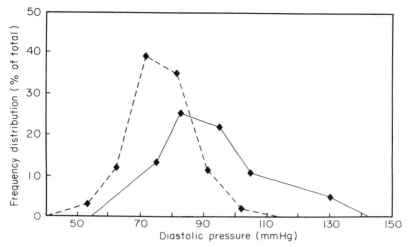

F<small>IG</small>. 7.1. Frequency distribution of diastolic pressures in young male adults. ◆——◆, Soldiers from an armoured brigade in Tripolitania; ◆————◆, 180 Englishmen recorded in London. (Cruz-Coke, 1960.)

recordings were made a few weeks after the battle, and a limited number of the hypertensives were followed up several months later. The high diastolic pressures had receded in 85 per cent of cases, despite the lack of changes in diet, climate or dehydration. A comparable pattern was observed in Finland (Ehrström, 1945). Of the male population 3·25 per cent manifest systolic pressures over 150 mmHg in peacetime surveys, while in 1943 the proportion rose to 9 per cent amongst civilians. The frequency was even greater in front-line soldiers: 28 per cent of healthy men had systolics above 150 mmHg, and the fraction increased to 49·5 per cent in those considered to be "mentally and vegetatively labile".

War brings a variety of emotional strains, chronic deprivations and restrictions, as well as direct threats to life. In contrast, the vast Texas City chemical explosion of 1947 was an isolated incident unexpectedly affecting a normal civilian population (Ruskin *et al.*, 1948). Blood pressures were monitored in 180 blast victims admitted for contusions, lacerations and damaged ear drums. Most were under 40, and less than 20 per cent had a history of hypertension. But half the group displayed systolic levels of 150 mmHg at some point, while diastolic pressures above 95 mmHg were recorded in 57 per cent. Black people may have been more susceptible, since the proportion with high diastolic pressure was 69·4 per cent, compared with 50·6 per cent of whites; it is possible that the pressor response to trauma was greater in those with a constitutional predisposition.

Less dramatic forms of perturbation also have potent effects on haemodynamics. Ambulatory monitoring techniques have confirmed that heart rate and blood pressure fluctuate widely over the day and night in people going about their normal activities. High variability is not confined to hypertensive individuals; for example, studies have been performed on junior physicians during case presentations to their seniors (Moss and Wynter, 1970; Taggart *et al.*, 1973). Increases from baseline of 80 bpm, provoking average rates of more than 150 bpm, were regularly observed. Taggart *et al.* (1973) also recorded ECG abnormalities in a number of cases, with six apparently healthy participants developing extensive ectopic contractions. Plasma noradrenaline rose significantly, together with free fatty acids and triglycerides. Many of these responses were attenuated by oxprenolol, suggesting the involvement of β-adrenergic mechanisms.

Another experience that has been studied for its impact on blood pressure is crowding. D'Atri (1975) compared the arterial pressures of prisoners housed in single cells and dormitories. Although the actual space occupied was not very different, dormitory accommodation led to greater social conflicts and threatening confrontations between inmates. In three prisons, blood pressures (recorded blind) were significantly higher amongst group housed men; however, in one case the dormitory inmates were also heavier and older. A more detailed evaluation was performed in a large maximum security prison, in which men were housed in two-, three- or six-person cells (Paulus *et al.*, 1978). The two-man cells provided 29 ft^2 per inmate, compared with 19 ft^2 in the other units. Analysis of systolic pressures, using age as a covariate, showed that average levels were significantly higher amongst men in the three- and six-person units (132·7 and 133·9 mmHg respectively) than in occupants of two-man cells (126·5 mmHg). Subjective ratings of crowding were also higher in the more populous units. These data further confirm the sensitivity of arterial pressure to chronic psychosocial stimulation.

Serum cholesterol

A pioneering study into the relationship between cholesterol variation and life experience was devised more than 20 years ago by Friedman *et al.* (1958). Blood samples were taken twice weekly from accountants throughout a five-month period. The men's weight remained constant,

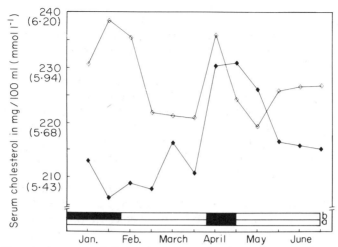

F<small>IG</small>. 7.2. Changes in serum cholesterol concentration in two groups of accountants. The groups differ in the type of work carried out, and thus in timing of work deadlines. Group a ($n = 18$) ♦———♦ ; group b ($n = 22$) ◊———◊ . Periods of severe work pressure are indicated by shaded blocks. (From Friedman *et al.*, 1958.)

and they admitted to no changes in exercise or diet. A number of "high stress" periods were objectively defined—these were the tax deadlines for the financial year, when the accountants were under extra pressure to complete work. Serum cholesterol increased reliably around these times with average changes of 15–20 mg/100 ml (0·38–0·51 mmol l^{-1}). Grouped data are plotted in Fig. 7.2.

Although these results are suggestive, there was no control group, nor could all the complicating factors be eliminated. It seems extremely unlikely, in view of the extra pressures and demands, that the accountants simply worked harder during office hours at stress periods, with no change in the rest of their lives; leisure pursuits, sleep patterns or speed of eating may have altered, with consequences for energy metabolism. Seasonal fluctuations in cholesterol may also occur, and these are not entirely predictable. Other surveys of serum cholesterol fluctuations in natural settings have only partially confirmed Friedman's observations. Variations in diet and exercise were strictly precluded in a small group of cardiac patients by admitting them to a metabolic ward under close supervision (Wolf *et al.*, 1962). Parallels between cholesterol change and the conflicts or harrassments of life were chronicled in a proportion, but behavioural data were not collected systematically or in a standardised way. Rahe's (1974a) intensive study of three individuals over several months of normal life revealed few striking cholesterol responses to everyday experience. Similarly, although serum cholesterol varied to a certain extent in the 10-week survey of students reported by Francis (1979), peaks were not associated with periods of objective distress, and correlations with reported mood were insignificant.

The evidence for cholesterol reactivity under more severe threat is also inconsistent. When US Air Force cadets were followed over 18 months, increases averaging 20 mg/100 ml (0.51 mmol l^{-1}) were recorded at the beginning of training (Clark *et al.*, 1975). High concentrations were also provoked around examinations and periods of intense military exercise. Training in underwater demolition might be considered an even more intimidating experience; the work is demanding, with physical conditioning, endurance tests, and the progressive introduction of new tasks (Rubin *et al.*, 1969). Each stage of the programme was associated with peaks in plasma cortisol, with secretion falling on mastery of those skills. Yet serum cholesterol was relatively insensitive, and did not respond to the different phases (Rahe *et al.*, 1971). Instead, a progressive increase was registered over the weeks of the course, probably a result of the ample meals provided. Serum cholesterol is unresponsive in other circumstances too. Carruthers *et al.* (1976) took blood samples from aircrews during a long transatlantic flight. The disorienting quality of this occupation was reflected in the reactivity of a number of neurohumoral parameters, but cholesterol was insensitive. A Swedish study of cardiac patients similarly produced negative results (Theorell *et al.*, 1972). Subjects attended the clinic every few weeks, and completed systematic questionnaires about incidents and disturbances in their lives. But the correlations between life adjustment and cholesterol were not significant.

The evidence for consistent changes of serum cholesterol in response to the experiences of everyday life is thus slight. This does not preclude the possibility that some individuals are reactive, but there is little reason to suppose that such changes are generally significant for atherogenesis. Unless chronic elevations in cholesterol concentration are provoked by disturbing environments, the importance of this pathway in the modulation of emotional or behavioural influences on cardiovascular disorders must remain doubtful.

Adrenocortical secretions

An extensive longitudinal study of adrenocortical responsiveness was performed on the parents of children with severe leukaemia (Friedman, S. *et al.*, 1963). They were monitored repeatedly during this harrowing hospitalisation period, as they lived on the ward or came to visit. Most were followed up for several months before and after their children died, but unfortunately no appropriate comparison group was devised. The participants showed a wide range in excretion of 17-OHCS, the corticosteroid metabolite, yet levels within individuals remained relatively uniform. When extra traumas such as infections or a death on the ward occurred, excretion rose above that seen during chronic distress (Tecce *et al.*, 1966). This long-term stressor did not therefore have a general activating effect on the adrenal cortex, a fact that was confirmed by measurements taken some time after the death of the children (Hofer *et al.*, 1972). In place of an overall decrease in corticosteroid excretion, as the parents adapted to their grief and loss, the mean output at six months and two years was no lower than that recorded before bereavement. Nevertheless, these grouped data disguise large individual variations, and some people were highly responsive.

Rahe *et al.*'s (1974a) longitudinal survey of the neuroendocrine correlates of everyday experience also revealed marked individual differences in cortisol response. Few gross changes were seen, however, except during the build up to an important swimming competition. Adrenocortical function has been monitored in pilots landing aeroplanes on aircraft carriers (Miller *et al.*, 1970). This manoeuvre is very demanding although not literally life threatening, since escape is possible with ejector seats. Blood and urine were collected on landing and non-flight days from pilots and their radar officers. In both groups serum cortisol and urinary 17-OHCS were higher on landing than on control days, with increases in cortisol of up to 270 per cent in pilots.

A rather different pattern was registered during studies of US soldiers in Vietnam (Bourne, 1970). Urine was collected from helicopter ambulance crew on flight days, when the men were extremely vulnerable, picking up casualties in the battle zone (Bourne *et al.*, 1967). These values were compared with corticosteroid excretion rates on days back at base. Despite this episodic danger, there were no systematic differences in adrenocortical activity between flying and non-flying days. Although there was no matched control group, output was generally considered to be rather low in comparison with normal levels; yet there were no signs of adrenal exhaustion. A second survey was performed on the officers and men of a Special Forces Unit, while they were under threat of attack in camp. The mean difference in 17-OHCS excretion between officers and men was significant, the higher rate amongst the former perhaps reflecting their special position of responsibility. It is interesting that on the day of attack, output fell substantially amongst the soldiers; they were able to use externally directed active responses (fighting) in coping with the threat, and such behaviours may be associated with reduced adrenocortical activity. The reverse was true of the officers, with 20 per cent increases in 17-OHCS, related perhaps to the relatively passive role they were forced to adopt in battle, spending most of their time liaising and interpreting orders from higher command.

Simple conclusions cannot therefore be drawn about chronic adrenocortical responses to behavioural stimulation. Although the system does react to extreme pressures, long-term hypersecretion has rarely been found (Mason, 1968). The output varies greatly between individuals, but whether this reflects psychological differences in appraisal or coping is not certain. The lack of matched control groups and the use of 24-hour excretion measures, which conceal important diurnal variations, are further bars to definite judgement.

Catecholamines

Surveys of adrenomedullary responses reveal rather more consistent patterns of activation. Frankenhaeuser and Gardell (1976) compared catecholamine excretion in different categories of workers in a sawmill. One group worked at machine-paced jobs, with short work cycles and continuous repetitive demands that were largely outside the men's personal control. In contrast, the maintenance workers performed more varied jobs and operated at their own pace. The groups were exposed to the same noise, had similar physical working postures, and were also equivalent on education, leisure activities and family conditions (Johansson *et al.*, 1978); increases in adrenaline excretion above no work control days were greater in machine-paced men, particularly early and late in the work shift. Noradrenaline output was also higher over the last part of the work period.

In another study of occupational pressures, workers in the confectionery industry were examined as they alternated between four-day periods with and without payment at piece rate (Timio *et al.*, 1979). The energy expenditure, assessed by oxygen consumption, was identical under the two regimens, yet noradrenaline excretion rose to 230 per cent, and adrenaline to 450 per cent on days with the added time stress. The pattern was duplicated in metal workers off and on the assembly line. Moreover, these effects are not transient, since differences persisted when the alternation of working conditions continued for six months. Adrenomedullary output is also disturbed when workers change from day to night shifts, although in this case there may eventually be adaptation to the new rhythm (Theorell and Åkerstedt, 1976).

Even the mild, but frequent, discomfort of crowding on a commuter train can provoke catecholamine responses (Singer *et al.*, 1978). Passengers who regularly travelled into central Stockholm on a long (79-min) journey were compared with those who took a shorter (43-min) but more crowded trip. The latter showed slightly greater increases in adrenaline excretion, although the differences were not large. Yet since the journeys were a regular feature of these people's lives, the survey indicates that catecholamine reactions may not disappear once conditions are familiar.

This possibility is borne out by other reports. Carruthers *et al.* (1976) found that urinary noradrenaline was elevated in passengers and crew during a long transatlantic flight from Argentina to London. The high concentration persisted after landing, while adrenaline output was also raised. Catecholamine excretion may be affected by periods of urban driving (Bellet *et al.*, 1969). Both healthy volunteers and cardiac patients were examined, and levels compared with those recorded after sitting quietly for the same length of time. In each case, catecholamine output was significantly greater after the car drive; patients with ischaemic heart disease had the higher concentrations in the urine, reacting more in this setting. The same pattern was seen in noradrenaline analysed from the plasma of racing car drivers (Taggart and Carruthers, 1971). Responses were very variable, but some individuals showed elevated catecholamines immediately after the race, falling to baseline within 15 minutes. Interestingly, plasma triglycerides peaked one hour after the event, while a rise in free fatty acids (FFA) occurred at an intermediate time; it is possible that FFA release was stimulated by catecholamines, followed later by conversion to triglycerides.

An innovative study by Theorell *et al.* (1972) documented the sensitivity of catecholamines even more precisely. Twenty-one survivors of heart attacks completed a Swedish version of the Schedule of Recent Events every few weeks. This questionnaire surveys a range of life events thought to require major adjustments — children leaving home, the death of a close friend and minor violations of the law are examples of the items included. Weighted scores, or life change units, were allotted to each incident according to its severity, as judged by a larger age and occupation matched sample. The average number of life change units per week calculated for each individual correlated significantly with mean adrenaline excretion. Thus people whose lives demanded greater adjustments have higher catecholamine outputs. This pattern has also been recorded over the acute recovery period in survivors of myocardial infarction (Klein *et al.*, 1974). The relationship was duplicated within individuals from repeated samples over several months; in seven patients the correlation between life change units per week and adrenaline excretion was over 0·60, and the association with noradrenaline was also significant. These surveys underline the value of regular investigations on the same people, with systematic scoring of psychological data. Catecholamines are amongst the most sensitive indices of prolonged disturbance, and psychosocial experience.

Blood coagulation and platelet aggregation

A naturalistic stressor that has frequently been used in the study of coagulation mechanisms is the case presentation by a junior doctor to superiors. In view of the haemodynamic and sympathetic nervous reactions that are observed, a heightening of platelet aggregation might be anticipated. Yet this has not been found (Haft and Arkel, 1976; Arkel *et al.*, 1977). Although most healthy subjects responded, they showed decreases of aggregation in blood samples taken immediately after performance. In several cases the second phase of the aggregation response to noradrenaline was lost altogether, while others produced slower aggregation rates. It is possible that this refractory response was due to partial aggregations induced by the naturally secreted catecholamines, making the platelets less sensitive to later challenges *in vitro*. However, the explanation is doubtful, since Arkel *et al.* (1977) observed increases in platelet ADP/ATP ratios.

On the other hand, enhanced platelet aggregation has been recorded from patients during the anticipation of minor surgery (Gordon *et al.*, 1973; Fleischman *et al.*, 1976). However, reactivity returned to normal soon after operations, and was not elevated even a day beforehand; the changes thus appear to be acute and short lived. Dintenfass and Zader (1975) assessed predominantly anxious psychiatric patients, considering them to be a group under chronic stress. A number of haematological factors were disturbed, with high plasma viscosity and reduced erythrocyte sedimentation rate. Changes in Factor VIII levels have also been described in patients undergoing surgery (Letheby *et al.*, 1974; Britton *et al.*, 1974).

The data on coagulation and thrombosis are thus conflicting, and there is disagreement about what stages of the mechanism are sensitive to behavioural influences. Russian investigators have suggested that coagulation systems may become either hypo- or hyperactive during emotional stress, and that the response depends on the type of individual studied (Sokolow and Volkova, 1977). It has been assumed that psychosocial stressors all have an equivalent impact on thrombotic pathways, so the form and intensity of noxious stimulation has seldom been well controlled. Nevertheless, further research in the area is likely to be fruitful, and the development of methods for *in vivo* assessment of platelet aggregation will permit more precise investigation of emotional and cognitive factors (Hornstra and Ten Hoor, 1975).

Patterns of adaption and alert behavioural responses

It will be apparent from this brief review that not all cardiovascular and neuroendocrine pathways show sustained hyperactivity in the face of prolonged stimulation or distress. A number of explanations can be put forward to account for the variation.

a. The absence of sustained reactions may reflect psychological coping amongst participants, so that they are able to tolerate the continued disturbance. This argument has been proposed in the case of parents of leukaemic children, discussed on p. 127; the low corticosteroid outputs may be related to successful psychological defence (Wolff *et al.*, 1964).

This explanation may be important, but its value is limited as yet, owing to the empirical deficiencies in assessing psychological defences. Thus Wolff's results were contradicted by Tecce (1966), using different tests. Moreover, there was no consistent association between defence and corticosteroid output in the Vietnam studies (Bourne, 1970). If all forms of psychological coping attenuate reactions, the hypothesis becomes meaningless, and can be replaced by this simpler generalisation:

b. Some neuroendocrine pathways may not be capable of sustained overactivity in response to the psychosocial disturbances experienced in naturalistic settings. Either there are physiological contraints on high output of these mechanisms, or the degree of psychological distress induced in naturalistic settings is never sufficiently great. If this is confirmed, the significance of short-term patterns for chronic cardiovascular dysfunction is doubtful. A third possibility can, however, be entertained.

c. The field settings studied, and the personal resources mobilised, may not be appropriate for the particular neuroendocrine or cardiovascular parameter being monitored. If the patterns of differential mobilisation outlined in Chapters 5 and 6 are reliable, then chronic hyperactivity will only be predicted when certain stimulus conditions and response demands prevail.

One way to tease apart these possibilities is by assessing a number of functions simultaneously. For instance, if pressor responses persist while adrenocortical output diminishes, it may be inferred that the potential for long-term overstimulation under those particular circumstances is different for the two systems. Unfortunately, few data of this type are available, since most investigators have interest in a restricted range of response parameters. But detailed examinations of parachutists have usefully elaborated the changes of reaction patterns over time (Ursin *et al.*, 1978). A group of healthy Norwegian soldiers were followed throughout their early training as parachutists. This involved jumping from a 12-metre tower, and later from aeroplanes. Blood and urine were collected for the analysis of several humoral factors, while cardiovascular indices were restricted to heart rate. The first jump from the training tower provoked the largest increases in cortisol, FFA and growth hormone, together with a reduction in testosterone below values recorded on pre-training days. These reactions had largely disappeared by the second day, and showed no further disturbance later in training. The rapid adaptation of adreno-

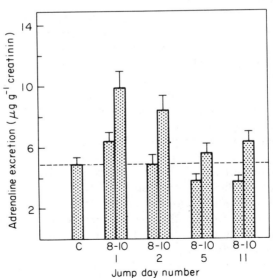

FIG. 7.3. Urinary output of adrenaline on control day at 8.00 a.m. (C), and before (8.00 a.m.) and after (10.00 a.m.) jumps from the training tower. (Hansen *et al.*, 1978.)

cortical secretions confirms the transient effect of overstimulation on this pathway, at least during actively enaging tasks. The brief fall in testosterone parallels the suppression of anabolic hormones in monkeys exposed to novel stimuli (Mason, 1975).

These adaptations contrast with the pattern of catecholamine excretion (Hansen *et al.*, 1978). Fig. 7.3 summarises the changes in adrenaline output. As with the other parameters, the large initial response habituated rapidly. Yet in addition, the post-jump levels were consistently higher than those recorded beforehand. There was a phasic activation with performance of the task itself, that did not habituate. The "basal" recordings were taken in the days before training, and cannot be considered as true baselines, since apprehension and anticipatory arousal was probably present; they may therefore be rather higher than those monitored under relaxed conditions. Noradrenaline reactions followed a similar course, although in this case, pre-jump levels did not fall below the average basal sample at any time.

These adjustments were elicited during training in a potentially dangerous skill, demanding alert and active coping. The adaptation following the first jump paralleled the decrease in reported fear; as the task became familiar, and soldiers gained experience, secretions from the adrenal cortex and other glands returned to normal. However, sympathetically mediated responses persisted, albeit at a reduced intensity, and may have been a crucial component of the active coping response. This is reflected in the "additional heart rates", increases in excess of metabolic demands, monitored during training (see p. 64). During the brief interval prior to every jump, large tachycardias rapidly developed to levels averaging more than 40 bpm above values predicted from oxygen consumption (Strømme, *et al.*, 1978). Moreover, the response did not habituate or diminish with training, but was maintained throughout.

The role of sympathetic pathways in the mediation of reactions during parachuting has been known for several years (Bloom *et al.*, 1963). Fenz (1975) showed that psychophysiological responses vary with the degree of task experience. Heart rate, respiration and skin conductance increased progressively in trainees right up to the actual moment of jumping. In contrast, the reactions of experienced parachutists to the initial stages of jump preparation were followed by a decline, so that the peak anticipatory responses were smaller (Fenz and Epstein, 1967). The distinction did not depend solely on the degree of familiarity with the task; poor performers, whether or not they had extensive training, tended to show the pattern of gradual rises in autonomic activity. Similarly, when a highly skilled performer had a jumping accident, his reactivity reverted to the type seen in novices.

The modifications in PRA recorded during parachuting are also interesting (Langos *et al.*, 1976). Measures were taken from beginners, men in training and experienced sports parachutists. There were no differences in PRA on rest days, yet differential reactions followed jumps (Table 7.1). All groups showed raised levels immediately after the jump, but the increase was smaller amongst the more experienced performers. Urinary adrenaline and noradrenaline were also elevated after the jump. The PRA peak was not only smaller in sportsmen, the recovery to baseline was more rapid. However, it is significant that these adjustments, modulated through β-adrenergic mechanisms, persisted even in people with considerable task experience. They may reflect the constant alertness required in active coping with demanding environments.

Another case in which emotionally based cardiovascular reactions persist is during ski jumps. Imhof and co-workers (1969) monitored heart rates from members of the Swiss and Yugoslavian teams during ascent to the platform, the countdown and the jump. A double-blind crossover of oxprenolol and placebo was performed, to determine the degree of cardiac sympathetic involvement. As the men climbed to the platform, the average heart rates of 130–134 bpm were reduced by only 15 per cent on β blockade: these tachycardias were predominantly due to the effect of the physical work. Yet during the countdown, when no motor activity was required, the traffic in cardiac sympathetic fibres heightened. The mean heart rate of 123·1 in the placebo condition was lowered by 34·2 per cent to 81·0 bpm with β blockade. Similarly a difference of 32·3 per cent was recorded on rundown, while rate after landing rose to 145·8 bpm under placebo. It seems

TABLE 7.1

Plasma Renin Activity and parachuting (Langos *et al.*, 1976).

PRA (mean $\pm$ s.e.) in ng/100 ml/12 h

| | | Time after parachuting | | |
	Control	5 min	30 min	90 min
Beginners ($n=10$)	145·0 ± 7·8	244·5 ± 9·4	209·0 ± 8·7	195·0 ± 7·7
Trainees ($n=9$)	149·0 ± 7·1	231·0 ± 8·1	203·0 ± 7·6	181·0 ± 5·7
Sportsmen ($n=6$)	148·3 ± 10·4	213·3 ± 10·9	191·7 ± 9·1	151·7 ± 9·1

likely that cardiac sympathetic neurons were selectively mobilised during these periods of emotional tachycardia, leading to a greater divergence between drug and placebo than in the physically taxing phases of the task.

These data are largely consistent with patterns recorded in the laboratory, showing persistent mobilization of sympathetic nervous pathways during active coping, and a corresponding attenuation of adrenocortical secretions. However parachuting and ski-jumping are unusual behaviours, where it is not easy to distinguish the physiological reactions due to physical and emotional demands. The identification of chronic patterns of adjustment must be even more tentative in sedentary settings.

Reaction patterns during severe crises

Life event techniques have unfortunately not been exploited in delineating the patterns of neuroendocrine and cardiovascular activation during disturbing experiences. However, the area has been explored by Cobb and Kasl in their investigations of factory closure, redundancy and re-employment in middle-aged workers (Kasl and Cobb, 1970; Cobb, 1974; Cobb and Kasl, 1977). Cardiovascular and neurohumoral data were first collected 4–7 weeks before shut-down, and then at intervals for two years after the event. Participants were long-term employees from two factories who had spent an average of more than 15 years in their jobs; they were contrasted with controls from comparable plants, whose employment was secure.

Changes were recorded in a variety of physical functions, only some of which are relevant to cardiovascular disorders. The primary augmentation of blood pressure occurred during anticipation, since in later phases, levels generally fell. However, a number of distinct patterns were recorded. A proportion of the workers from one factory suffered little unemployment, while their colleagues were redundant for longer. The re-employed showed more rapid decreases in pressure, and the inverse correlation across individuals between the overall drop in systolic pressure and the number of weeks of unemployment was significant.

There were also trends towards lower serum cholesterol concentrations over time. Nevertheless, differential changes with varying work experience again emerged. The men who became unemployed on factory closure showed small but reliable average increases in cholesterol of 9 mg/100 ml (0·23 mmol l^{-1}) compared with 2 mg/100 ml

(0·05 mmol l^{-1}) falls in those going directly to new jobs. Interestingly, the unemployed who subsequently found jobs produced larger decreases (24 mg/100 ml or 0·62 mmol l^{-1}) between job termination and 6-month follow-up, than the group who remained redundant (11 mg/100 ml, 0·28 mmol l^{-1}).

Yet another response pattern emerged from catecholamine analyses, since this pathway manifests sustained overactivity. Noradrenaline excretion rates are compared in Fig. 7.4 with the mean output of men in control companies. Levels were reliably elevated on all occasions except two-year follow-up, so reactions were very persistent. Noradrenaline was also associated with coffee drinking, although caffeine did not consistently provoke rises in excretion rates.

It seems that while cholesterol and blood pressure fluctuated with the uncertainties of factory shut-down and seeking re-employment, noradrenaline was sensitive to rather different factors. Excretion remained high even after new occupations were found. During this time, men may have been heavily involved in adapting to their new environments and work positions, mobilising flexible response strategies with un-

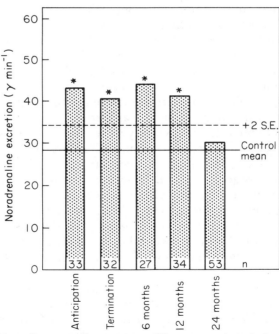

Fig. 7.4. Noradrenaline excretion rate on different occasions before and after redundancy. *significant difference from controls, $p < 0.05$. (Cobb, 1974.)

certain outcomes. It is interesting that firm psychological defences, generally considered to be of value in the face of hostile conditions, were associated with low noradrenaline output during the anticipatory phases. But at 6 and 12 months, when the day-to-day coping demands were more salient, no relation was found with defences.

Although it is tempting to integrate these findings into a broader conceptual scheme, care must be exercised. Unemployment may bring about many changes in sleeping, exercise and dietary habits, that are difficult to control. It can also be associated with a variety of psychological responses from fatalistic despondency to continual active searches for new opportunities. Each of these strategies may lead to different patterns of cardiovascular and endocrine modification. However, one of the hazards of field surveys is that variables are seldom identified with ideal precision.

Summary and conclusions

Much of the evidence gathered in naturalistic settings is consistent with the response patterns observed in the laboratory. Yet not all parameters of endocrine and cardiovascular function show augmented activity in the face of prolonged psychosocial stimulation. Some apparently habituate rapidly, others remaining reactive, while tonic changes in level of function may also be recorded.

Thus blood pressure and circulating catecholamines are persistently stimulated under a variety of conditions. In contrast, adrenal cortical output generally adapts even to sources of major threat, although the gland may remain responsive in field settings. The evidence for disturbances of serum cholesterol and blood clotting mechanisms is less consistent.

Variations in reaction patterns may reflect the modest capacity of certain pathways for hypersecretion, the ability of people to defend psychologically against life events, or the type of cognitive and behavioural responses demanded under different conditions. Sympathetically mediated activation is more prominent when skilled actions with uncertain outcome are required. Reactions will be heightened by poor performance, but persist even in the proficient. However, many naturalistic studies involve so many uncertain interacting factors, that close parallels cannot be drawn with the effects of experimentally imposed stimuli.

8
Psychological Factors in Essential Hypertension

Earlier chapters have been concerned with the details of cognitive and behavioural influences on the cardiovascular system, as seen in the laboratory and naturalistic settings. Effects are profound under some circumstances, and sufficiently intense to provoke sustained pathological responses. However, it has not yet been shown that these mechanisms actually operate in human cardiovascular disorders; the final links in the aetiological chain must concentrate on the development of the disease states themselves. Essential hypertension is discussed in the present chapter, with ischaemic heart disease and stroke in the remaining sections.

Psychosocial analyses of individual patients with essential hypertension are scattered over the medical literature of the last century. Unfortunately, their value in identifying causal associations is somewhat limited. Two of the largest series were collected under the direction of Reiser (1951) and Wolf (1955). Patients were followed over several years, and assessed with the range of haemodynamic techniques then available. Emotional factors and life stresses clearly emerged from these surveys as having powerful effects on the course of dysfunction in some cases. Many patients showed exacerbation of hypertension during periods of strain and worry, with comparatively low pressures under calmer conditions. No special personality characteristics emerged from these cohorts, since subjects differed widely in temperament. Wolf *et al.* (1955) suggested that most of their patients were non-reflective, showing a "taste for dealing with problems by action"; but at the same time, difficulties in self-expression and assertion were inferred from indirect sources such as dream analysis.

In a more recent exploration of the relationship between emotional state and hypertension, 25 volunteers were taught to monitor their own blood pressure (Whitehead, *et al.*, 1977). Readings were taken four

138

times each day, and simultaneously patients were asked to rate anxiety and anger. Although the strength of the association between reported tension and blood pressure varied considerably between people, anxiety correlated on average 0·36 with systolic and 0·27 with diastolic pressure. Thus despite the presence of numerous other factors affecting arterial pressure during the day, high levels tended to occur in parallel with extreme anxiety. The correlations were as great as 0·79 in some individuals, while the association between haemodynamics and anger was slightly less consistent. Regrettably, the fact that subjects recorded both blood pressure and emotional state leaves open the possibility of direct contamination of the self report data. Nevertheless, similar patterns led Singer and her associates to emphasise the role of involvement or engagement in hypertension (Singer, 1974). They observed that patients exhibited high pressures when emotionally aroused and actively involved in interviews; in contrast, lower pressures were recorded while subjects replied in a detached or evasive fashion.

Although such investigations suggest that the hypertensive's blood pressure may vary with psychological state, they provide little evidence on causal links. The participants must have displayed elevated arterial pressures of a sufficient magnitude and durability to be classified as essential hypertensives before their emotional condition was explored. Retrospective descriptions of childhood experiences indicated that many patients were raised in deprived or troubled circumstances; yet the absence of early haemodynamic data or control groups makes an aetiological interpretation impossible. In an effort to solve this problem, Reiser *et al.* (1951) selected cases in which hypertension onset could apparently be pinpointed in time, and assessed whether it coincided with an emotionally charged life crises. The incidence of such associations was directly proportional to the depth of psychological examinations performed. Thus amongst patients given minimal medical and psychiatric evaluation, a link between hypertension onset and emotional disturbance was shown in only 9 per cent. This figure rose to 100 per cent in those who underwent prolonged psychological investigation. These trends suggest that patience is needed to identify idiosyncratic cognitive factors, but may also reflect the influence of selection, and conscious or unconscious bias, on the evidence extracted—if an emotional trigger is sought with sufficient diligence, it is almost certain to be found. It is also extremely doubtful that a point in time can be identified, at which the continuously fluctuating arterial pressure "becomes" hypertension.

Series of individual cases are generally chosen to illustrate certain

points, and there are problems in the collection of genuinely representative groups. It is therefore difficult to decide whether the associations
reported are typical of hypertensives at large. Wolf *et al.* (1955) attempted to gather an unselected cohort, but realised that referrals from
other physicians would probably include a high proportion of "interesting" patients. Furthermore, in these uncontrolled surveys, it is not
known whether the psychological disturbances differ from those of
comparable normotensives.

A greater element of control was introduced by Friedman and
Kasanin (1943) in their study of a pair of identical twins. The hypertensive had a resting blood pressure of 180/110 mm, without any other
gross cardiovascular disorder, while his twin was a healthy normotensive with a pressure of 135/80 mm. The patient was described as
dynamic, excitable and extrovert. He was sociable and a member of
many clubs, but was extremely conscientious and concerned about the
quality of his work. The normotensive twin seemed steadier and more
easygoing, leading a calmer life with less tension. Since no other factors
appeared to account for the difference in blood pressure, behavioural
aspects were considered to be primary. Yet although the conclusion
may be valid for this particular case, it is unwise to generalise about the
nature of the psychological differences recorded; almost precisely the
reverse pattern emerged in a survey of Norwegian twins, higher blood
pressures being characteristic of the more submissive, obedient and
withdrawn member of each pair (Torgersen and Kringlen, 1971).

Individual case studies illustrate the manner in which blood pressure
may be responsive to psychosocial influences, and it is interesting that
high levels have regularly been recorded during periods of anxiety or
active involvement (reflecting the patterns identified in earlier chapters). Nevertheless, the individual case strategy provides little information on the development of essential hypertension.

The role of personal characteristics has also been analysed with
formal tests, but here too confounding factors severely limit general
conclusions, as will be seen in the next section.

Personality traits in essential hypertension

The psychosomatic tradition that grew up in the wake of the Second
World War was principally concerned with identifying underlying
traits or personal characteristics in disease groups. Alexander's (1952)
approach to essential hypertension was influential. On the basis of
psychoanalytic explorations, he suggested that the hypertensive

typically inhibited hostility, and was unable to express aggression. Other authors found neurotic traits in patients with high blood pressure. A large literature accumulated, trying to isolate the intrapsychic factors special to essential hypertension; this work has been reviewed extensively, and need not be recounted in detail (Davies, 1971; Weiner, 1979).

Unfortunately, few reliable conclusions can be drawn from these investigations. The assumption of stable traits that underpins the whole effort to generalise about patients' personalities has been under severe attack (Mischel, 1968). The responses to many personal assessments depend as much on the circumstances in which they are elicited, as on the predispositions of the individual. Global judgements are especially vulnerable to the investigator's biases or preconceptions, and have low reliabilities in comparison with measurements of specific behaviours.

Even when these problems are reduced by the use of established psychological tests, there are further difficulties in essential hypertension. High blood pressure is widespread in the population at large, and a considerable proportion of victims do not seek or attract clinical attention. The elevated hostility or neuroticism levels reported amongst diagnosed hypertensives may not be typical of the group as a whole, but characterise only those who have contact with medical services. Thus Robinson (1964) collected psychological ratings from hypertensive outpatients, people attending a psychiatric outpatient clinic, and participants in a blood pressure screening survey. The patients with diagnosed essential hypertension had higher neuroticism scores than the population sample, but did not differ from the psychiatric group. Within the screened population, there was no significant correlation between neuroticism and pressure.

The medical attention factor may be controlled by discovering hypertensives through screening, rather than relying on diagnosed groups; under these circumstances, individuals with high blood pressure do not usually emerge with distinctive personal profiles (Balter and Levine, 1977). Cochrane (1973) studied the participants in a heart disease prevention programme, matching high, medium and low pressure groups on age, class and marital status. No correlations were recorded between personality measures and arterial pressure. In another screening survey, Mann (1977) failed to uncover firm associations between psychiatric tests and diastolic levels, although some people with high blood pressure rated above average in "acting out hostility"; this may however, have been a chance result in the large series of statistical comparisons.

Situational variables and the sensitivity of blood pressure to recording conditions, should also be borne in mind. Even a tentative diagnosis of essential hypertension can be psychologically disturbing. These factors may underlie the correlation between anxiety and blood pressure identified during screening by Banahan *et al.* (1979). Anxiety questionnaires were administered to hypertensive individuals only after their blood pressures had remained elevated on more than one occasion, and they had been referred to their physicians for follow-up; anxiety over these disclosures may have affected the psychological assessments directly.

The question of whether essential hypertension is related to specific personality disturbances can be reversed, by monitoring blood pressure in psychiatrically morbid groups. Heine and Sainsbury (1970) reported that systolic pressures correlated significantly with the number of diagnosed depressive episodes, independently of age. Yet when psychiatric ratings were examined more precisely, pressure was linked not with depression but anxiety. Friedman and Bennet (1977) drew a similar conclusion from a survey of 1100 depressed outpatients, since diastolic pressure correlated with anxiety rather than depression ratings. These positive links with anxiety must, however, be set against failures to find any such connection (Wheeler *et al.*, 1950; Rudolff, 1955).

Even when differences are reliable, the interpretation of cross-sectional data is hazardous. McFarland and Cobb (1967) pointed out the alternatives to a causal explanation, and their general argument is worth repeating. The higher prevalence of a psychological or biological characteristic amongst people with a particular complaint, may be consistent with three different hypotheses. The factor may have a harmful effect, speeding the development and progress of the disorder. Alternatively, it may be beneficial, so that people lacking this quality succumb to the illness more rapidly — leading to an increase in the proportion of survivors displaying the attribute. Thirdly, it may have no effect at all, but arise purely as a result of the disorder.

The alternative hypotheses can best be distinguished prospectively, yet few such surveys have been performed in essential hypertension. The longitudinal perspective is especially pertinent in view of the role of autonomic factors in the initial stages of aetiology; the heightened emotional lability observed amongst people with hyperkinetic circulations underlines the importance of shifting attention from established to early and borderline phases (Safar *et al.*, 1978). Personal assessments that have failed to take the diversity of the condition into consideration have added little to our understanding of the psychosocial contributions to high blood pressure.

Population differences, migration and essential hypertension

Large-scale surveys that link behavioural factors to disease are forms of psychosocial epidemiology. Such investigations are directed at broad issues with population-based field samples, and allow for confounding variables through statistical manipulations rather than experimental controls. Interesting information on the association of ischaemic heart disease with psychosocial experience has been collected with these methods, and patterns of blood pressure distribution may be analysed in the same way.

Perhaps the grossest use of this research strategy is in the comparison of blood pressure levels in different societies and cultures. Some relevant data have already been described in Chapter 3; surveys indicate that not all populations in the world have the same incidence of hypertension, nor do blood pressures universally rise with age (Fig. 3.2, p. 41). It has been suggested that a proportion of the variance may be ascribed to cultural ambience, the groups with lower blood pressure leading less "stressful" lives, perhaps maintaining more stable traditional social systems (Henry and Cassel, 1969). Thus Puerto Ricans living in relatively primitive rural environments have lower pressures than their urban counterparts (Benson *et al.*, 1966). Tseng (1967) reported that hypertension was more prevalent in a Taiwanese fishing population than a neighbouring agricultural society. Although both followed traditional customs and diets, the fishermen lived in crowded towns while the farmers were rural. In the US, cultural isolation has been examined in religious sects such as the Amish of Pennsylvania (Jorgenson *et al.*, 1972). Subgroups of the community vary in their contact and participation in contemporary lifestyles. The age-related systolic pressure increases are smallest in those who maintain the greatest separation and independence. Comparisons of a similar type have been made between populations differing in blood pressure distribution from most racial groups of the world (Henry and Cassel, 1969).

One difficulty with interpretation is that many other factors may distinguish groups, and these can have direct influences on arterial pressure. Body weight, salt intake, exercise, diet, medical care and the mortality rate in different age strata can all affect the pressure distribution, and one can rarely account for all such factors. Exceptions can of course be found, as in the instances of high salt/low pressure groups cited in Chapter 3 — but these do not provide adequate grounds for dismissing the involvement of variations in physical makeup and diet.

Furthermore, population contrasts have not all been consistent. Norman-Taylor and Rees (1963) found no differences in the pressure spectra of three New Hebridean communities, despite considerable divergence in urbanisation and contact with Western civilisation. The blood pressures of Japanese men living in California and adopting a Western lifestyle were similar to those in more traditional groups (Marmot and Syme, 1976). The separation of urban and rural populations is not universal either (Miall *et al.*, 1962; Langford *et al.*, 1968). An added problem is that many explanations of population differences may be devised *post hoc*, and not tested predictively. For instance, it is possible that a rural community, struggling to maintain traditional practices in the face of encroaching mechanisation and outside influence, will experience a great deal of internal conflict and social stress. Thus traditional customs may buffer and protect, or alternatively augment culture shock. Some investigators fail to define their expectations before collecting data, and are thus able to "explain" almost any difference.

Firmer predictions can be made in the case of migration, since it is agreed that transfer to a new culture may lead to profound psychosocial upheavals, as novel customs are confronted. Since behavioural and emotional factors may have their greatest impact in the development rather than maintainence of essential hypertension, migration is especially interesting in that the cultural change can be pinpointed in time.

A good deal of evidence supports the general hypothesis that high blood pressure is associated with migration (see Stamler *et al.*, 1967). Cruz-Coke (1960) compared two groups of trainee policemen from Cuzco in highland Peru. One group had lived in urban Lima for several years, and their pressures were higher than those of recruits newly arrived from the country. Scotch's (1963) studies of Zulus on rural reserves and in urban communities also implicated rapid cultural change in the aetiology of essential hypertension.

Of course, migration often results in changes of diet and exercise. Unfortunately, the movement is almost invariably towards higher risk on these parameters, although the appearance of alternative cultural migration back to rural self-sufficiency may afford an interesting test of the psychosocial explanation. Ostfeld and D'Atri (1977) have argued that blood pressure modifications are largely due to increases in weight amongst migrants. Florey and Cuadrado (1968) reached a similar conclusion, when comparing communities of Cape Verde Islanders in their native land with those living in the US. Furthermore, migrants are never picked at random from their original populations. They are generally self-selected, and the same factors might underlie both blood pressure change and the tendency to migrate.

In some senses, it is immaterial whether the pressure modifications are mediated by diet, weight, exercise or psychological distress, since all of these are elements of behaviour, and not organic pathologies. They may themselves reflect emotional distress, albeit in different ways. Thus the fact that weight contributes to pressure change does not diminish the importance of psychological factors, since overeating can be a response to personal problems (Brunswick and Collette, 1977). Nevertheless, these links undermine the relevance of direct connections between cardiovascular responses and the higher central nervous system. It is therefore interesting that the detailed studies of Polynesian migrants to New Zealand suggest arterial pressure distributions cannot be accounted for solely by weight variations. These investigations have focused on the inhabitants of the Tokelau Islands (Prior, 1977). Prospective surveys, encompassing the whole migrant group (2000 people), and 1560 left on the Islands, have been performed. The blood pressures of male migrants rose, along with weight, salt intake and carbohydrate diet. Social interactions with New Zealanders in work, church and leisure activities, were also assessed by questionnaire (Beaglehole *et al.*, 1977).

Fig. 8.1 summarises the average systolic pressures of men in the upper and lower tertiles of social interaction, stratified according to age. The overall difference was significant, with higher pressures recorded from those who interacted extensively, in comparison with the more exclusive Tokelauans. Moreover, the difference persisted after controlling for body weight, age and length of stay in New Zealand. Surveys of Tokelauan migrant children indicated that blood pressures may diverge at an early age (Beaglehole *et al.*, 1978). Levels amongst 2–14 year old boys were higher in New Zealand, despite appropriate numerical adjustments for weight and height. Sodium excretion failed to correlate with pressure after controlling for other factors, suggesting that salt did not account for the difference.

Migration is a complex and variable phenomenon, and simple predictions cannot necessarily be made. Hypotheses must be tailored to the particular study population. The impact of migration is modulated by the strength of group supports, the expectations the individual has about change, and the amount of preparation that goes into the move (Prior, 1977). Effects may also fluctuate with the person's original social position, and subsequent role in the new structure. It is not surprising that many discrepancies in blood pressure responses have emerged. For instance, Scotch (1963) found that levels were higher

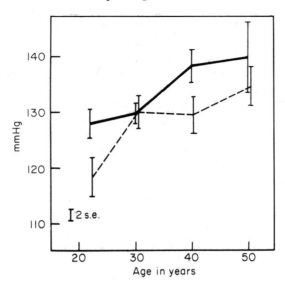

Fig. 8.1. Relationship between systolic blood pressure and social interaction pattern in adult Tokelauan men resident in New Zealand. ——, Tertile with greatest New Zealand interaction; – – – –, tertile with greatest Tokelau interaction (Beaglehole *et al.*, 1977.)

amongst urban Zulus who maintained traditional practices; in other cases, this segment of the migrant population seems to be the least vulnerable. In the carefully controlled Tokelauan studies, the amount of variance attributable to the social interaction factor in adults was not large (Beaglehole *et al.*, 1977). Yet the data on migration does lend some support to the hypothesis that psychosocial factors are significant.

High blood pressure and exposure to taxing conditions

The measurement of distress in everyday life has become a good deal more objective with the introduction of systematic life event techniques. The relation of life events to catecholamine excretion has been mentioned in Chapter 7, and many investigators have focused on the association with ischaemic heart disease. Yet in general, life events have not emerged as salient factors in essential hypertension. For example, Rahe *et al.* (1976) failed to uncover positive links between life change scores and systolic pressure amongst rural Finns. Newly diagnosed hypertensives, normotensive controls, and patients with established high blood pressure were compared by Balter and Levine

(1977). Again, no consistent differences appeared in the rate of severe or mild events.

However, a close connection between life events and high arterial pressure should perhaps not be expected. If persistent attempts at active coping are important, then people under chronic threat will be at greater risk. A severe, uncontrollable event such as an accident or death may be deeply disturbing, but will not necessarily provoke the appropriate cardiovascular reactions. Some interesting trends have emerged from the study of work settings, implicating sustained psychosocial stimulation in the development of essential hypertension.

The criterion of environmental stress adopted by Jonsson and Hansson (1977) was the degree of hearing impairment suffered by industrial workers; it was assumed that men with severe losses worked in noisier and hence more unpleasant conditions. The differences in blood pressure distribution were not significant, but the mean level of those with impaired hearing was 145·2/88·6, compared with 132·6/80·6 in controls. Unfortunately, the hard-of-hearing were on average slightly older than controls, so an age factor may have accounted for some of the effects. A more recent and sophisticated analysis of adverse working conditions focused on perceived stress, rather than the objective environment (House *et al.*, 1979). Industrial blue collar workers completed extensive questionnaires relating to perceived responsibility, work load, role conflict and aspects of job satisfaction. After controlling for age, smoking, education and other factors, hypertension was reliably associated with a number of questionnaire responses. For example, the estimated prevalence amongst men reporting the highest degrees of job satisfaction was 3·5 per cent, compared with 14·4 per cent in the lowest category; the levels in groups with the highest and lowest amount of role conflict at work were calculated to be 27·5 per cent and 4·9 per cent respectively.

Further information can be collected by contrasting whole groups who share similar incomes and domestic conditions, while differing in pressure at work. For example, air traffic controllers are engaged in a taxing occupation that requires constant alertness and carries heavy responsibilities. Cobb and Rose (1973) compared over 4000 controllers with nearly twice as many second-class airmen, and showed that essential hypertension was some four times more prevalent amongst the former. It is thought that some of this effect was due to discriminant licensing practices, since airmen were more likely to fail medical examinations because of hypertension. Therefore, data from two annual checkups were collected, and an incidence rate calculated that was not biased by licensing variations. These values are summarised in Table

8.1; the annual incidence was nearly six times higher in the traffic controllers, being augmented in all age strata. Furthermore, the mean age of onset was 41 in controllers, compared with 48 in airmen. Thus more men in the demanding occupation tended to develop hypertension, and they did so at an earlier age. An additional analysis was performed on controllers working at airfields with high and low traffic densities — these were designated high and low stress towers. The prevalence rates in Table 8.1 suggest that men working at busy terminals were prone to develop essential hypertension at a younger age. Despite problems in the collection and interpretation of these data, the differences lend substantial support to the psychosocial hypothesis, although trends have been less striking in other analyses (Caplan *et al.*, 1975).

A rather different methodology was employed in a survey of middle-aged Swedish working men (Theorell and Lind, 1973). Two psychosocial factors, job responsibility and educational achievement, emerged from detailed interviews as potentially significant in high arterial pressure. Discrepancies between responsibility level and education seemed particularly important, and were therefore standardised into five categories. Hence an individual who had achieved a high social and occupational position but had little formal education scored 5,

TABLE 8.1

a. Air traffic controllers versus second-class airmen.
Annual incidence of hypertension per 1000 men

Age	Controllers	Airmen
20–29	2	1
30–39	12	2
40–49	17	4
50+	15	4

b. Controllers at high and low stress towers. Prevalence of hypertension per 1000 men

Age	High stress	Low stress
20–29	4	1
30–39	18	12
40–49	77	36
50+	—	36

From Cobb and Rose (1973).

TABLE 8.2
Discrepancy index in relation to mean systolic blood pressure
(Theorell and Lind, 1973)

Discrepancy	n	Mean systolic BP mm Hg
1	15	130 ± 4·2
2	19	133 ± 3·2
3	39	140 ± 3·1
4–5	12	144 ± 6·9

whilst those with congruent occupation and education were given a rating of 1. Table 8.2 shows the average systolic pressures of each group. Although there were some variations within strata, pressures tended to be higher amongst men with the largest discrepancy ratings. Such self-made men, rising from relatively humble origins, may be particularly vulnerable to social uncertainties and confusion.

All these results are consistent with the suggestion that people living or working in especially arousing conditions are prone to develop essential hypertension. But an additional problem is whether effects are specific to blood pressure, or reflect general illness susceptibility. Syme and Torfs (1978) have pointed out that socio-economic variables are linked with many different diseases and causes of death, so no special relationship with the cardiovascular system may be present. Thus Cobb and Rose (1973) found that peptic ulcer, another "stress-related" disorder, was also commoner amongst air traffic controllers than airmen. Similarly, excessive geographic mobility early in life may promote wide ranging physical morbidity in adulthood (Metzner *et al.*, 1977). Cobb and Kasl (1977) not only identified a heightened incidence of hypertension in men being made redundant, but also increases in arthritic joint swelling and alopecia. On the other hand, few objective aspects of poor health, apart from hypertension, were associated with perceived stress at work in the House (1979) study. The relationship between educational–occupational discrepancies and blood pressure recorded by Theorell and Lind (1973) was also relatively specific, since correlations with serum cholesterol were not significant.

At present, little is known about the specificity of associations between psychosocial parameters and blood pressure, since few investigators assess more than a single clinical endpoint. The same problem looms over research into ischaemic heart disease, as will be seen in the next chapter. However, there may be circumstances in which more precise connections can be made.

The environment, behaviour and physical predisposition

The hypotheses discussed thus far have been based on the influence either of internal characteristics (and personality), or of external stimuli. Although both may account for some of the variance in hypertension incidence, neither appears pre-eminent in isolation. It is probable that a more interactive model should be considered, since cardiovascular reactions may only be important when associated with appropriate behavioural dispositions or response styles.

Theorell (1976) has provided an indication of the nature of the inter-relationship. Data were derived from a prospective survey of ischaemic heart disease amongst middle-aged Swedish men in the construction industry. Participants completed two questionnaires; the first was a schedule of life events and adjustments, from which life change scores were calculated. The second related to perceived work responsibility, hostility and work satisfaction, and may have tapped habitual psychological response styles. Each individual was given a "discord" score, in which a high rating reflected dissatisfaction with home and working life, feelings of hostility when faced with slow people or queues, and difficulties with relaxation. From more than 5000 respondents, groups were selected with high and low scores on each scale. Thus the contribution of acute events and longer-term habits could be evaluated alone or in combination.

Systolic and diastolic pressures were significantly greater amongst high scorers on both scales, than in all other groups. People with large scores on only one scale did not show high average pressures, emphasising the importance of the interaction between external events and behavioural reactions. The difference was particularly marked amongst the younger (41–46 year) cohort, where the mean difference in systolic pressure was 11 mm. The prevalence rates of hypertension were also distinguishable. The acute life changes most frequently reported included trouble with employers, a decrease in income, and changes in sexual habits. Passive stressors, such as the death or serious illness of close relatives, were equally common in the double high raters, and in men with large life change but low discord scores.

Again, the possibility of a heightened general vulnerability in those who suffer frequent life events, and have high discord scores, must be entertained. In fact, these people did not show elevated concentrations of serum cholesterol or triglycerides, although more cases of chronic neurosis were identified. The physical or biological vulnerability of the individual should also be considered, since this may modulate reactions to psychological stimuli.

The triple interaction between physical predisposition, behavioural style and external harassment has been explored cross-sectionally amongst residents in Detroit (Harburg *et al.*, 1973, 1979). Different levels of constitutional risk were compared by assessing black and white members of both sexes. Two levels of environmental disturbance were included by selecting high and low stress areas of the city, defined according to population density, mobility, crime and economic status; the high stress areas were poorer, with higher juvenile and adult crime rates, less home ownership and more marital instability. Thirdly, personal coping style was delineated through responses to imaginary scenes of confrontation with the police, employers or houseowners. Reactions were scored for the amount of resentment, anger or hostility displayed.

These comparisons are highly complex, so few of the results were straightforward. However, it appeared that all three dimensions were associated with blood pressure. Hence, blacks tended towards higher pressures than whites, whilst men of either group living in the high stress zones had elevated levels in comparison with low stress residents. These effects were significant even when age and weight were taken into account. Race and external conditions interacted, so that black high stress males displayed the greatest arterial pressures of all. But the cardiovascular status was also influenced by psychological response style. Table 8.3 summarises one such comparison, in which subgroups were distinguished according to their responses to imagined police harassment. Anger out/no guilt men said they would express their anger or annoyance openly, and not feel guilty afterwards. The Anger in/guilt group claimed they would either experience no annoyance, or feel but not express it, and that they would subsequently regret their responses. Replies were related to blood pressure only for men living in high stress zones. Amongst both black and white residents, the Anger in/guilt respondents exhibited significantly higher mean diastolic pressures, and a greater prevalence of hypertension than the Anger out/no guilt subjects. Race was also important, since black high stress males reporting the Anger in/guilt pattern displayed the highest average diastolic pressure.

A subsequent study divided subjects on the basis of coping styles into resentful (feeling anger, either expressed or inhibited) and reflective (adopting a rationalising stance) categories. Again, behaviour inter-

TABLE 8.3
Associations between blood pressure, race, chronic stress and psychological response
(Harburg *et al.*, 1973)

Race	Response style	Residential stress	Mean diastolic pressure	Percentage with diastolic >95 mmHg
Black males	Anger out/ no guilt	High	84·0	16
		Low	83·6	16
	Anger in/ guilt	High	93·7	33
		Low	81·8	15
White males	Anger out/ no guilt	High	78·6	8
		Low	82·1	12
	Anger in/ guilt	High	83·2	19
		Low	83·2	18

acted with other factors (Harburg *et al.*, 1979). Resentful males living
in high stress areas exhibited a higher incidence of diastolic pressure
over 95 mm (17 per cent) than reflective males (8 per cent), while no
difference was recorded in low stress conditions, or in females. These
investigations illustrate the diversity of psychosocial associations with
hypertension. Although the psychological reaction patterns and coping
styles were assessed in somewhat rudimentary fashions, it seems that
disturbing external conditions, behaviour and biological factors
operate interactively in modulating arterial pressure levels.

Summary and conclusions

Investigations of essential hypertensive patients have frequently produced ambiguous results. There are major limitations to the study of
psychosocial factors in isolation, since many mechanisms are involved
in high blood pressure. No single element, be it weight, age, salt intake
or psychosocial stimulation, consistently accounts for more than a
fraction of the variance in pressure between populations or large
groups. Furthermore, essential hypertension is not a unitary state; as
was emphasised in Chapter 3, different mechanisms become important
as the disorder progresses. It is probable that behavioural factors are

more salient in the development than maintenance of the dysfunction. Thus it is unlikely that many general trends will be found across an unselected spectrum of patients. Additionally, behavioural stimuli are not equivalent or interchangeable, and sustained pressor responses are found only in limited circumstances.

The psychosocial influences on essential hypertension can best be understood in an interactional framework. Some of the important elements are summarised in Fig. 8.2. It goes without saying that for particular patients, different factors will vary in their salience. Pickering's (1961) stricture should also be borne in mind: "The genetic and environmental factors that determine the higher levels of arterial pressure characteristic of the disease are not different in kind from the factors resulting in lower pressure, they are different in degree."

It is apparent that behaviour may be involved in two quite different ways. Voluntary actions determine the levels of many "physical" risk factors. For instance, the variations in body weight that are significant for essential hypertension are not pathological abnormalities, but responses to differences in eating habits, diet and energy output. Clinically, it is appropriate to tackle these elements as undesirable behaviours, and not as medical problems.

Secondly, disturbing psychosocial conditions may promote hypertension directly. It is uncertain whether the cardiovascular system is uniquely fragile, or whether other aspects of health are also put at risk. Not all distressing environments will affect hypertensive mechanisms however. These influences are likely to operate through a pathway that

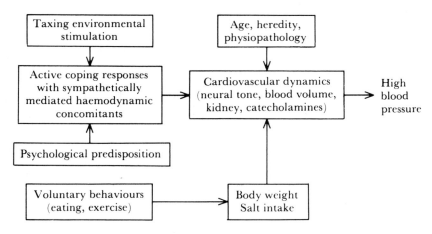

Fig. 8.2. Behavioural and psychological contributions to essential hypertension.

resolves on to the sympathetically mediated cardiovascular components of active behavioural coping. The mechanism is stimulated only when the appropriate behavioural responses are elicited. The part played by personal traits in modulating these reactions is not yet clear.

Such processes are important in the production of transient high pressure episodes. If reactions persist, they may trigger the physiological adjustments that contribute to the maintenance of hypertension. Laboratory research suggests that psychological stimuli may influence renal function directly, but this remains to be clarified in clinical groups. Finally, constitutional predispositions to high pressure cannot be ignored, and will on many occasions override other factors.

The salient individual differences in reactivity are still poorly characterised in essential hypertension. Longitudinal studies are rare while few prospective investigations have been performed. Nevertheless, progress will be made provided categories of hypertension are defined, and researchers acknowledge the complexity of the dysfunction.

9
Personality and Experience in Ischaemic Heart Disease

The study of psychological aspects of ischaemic heart disease has burgeoned over the last 20 years, exploiting the battery of techniques discussed in earlier sections. Much work has been done with the victims of the disease themselves. Yet paradoxically this direct approach to the problem of psychosocial involvement has perhaps the greatest methodological problems. This can best be illustrated by outlining a survey carried out a generation ago. No special criticism of the report is implied; rather it exemplifies general difficulties of interpretation.

In 1958, Russek and Zohman looked at the significance of heredity, diet and occupational stress in young adults with ischaemic heart disease. One hundred 25–40 year old patients were collected, most of whom had suffered myocardial infarction but did not have hypertension. Controls of similar age, occupation and ethnic origin were selected, and all participants were subjected to an interview concerning health. diet, sources of tension, and family medical history. A larger proportion of the patients had a familial history of cardiovascular disorders, and they reported more smoking and higher fat diets. Of these 91 per cent were also said to be under inordinate occupational stress, compared with 20 per cent of controls. The authors concluded that job-related emotional strain was far more significant for the aetiology of heart disease in this group than the other recorded variables.

Retrospective investigations of this kind run into several difficulties. Firstly, only survivors of cardiac events are interviewed, and there is no guarantee that they share characteristics with those who die. Prospective surveys have actually suggested a number of psychological differences between survivors and fatalities (Lebovits et al., 1967; Bruhn et al., 1969). The second problem is that patients may ascribe their illness to occupational stress retrospectively. Being perhaps aware of the popular link made between stress and the heart, patients may over emphasise and exaggerate minor aggravations, biasing their reports.

The presence of work-related emotional strain cannot be taken as evidence of a causal link with ischaemic heart disease. An alternative explanation is that the illness caused the difficulties at work. Cases rarely come to clinical attention until a very late stage, by which time the pathological process may have continued for decades. It is possible that as the physical capacity of the men diminished with progressive atheroma, they lost the ability to cope with their work loads, and experienced more and more strain. The evidence available from this type of research design is not sufficient to choose between the different explanations.

Interpretation is also limited by the selection of control groups. In Russek and Zohman's study, controls were in good health, while patients had recently suffered a distressing, life-threatening crisis. No special connection can therefore be made between the psychosocial dimension and cardiac disease; the presence of occupational stress might imply vulnerability to illness in general. Moreover, the two groups may have varied on unrecorded variables, such as serum cholesterol, that relate to the disease state independently. It is necessary to match on other physical and social indices, and to make comparisons with other sick groups, before inferences can confidently be made.

More serious weaknesses lie in the techniques of measurement. Data on psychological characteristics or the pressures of living are notoriously difficult to assemble, particularly when they are collected during personal interviews. The patient may be influenced by situational variables, and tailor replies to tally with the examiner's biases. The investigator too may be swayed by preconceptions about respondents that are independent of their actual behaviour. Reliability tests on data collection or interviewing technique are rarely reported, and the assessors may not be blind to the status of individuals as patients or controls. These limitations are exacerbated when the psychosocial factors being investigated are vague and loosely defined. Occupational stress is a complicated phenomenon, with diverse ramifications, and results may differ according to assessment procedures (Kasl, 1978; House *et al.*, 1979). Since methods are adjusted to suit particular study groups, and may not even be described in detail, failures to replicate previous patterns may reflect genuine variability, or only technical differences. It is not surprising that twenty years ago, when risk factors such as arterial pressure were being recorded with more care than ever before, studies on psychological parameters had little impact. The behaviours which can readily be quantified, including smoking and eating habits, were the first to be accepted as identifiable risks.

In the present day, Russek and Zohman's report would be considered anecdotal. Although work with similar limitations is still done, more sophisticated methodologies incorporating prospective designs are now common. Almost all the research linking the psychosocial environment with atherosclerotic disorders has been concerned with ischaemic heart disease; the small number of systematic studies into the precursors of stroke will be discussed in Chapter 11.

Three fundamental approaches to cardiac disorders can be identified. Firstly there are demographic or epidemiological surveys, in which broad characteristics such as socioeconomic status, education or mobility within the social spectrum are measured in large populations. The significance of positive correlations between such features and heart disease may vary considerably. At the least, they can help to identify the subgroups of the population with the greatest risk, so that preventive measures can be appropriately directed. At their best, they may suggest links which have implications for aetiology.

The second strategy is to examine the personality and behaviour of individuals who suffer from, or are predisposed to, ischaemic heart disease. Certain characteristics may be common to a large proportion of patients, or they may share tendencies to respond in particular ways to environmental demands. Type A coronary-prone behaviour is a product of this approach, and its role is described in Chapter 10. However, other aspects of personal behaviour have been studied, and these will also be considered.

A third type of investigation examines what has actually happened to people before the onset of clinical heart disease. Do future victims experience major crises or chronic harassments in their lives, and do these incidents precipitate infarction or clinical symptoms? The research on acute life events, and their relation to ischaemic heart disease and stroke, is discussed in Chapter 11. Important results are emerging from all these methodologies, and together they strengthen the case for considering behavioural and psychosocial variables very seriously.

Social-demographic factors in ischaemic heart disease

The large amounts of research into the social epidemiology of ischaemic heart disease have been thoroughly reviewed by many authorities (Marks, 1967; Jenkins, 1971; 1976). The inconsistencies in the data may reflect real differences in the composition of populations, and in the indices of social function employed. Furthermore, associations may not be static, but fluctuate as domestic and work roles change, and affluence spreads. For example, early investigations based on prevalence and mortality statistics in Britain tended to reveal greater rates among men in the higher social categories (Logan, 1952; Brown *et al.*, 1957). Cardiovascular disorders were regarded as middle-class diseases. But more recent surveys have shown a reversal in this pattern (Marmot *et al.*, 1978). Since 1961, the mortality rate for cardiovascular disease in Classes IV and V has exceeded that of Classes I and II. The trend is particularly striking in younger men; thus in the 35–44 age range, 10 men in the lower social strata die from these causes for every 6 in Classes I and II.

Temporal trends make comparisons between surveys difficult. Additional discrepancies derive from studying populations with smaller spans. Thus employees of industrial and commercial companies are not distributed to all social classes in proportions that reflect the general pattern in the population; rather they range across a restricted portion of the spectrum. Associations between heart disease and status have consequently fluctuated (Lehman, 1967).

Furthermore, criteria such as occupation and income are confounded with serious illness, so the unhealthy may be under-represented in the higher brackets. Kitagawa and Hauser (1973) suggested that education might be a more reliable socioeconomic index, and calculated a broadly inverse association between ischaemic heart disease and educational achievement in the USA. For instance, adult (25–64 year old) women with less than eight years schooling have a relative mortality risk of 2·40 over college educated females. Similar patterns were recorded in a survey of 270 000 employees in the telecommunications industry; the incidence of heart disease over a three year period was greater amongst workers than executives, and this was accounted for by educational rather than occupational differences (Hinkle *et al.*, 1968). In the Western Collaborative Group Study (WCGS) of middle-aged men in California, heart disease over the $8\frac{1}{2}$-year prospective period was inversely linked to educational achievement, but unrelated to income (Rosenman *et al.*, 1975). For men aged 50–59 on intake, the average annual rate per 1000 was 9·1 in college graduates, and 16·8 for those without higher education.

Yet these trends are not universal. A retrospective case control study was carried out on a series of middle-aged white women admitted to hospitals in Maryland with their first infarction (Szklo *et al.*, 1976). Each was matched on age and admission date with two hospitalised non-cardiac controls, and sociodemographic data were collected. There were no differences in the proportion of women in the various groups with college education, nor were such indices as number of marriages, urban–rural background and reported rate of church attendance significant. Likewise the Israeli prospective study of 10 000 civil servants found no extra risk attached to low educational status (Goldbourt *et al.*, 1975). An additional problem with educational comparisons may lie in the manner heart disease is brought to clinical attention. Croog and Levine (1969) have documented variations in the reporting of symptoms with education, irrespective of the severity of heart disease. The better educated were more likely to complain of chest pains before the onset of acute coronary episodes. Those without higher education seldom identified symptoms of this type, preferring to label them as gastro-intestinal complaints. Thus differences in illness behaviour may conceal real variations in prevalence.

The lack of conformity in educational associations with cardio-vascular disease is shared by other aspects of medical ecology. For example, Levy and Herzog (1974) uncovered a positive relationship between cardiac mortality and population density in the Netherlands, but this was not replicated in Chicago (Levy and Herzog, 1978). Again, it is difficult to distinguish genuine variations from correlations that are only fortuitously significant in some populations. Moreover, even when the patterns are robust, interpretation is hazardous. Many aspects of living, apart from psychosocial pressures or behaviour, separate members of social or educational groups, and these may account in part for cardiovascular effects. Confounds have been ruled out in some cases; the class variations in mortality rate in Britain, for example, are not paralleled by differences in fat intake (Marmot *et al.*, 1978). But the multifactorial nature of cardiovascular disorders, together with fluctuations in other risks, is likely to cloud associations with broad sociodemographic categories. Specific hypotheses can be tested more precisely, since they permit closer control of confounding variables. One such concept is status inconsistency.

Status inconsistency and social mobility

Status inconsistency has been considered widely in the sociological literature, in relation to political attitudes, prejudice and social participation (Horan and Gray, 1974). It applies to people whose class of origin and adult status differ, or who show inconsistencies between their positions on various status criteria. Thus individuals may have achieved high educational standards but have comparatively low income, or may have been brought up in circumstances which differ from those of adult life. Such experiences are thought to promote conflicting cultural expectations, disruption of interpersonal relationships, and confusion about social roles (Blalock, 1967). People displaying status inconsistency are thought to be in a vulnerable position, since an extra element of uncertainty is introduced into their lives. The theory has appeal because it can be reduced to a series of predictions about personal history and life style, and tested systematically. It has been applied fruitfully to the study of social risks in ischaemic heart disease.

Shekelle and his colleagues (1969) carried out an extensive prospective investigation of social incongruity in 1472 married men, employed by the electrical industry in Chicago. During a five-year period, 103 exhibited ischaemic heart disease in various forms, and incidence was related to the presence of status inconsistencies. Several categories of incongruity were recorded, based on differences between status on various criteria (education, income, occupation), discrepancies either in men or their wives between present status and their class of origin, and lower educational achievement or class of origin in men compared with their wives. Four of these five categories were significantly associated with heart disease, and the number of inconsistencies increased the risk. Table 9.1 summarises some of the effects. Both for the "soft" endpoint of angina, and for myocardial infarction, the risk was some three times greater in people with four or five social discrepancies, compared with those who had only one. Cross-categorisation on risk factors such as serum cholesterol concentration failed to account for the sociodemographic pattern. It is interesting that the bulk of individuals who showed changes between childhood and present class were upwardly mobile, since few gravitated towards lower status in the population.

TABLE 9.1

Relationship between number of social incongruities and ischaemic heart disease incidence (Shekelle *et al.*, 1969)

Number of incongruities per subject	Number of IHD cases	Average annual incidence per 1000		
		Angina pectoris	Infarction or death	All cases
0	355	6	1	7
1	355	9	5	14
2	416	9	5	14
3	210	13	6	19
4 or 5	33	28	19	46

The incidence of heart disease amongst former Harvard students has also been connected with sociocultural mobility (Gillum and Paffenbarger, 1978). Men who suffered sudden cardiac death or non-fatal myocardial infarction scored higher on intergenerational mobility than their classmates. In particular, there was an inverse association between these clinical manifestations and the father's status, so that those who came from relatively humble backgrounds yet graduated from Harvard were especially vulnerable. The relationship persisted in multivariate analyses that accounted for the conventional physical risks. Likewise Szklo *et al.* (1976) noted large discrepancies between the educational level of female cardiac patients and their husbands, and the pattern is reflected in a number of other retrospective surveys (Jenkins, 1971; 1976).

The reverse of the social inconsistency hypothesis is that stable, cohesive cultures, in which the individual's status is clearly established, may be protective against myocardial ischaemia. This is illustrated in a comprehensive study of heart disease amongst Japanese-Americans (Marmot and Syme, 1976). The mortality and prevalence of ischaemic heart disease in this group is much higher than that in Japan, while Japanese male residents of Hawaii sustain an intermediate rate (Marmot *et al.*, 1975). The gradient is not accounted for by standard risks such as serum cholesterol, high arterial pressure or smoking. However, Japanese culture places particular emphasis on cohesion, group achievement and stability, while individual ambitions and abilities are promoted in the USA. It is possible therefore that discrepancies between the social and cultural values of Japan and the USA are responsible.

Marmot and Syme compared men who had been brought up in traditional ways, maintaining contact with Japanese language and habits, and those raised in a more Western manner. The latter showed a higher prevalence of clinical ischaemic heart disease, and the difference in rate was particularly striking in younger men (Fig. 9.1). The pattern persisted after controlling for blood pressure and serum cholesterol, and did not appear to be due to dietary variation. The prevalence of cardiac disease amongst men who persisted with traditional customs was comparable with that found in Japan, while the Westernised group approached Caucasian American rates. It is interesting that those brought up in the Japanese manner, who later assimilated with Western lifestyles, sustained an intermediate rate; such people might be at highest risk in terms of status incongruity, but at the same time appeared to have benefited from the protective effects of Japanese culture in early life.

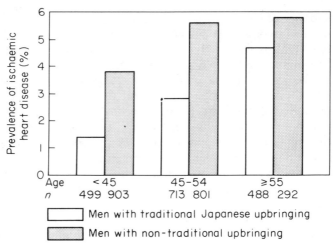

Fig. 9.1. Prevalence of ischaemic heart disease amongst men of Japanese ancestry living in California. Three different age cohorts are identified. (Marmot and Syme, 1976.)

There are other examples of traditional social networks buffering against ischaemic heart disease. The small, tightly-knit town of Nazareth in Pennsylvania has been examined in detail (Bruhn *et al.*, 1968). The bulk of the population derive from German Protestant stock, although people with other backgrounds have moved into the area during the present century. However, family origin seems especially influential in modulating the degree to which individuals are accepted socially. Patients with heart disease were more likely to be of minority (non-German) origin than controls and had lived in Nazareth for a shorter time. Striking differences were also recorded between the Catholic Americans of Italian origin in Rosetto, Pennsylvania, and neighbouring communities. The cardiovascular death rates were significantly lower in Rosetto during the late 1950s than in nearby Bangor, despite the high levels of animal fat in the diet (Stout *et al.*, 1964). The inhabitants of Rosetto formed a closely meshed, cohesive population compared with the ethnically mixed Bangor.

However, these associations between ischaemic heart disease and status inconsistency have not been universally observed. Hinkle *et al.*'s survey (1968) of employees in a large industrial concern showed no greater risk amongst the upwardly mobile, compared with people in static occupational positions. Correlations between intergenerational mobility or class incongruity and heart disease did not emerge at Framingham, nor in a retrospective study in South-eastern Connecticut

(Haynes *et al.*, 1978a,b; Wardwell and Bahnson, 1973). Given the complexity of social pressures bearing on people in adult life, the variability of links with atherosclerosis are not surprising. Within each culture, the salience of cues relating to social functioning will differ, so an objective criterion of status inconsistency, such as educational and occupational discrepancies, may be highly important in some cases, and trivial in others. The investigator must begin with an understanding of the study population, recognising the idiosyncratic social norms, aspirations and sources of tension, before hypotheses about incongruity can be formulated.

Similar arguments apply to the study of links with residential or occupational mobility. Both in California and North Dakota, Syme *et al.* (1966) found that ischaemic heart disease was more prevalent amongst men who had occupied several different posts, in comparison with those who kept the same job for most of adult life. But support for this pattern is mixed (Medalie *et al.*, 1973b; Haynes *et al.*, 1978b). Again it is probable that the mobility factor has no universal significance; in the aspiring middle classes, moving between jobs and neighbourhoods may be a positive aspect of career development, reflecting successful material advancement. In other cases, it will be indicative of poor social integration and restlessness. The notion of mobility must be embedded within an appropriate population framework.

The absence of robust, global social inconsistency and mobility effects is explicable by the heterogeneity of contemporary cultures. It creates an important methodological problem, however, since risk factors identified in some surveys may not generalise to other groups. The solution may be not to consider global demographic characteristics, but the way in which the individual responds to pressures in the immediate environment. This strategy itself has two components, and involves the study both of personality or behavioural styles, and the presence of everyday occupational and social life.

Ischaemic heart disease and personal characteristics

With the exception of work on Type A coronary-prone behaviour, discussed in detail in Chapter 10, research into personality and clinical heart disease has been inconsistent and methodologically weak. The problems of using retrospective techniques are even more marked than in the case of hypertension (see pp. 140–142). Infarction, angina and other signs of cardiac disorder are distressing and life-threatening experiences, having an enormous psychological impact on patients.

They can lead to major changes in lifestyle, reappraisal of aims and ambitions, and drastic revisions of attitudes to health. Thus the responses to psychological assessments in diagnosed cases may have little or no relation to prior state. The reporting biases òr genuine changes in outlook of those who know they have heart disease confound almost all retrospective surveys. Segers *et al.* (1974) highlighted these drawbacks in a screening study of 1695 men. The 176 who were identified clinically or electrocardiographically as having ischaemic heart disease scored higher than healthy men on manifest and covert anxiety scales. But the differences were due entirely to the sub-group who had previously consulted a doctor about cardiac problems; those without earlier positive diagnoses were indistinguishable from the remainder of the cohòrt. The special psychological profile was either restricted to those who perceived earlier symptoms, or arose after diagnosis.

The second of these explanations was supported in a comparison between personality ratings made prospectively and retrospectively in the Chicago Heart Study (Lebovits *et al.*, 1967). Survivors of myocardial infarction showed a number of changes on MMPI scales related to neuroticism, when compared with pre-illness scores. They also reported increases in awareness and concern for bodily symptoms. Furthermore, the psychological profiles of those who died after infarction were different from those of survivors (Lebovits *et al.*, 1967; Bruhn *et al.*, 1969). Thus two important assumptions underlying retrospective surveys of personality are untenable in the case of ischaemic heart disease. Additional problems in the interpretation of these data were discussed on p. 155.

Retrospective investigations may still have an heuristic value if they uncover consistent, robust relations between personal traits and clinical heart disease. But this has not been the case; to take publications of the last decade only, several positive associations between neuroticism or anxiety and heart disease have been reported (e.g. Bengtsson *et al.*, 1973; Thiel *et al.*, 1973; Finn *et al.*, 1974). Yet others have failed to confirm this relationship (Wardwell and Bahnson, 1973). Langsoch (1976) concluded that cardiac patients at a German spa had no special personality profile, beyond a reduction in aggressiveness, which may have been a consequence of the illness. Blumenthal *et al.* (1979) found little to link arterial stenosis with anxiety-proneness in a survey of patients undergoing coronary angiography.

Prospective studies of personality are not subject to the same doubts about changes after diagnosis. Some evidence suggests that neurotic traits predispose to angina (Floderus, 1974). The incidence of angina in the Israel prospective survey was twice as high amongst individuals who endorsed the three anxiety questions positively, compared with negative responders (Medalie *et al.*, 1973a). In contrast, no association was found between anxiety and infarction (Goldbourt *et al.*, 1975). The Kaiser–Permanente study compared patients hospitalised for myocardial infarction with control groups matched either on sex, age and race, or on these characteristics plus serum cholesterol, blood pressure, smoking and serum glucose (Friedman *et al.*, 1974). The cardiac patients had completed a lengthy questionnaire some 17 months before infarction, so the survey was prospective for acute stenosis. Although some differences in patterns of response were uncovered, few related to anxiety or depression. Furthermore, when subjects who had displayed non-acute signs of heart disease at the beginning of the prospective period were excluded, the correlates of infarction became even more slight.

The evidence in favour of neurotic characteristics predisposing to ischaemic heart disease is therefore weak. The association with angina may be non-specific; neurotic individuals are more likely to report symptoms of any origin, and their heart disease will consequently be identified at an earlier stage. However, this negative conclusion may be a consequence of considering personality factors in isolation. The emphasis in earlier chapters has fallen on the reactive component, and the ways in which people respond to the challenges and hazards of life. Similar elements may be involved in the development of atherosclerotic diseases.

Work and family circumstances in clinical heart disease

There are two approaches to the study of adverse environmental conditions in ischaemic heart disease. The first is to identify discrete incidents or life events that may have an impact on clinical symptoms. This research is discussed in Chapter 11, since the strongest associations have been found with the precipitation of triggering of acute ischaemic attacks. Additionally, the individual's occupational or social environment may have chronic effects on cardiovascular disease. It has been argued in Chapters 6 and 7 that the neuroendocrine pathways influencing the course of atherosclerosis show more sustained mobilisation when behavioural demands are continuous. The relation of such factors with disease may differ from that articulating the response to acute trauma. Thus it is possible that the distress of redundancy or divorce will precipitate severe clinical events in the patient with stenosis; but the slow, progressive development of atheroma is less likely to be affected by an isolated event of this kind.

The technique, used in hypertension research, of selecting groups that differ in their experience of chronically disturbing conditions, can also be applied to ischaemic heart disease. The unpleasantness of living or working environments may be defined either by the occupants themselves, or by objective criteria. Russek and Russek (1976) sampled prevalence rates of ischaemic heart disease in different medical and legal specialities thought to vary in their stressfulness. General practitioners and anaesthetists, who are considered to work under considerable pressure and tension, reported higher levels of heart disease than the less harried dermatologists and pathologists. Unfortunately, health information was solicited from the subjects themselves without independent confirmation, and reply rates were low. There may be variations in the probability of different professionals recognising cardiac symptoms in themselves.

Another very competitive field of work is the aerospace industry, and workers at Cape Kennedy have been intensively studied (Reynolds, 1974; Eliot *et al.*, 1977). The occupational environment encourages ambition and hard work, but is clouded by the threat of redundancy; the 65 000 workers on the payroll in 1965 were reduced to 8000 by 1976. The strain is reflected in the high rates of alcoholism, divorce, behaviour disorders amongst the children, and psychiatric symptomatology as revealed through questionnaires (Warheit, 1974). Despite the low average age of personnel, the incidence of sudden cardiac death and non-fatal infarction is high. In a cross-sectional survey, Reynolds (1974) found that the prevalence of ECG abnormalities was significantly higher than that in controls, running at some 30 per cent amongst men involved in controlling lunar missions. The ischaemic patterns were not associated with elevated arterial pressure or serum cholesterol.

It cannot be inferred that this taxing environment is conducive to ischaemic heart disease, however, since people generally select their own occupations. Some underlying characteristic may not only lead certain types to choose demanding careers, but simultaneously put them at risk for atherosclerosis. If this is the case, the adverse environment may be a by-product rather than a cause. House (1975) noted that people with "extrinsic" motivations for work, such as the desire for status or money, are likely to select stressful jobs for the prestige they carry. In contrast, those who are interested in the work itself are less swayed by external factors. Furthermore, it is clear that many elements contribute to the subjective appraisal of a particular work environment. Objective conditions, such as heavy workload or greater responsibility, may be harassing, but can also be perceived as challenging. Similarly, overwork is not simply a function of load, but may result from a disorganised work strategy or failure to delegate. In each case, the personal dimension must be added to the measurement of external demands.

This is reflected in the emphasis placed by many investigators on perceived workload and job responsibility (House *et al.*, 1979). Van Dijl (1974) showed that Dutch cardiac patients rate themselves as more involved in their jobs, more responsible and active than controls. Using mortality statistics and information on work satisfaction, Sales and House (1971) identified consistent negative correlations between job satisfaction and fatal ischaemic heart disease across occupational groups. The speed of recovery and rehabilitation after an infarction may also be delayed by problems at work (Pancheri *et al.*, 1978).

Self-report data on aggravation and distress may be relevant to the study of family and social conditions as well. In the Israel heart disease survey, participants were questioned about problems in five psychosocial spheres — the family, finance, work, relations with co-workers and with superiors. Ratings in all problem areas predicted the incidence of angina at 5-year follow-up. Illustrative data are shown in Table 9.2. The incidence of angina increased with the severity of difficulties reported in each area of life (Medalie *et al.*, 1973a). The relationship with future infarction was less strong, since only scores on work-related items predicted incidence (Medalie *et al.*, 1973b). Once again, therefore, it is possible that dissatisfaction with life might increase symptom reporting, leading indirectly to the identification of more angina.

As with so much of the work described in this chapter, contradictory data can also be cited (Wardwell and Bahnson, 1973; Haynes *et al.*, 1978b). Failures to pick up associations between family or work-

TABLE 9.2

Association between incidence of angina pectoris and problems in the family area (Medalie *et al.*, 1973a)

Severity score for family problems	Number of subjects	Number of cases	Age adjusted rate per 1000 men per year
0	1636	50	6·2
1	3972	125	6·6
2	1836	68	7·6
3	865	41	9·8
4	219	16	17·2

related problems and heart disease may reflect methodological variations. Patients may be reluctant to disclose these personal feelings, and the areas of experience covered are clearly very sensitive. Subtle differences in the wording and presentation of requests for information may have profound effects on replies. Moreover, there is little uniformity in the ways people describe their dissatisfactions with life. Some blame problems on employment, while others implicate the family. Romo and his associates (1974) gave these considerations some force in a comparison between cardiac patients in Finland, Sweden and the USA. Although a degree of consistency was recorded, national reporting characteristics also emerged. The Finns were dissatisfied with achievements and goals in life, but did not complain of undue responsibility or overtime at work. Grumbles about the latter were more prevalent amongst the Americans, who also emerged as the least unhappy with their achievements. Thus variations in cultural mores and social demands may further cloud relationships.

The evidence relating chronic strain and harassment to ischaemic heart disease is firmest when selected groups are studied in depth. A prospective survey has been carried out on workers in the construction industry in the Stockholm area (Theorell *et al.*, 1975). Over 6500 middle-aged men filled in questionnaires, and were traced through state registers for heart disease or other illness during the next two years. Unfortunately, no physical examinations were performed at the start, and since the questionnaires were administered postally, they were not completed under controlled conditions. However, robust relationships between cardiovascular risk factors and psychosocial variables were uncovered, some of which were described earlier (see pp. 148–150). The 51 men who subsequently experienced infarction could be disinguished on questionnaire ratings. A "Discord index" was devised that included items concerned with work conditions and level of responsibility. The scores of the cardiac group were significantly greater than their age-adjusted control level, and thus predicted cardiovascular risk. Subjects hospitalised with neurotic disorders also scored above expected rates, suggesting that the association with heart disease was not unique.

Further investigations of the same population indicated that heart disease was associated with work problems rather than with adverse family conditions (Theorell and Floderus-Myrhed, 1977). By contrast, difficult family circumstances were linked prospectively with degenerative joint diseases. A subgroup of Swedish building workers seems to be at especially high risk for atherosclerotic disorders. The older "concrete" workers sustain more myocardial infarctions than other workers of the same age (Theorell *et al.*, 1977). They are distinguished by having less education, coming from larger families or broken homes, and being at risk for violent accidental death. Concrete workers are also subject to other psychosocial pressures, as may be seen in Table 9.3. The psychosocial risks included in this analysis were: cigarette smoking, family background (presence of six or more siblings and/or broken parental home), crowdedness at home, psychosocial workload (changes in job responsibility, redundancy, etc.), and income. Presence of these factors increased infarction incidence in both concrete and other building workers, but at each level the rate in older concrete workers was higher.

The physical demands of concrete workers are considerable, while the piecework system present in earlier decades imposed strong time pressures. Concrete workers operate in teams, and when older members become unable to sustain the work rate, they hold back the whole group's productivity. Consequently, the work pressures may be complemented by friction with younger colleagues. Myocardial infarction may be just one way in which members of this group break down under the strain. These studies indicate how general hypotheses about adverse living conditions can be refined through detailed analysis, and thus provide more substantial evidence linking behavioural factors to clinical heart disease.

Summary and conclusions

The aim of this chapter has been to identify links between psychosocial factors and ischaemic heart disease that are of significance in aetiology. Cross-sectional, sociodemographic surveys indicate that certain groups in the population sustain more heart disease than others; such investigations do not necessarily imply a causal relationship, but may be valuable in directing preventive resources more economically. Like

TABLE 9.3

Psychosocial risks in concrete and other building workers (aged 52–61) in relation to incidence of myocardial infarction (Theorell *et al.*, 1977)

Number of risks	*n*	Concrete workers Annual incidence per 1000 men	*n*	Other building workers Annual incidence per 1000 men
0–1	268	5·6	598	4·2
2	353	5·7	741	3·4
3	293	10·3	651	3·9
4–5	127	15·8	309	9·7

other elements of risk, behavioural aspects are best studied prospectively, since the diagnosis of clinical heart disease causes substantial changes in psychological outlook, and these may obscure the premorbid profile.

A number of psychosocial hypotheses have been confirmed in prospective surveys, and more will be described in the next chapter. Thus it is probable that the cardiovascular and neuroendocrine reactions outlined in earlier sections may have direct significance in clinical heart disease. However, many of the psychosocial data are inconsistent, in that factors of importance in some populations do not transfer to others. Such variability is not surprising: attempts to put different cultural groups on the procrustean bed of a global sociological or psychosocial concept will seldom succeed. Simple associations with complex social factors should not be expected, since individual responses are flexible. In each population, the elements of social function will be weighted differently.

Thus social role incongruity and group cohesiveness are of demonstrable importance to the development of ischaemic heart disease in certain populations. But these concepts cannot be reduced to a universal set of empirical constructs that will be applicable in all cases. Indices such as occupational or residential mobility may reflect social inconsistency in one culture, while being predictable consequences of career role and successful social integration in another. Without an understanding of the social framework articulating each study population, dimensions of psychosocial dysfunction will not be correctly identified. It is notable that when the investigator formulates hypotheses directly relevant to the cohort being scrutinised, as with the Japanese-Americans and Swedish building workers, associations with ischaemic heart disease emerge more clearly.

Many of the factors emerging from psychosocial surveys seem responsible not only for cardiac disease, but other dysfunctions in the physical and social spheres. There are a number of mechanisms by which the cardiovascular system will be put at greater risk. Some effects may be translated through standard risk factors, in particular high blood pressure — evidence in Chapter 8 implicated aspects of social functioning of a similar type to those explored in ischaemic heart disease. For example, job dissatisfaction has been linked both with hypertension (p. 147) and clinical heart disease (p. 167). However, standard risks do not account for increased vulnerability in all cases. Thus in the Japanese-American study, the prevalence of heart disease in men brought up in non-traditional and traditional cultures differed by a ratio of 1·83 to 1, even after controlling for age, serum cholesterol and blood pressure.

A second possibility is that subtle differences in behaviour modulate cardiovascular effects. For example, plasma catecholamine levels may be augmented in people with a high caffeine intake, so regular tea and coffee drinkers may be more vulnerable. The social tensions identified in epidemiological surveys may lead future cardiac patients to greater levels of risk on diet, drinking habits, smoking or exercise. It is difficult to distinguish such mechanisms from direct effects of central nervous stimulation on autonomic and endocrine function, since both will tend to be elicited under similar conditions. The evidence against coffee drinking is inconsistent. Correlations have been found between coffee drinking habits and noradrenaline levels, while pathological responses may emerge in animals (Cobb, 1974; Henry and Stephens, 1977). On the other hand, a prospective survey in Sweden did not confirm the association between future infarction and reported coffee consumption, although it is possible that intake may increase in the period immediately prior to the heart attack (Wilhelmsen *et al.*, 1977).

Finally, psychosocial disturbances may be mediated through the psychophysiological reaction patterns described in earlier sections. This possibility is of great interest, since it would suggest that the dimensions of coping and behavioural demand discussed in Chapters 6 and 7 might be relevant in clinical heart disease. Little direct evidence is available, although a ballistocardiographic study of coronary patients has provided some relevant information (Theorell *et al.*, 1974). Cardiac patients were studied with the ballistocardiogram, and on each occasion descriptions of emotional state were collected. These were rated blindly and classified into three groups. Emotional withdrawal and passivity were thought to follow uncontrollable events such as a death in the family, a gaol sentence or insuperable frustrations. The emotional state was judged to be aroused or excited when the patient displayed open aggression, showed new interests or had experienced unexpected success. In other cases the emotional tone was rated as neutral. These assessments were supplemented by observations during stress interviews in a smaller number of patients. Cardiac contractility, indexed by IJ velocity on the ballistocardiogram, was significantly higher on average when the emotional tone was excited. On the occasions that the patients were rated as passive and despondent, contractility fell below levels recorded in neutral sessions. Cardiac sympathetic tone may thus have been higher during excitement, diminishing when the patients displayed passive withdrawal.

These mechanisms are not mutually exclusive, and may all contribute to the final pattern. The position will become clearer when premorbid groups can be studied with laboratory techniques. Such research is already being carried out in the case of Type A behaviour, as will be seen in the next chapter.

10
Type A Coronary-prone Behaviour

The constellation of behavioural characteristics designated as Type A or "coronary-prone" was first described in cardiac patients by Friedman and Rosenman (1959). Generalising from clinical impressions, they identified a group of properties including sustained aggression, ambition, competitiveness and a chronic sense of time urgency. Type As were further described as impatient, intensely committed to vocational goals and behaviourally alert. The contrasting, more relaxed people who did not display these features were labelled Type B. The assessment of the behaviours was made from global impressions of patients' performance in a structured interview, designed to evoke Type A responses. Alternative methods of identifying the groups include a number of questionnaire techniques.

Despite inconsistencies, there is a considerable amount of evidence relating Type A behaviour with ischaemic heart disease. The most substantial results have emerged from a prospective survey, the Western Collaborative Group Study (WCGS). This investigation began in 1960–61, and traced over 3000 employed middle-aged Californian men for $8\frac{1}{2}$ years (Rosenman et al., 1964). Half of the population were classified as Type A on interview assessment, and the remainder as Type B. During initial screening, 113 cases of ischaemic heart disease were identified, of whom 68·3 per cent in the 39–49 year and 73·6 per cent in the 50–59 year age groups were labelled Type A. The WCGS did not survey men from the whole social spectrum, but was heavily biased towards the middle classes. Thus more than half the men earned over $10,000 on screening in 1960, while the majority had some college education.

Two hundred and fifty-seven individuals developed coronary disease during the prospective period, and 50 did not survive. In both younger (39–49) and older (50–59) age cohorts the rate amongst Type As was twice that of Type Bs; the standardised incidences per 1000 for the older group for instance, were 18·7 against 8·9 (Rosenman *et al.*, 1975). As might be expected, the standard risks, including high arterial pressure and serum cholesterol, were reliable predictors of ischaemia in this survey. But even after stratification on these factors, the link between Type A and cardiac disease persisted. Multivariate analyses confirmed systolic pressure, serum cholesterol, behaviour pattern and smoking, as the most important independent predictors of incidence (Rosenman *et al.*, 1976). Other parameters such as diastolic pressure, plasma triglycerides and ponderal index did not contribute separately, owing to their associations with the main risks. After controlling for all other variables, the relative vulnerability of Type A compared with B men was 1·87 in the younger, and 2·16 in the older cohorts.

The standard risks emerged with a predictive power similar to that observed in Framingham; thus when the Framingham multiple logistic model was applied to the WCGS population, the predicted number of cases did not differ from the rate actually present (Brand *et al.*, 1976). The WCGS sample thus appears comparable with other

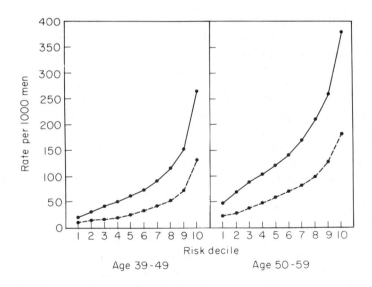

Fig. 10.1. The expected incidence of ischaemic heart disease over 8·5 years in Type A men (solid line) and Type B men (dotted line). The younger cohort (39–49 years) is shown on the left, with the older group (50–59 years) on the right. The groups are stratified by decile (10 per cent segment) of risk on other major risk factors. (From Brand *et al.*, 1976.)

prospective groups. The expected rates of ischaemic heart disease in Type A and B men are stratified at different levels of multivariate risk in Fig. 10.1. Those in decile 1 are the 10 per cent with the lowest combined risk on other predictive factors. It can be seen that in all risk deciles, higher rates are sustained amongst Type As.

The WCGS has implicated Type A behaviour as a characteristic predisposing to heart disease, at least in part independently of blood pressure, serum cholesterol, cigarette smoking and other factors. This association goes some way towards accounting for the problem outlined in Chapter 1 — why many individuals, apparently predisposed towards ischaemic heart disease, fail to develop coronary stenosis. Yet even amongst Type A men at highest risk on all factors, some 74 per cent would be expected to remain disease free over $8\frac{1}{2}$ years (Rosenman *et al.*, 1976). Thus although this assessment of behaviour may refine the prediction of cardiac disease, much of the variability still remains unexplained.

Participants in the WCGS were also administered a questionnaire, the Jenkins Activity Survey (JAS), thought to tap Type A characteristics. Pencil-and-paper methods have clear economic advantages, since the presence of a trained interviewer is not required. But although incidence of ischaemic heart disease was greater amongst high JAS scorers, the difference in numerical terms was not large. The scales of the JAS are adjusted to have a mean of 0 and standard deviation of 10. Over a four-year prospective period, the overall Type A score in men who developed heart disease averaged 1·70, compared with −0·60 in controls (Jenkins *et al.*, 1974). The differences were statistically significant in this large sample, but the predictive power for individuals was small; if JAS scores were translated into IQ levels (mean 100, s.d. 15), controls and patients would be separated by only 3·5 points. The association of ischaemic heart disease with extreme questionnaire scores was more powerful. Thus the annual rate for those with JAS ratings of +5·0 or more was 14·3 per 1000 men, compared with 8·0 per 1000 in people scoring at −5·0 or below.

JAS scores predicted recurrent infarctions with greater consistency (Jenkins *et al.*, 1976). These data are summarised in Table 10.1, where a division is made according to the stage at which the questionnaire was administered. For all groups, Type A ratings were higher in men suffering repeated infarcts, while being close to the population mean for single event patients. The association was similar whether the JAS was given prospectively or retrospectively; this suggests that the high scores were not products of manifest heart disease, and were not biased by assessment after the emergence of clinical symptoms. The differences

TABLE 10.1

Mean JAS scores in patients with single events and recurrent myocardial infarction. The JAS was administered to all subjects in 1965 (Jenkins *et al.*, 1976)

Group	Timing of coronary events	Relation of JAS assessment to events	*n*	Type A score
Single event	Before 1961	Retrospective	77	−0·73
(angina, silent	1962–1965	Retrospective	66	0·75
or acute	1966–1968	Prospective	77	1·66
infarction)				
Recurrent	Both before 1965	Retrospective	23	4·78
events	One before and	Retrospective	36	4·38
(infarction	one after 1965			
only)	Both after 1965	Prospective	6	3·48

between the single case groups may reflect random fluctuation, but alternatively those studied retrospectively may have made efforts to alter their behaviour, following their first cardiac crisis.

Type A behaviour has been associated with ischaemic heart disease less consistently in independent prospective surveys. The Kaiser–Permanente study, with its formidable matching procedures, was described on p. 165 (Friedman, G. D., *et al.*, 1974). Participants filled in a long questionnaire, from which items likely to discriminate coronary-prone behaviour were selected. The replies to these questions did not predict myocardial infarction, and indeed some negative correlations were recorded. The survey population differed in many demographic features from the WCGS sample. The negative result may also reflect the relative weakness of questionnaire measurement. The Swedish building industry project outlined on p. 168, included Type A items in the "discord index" that forecast myocardial infarction and neurosis (Theorell *et al.*, 1975). However, questions relating to dissatisfaction and responsibility at work were also included, and the relative contribution of specific Type A items was not distinguished. More recently, responses to Type A questions have been found to predict ischaemic heart disease incidence in Framingham independently of other risks (Haynes *et al.*, 1980). Over the 8-year prospective period, Type A males were more than twice as likely to develop angina or acute heart disease, and differences were also recorded amongst women.

Much retrospective and cross-sectional work has also been reported, comparing cardiac patients with sick or hospitalised controls rather than with healthy population samples. The relationship between Type A and heart disease has again been variable (e.g. Wardell and Bahnson,

1973; Bengtsson *et al.*, 1973; Kenigsberg *et al.*, 1974). In a Swedish study, Type A scores were greater amongst men admitted to a coronary care unit, who later proved to have no ischaemic heart disease, than in genuine cases of infarction. This suggests an association with acute chest pain rather than stenosis (Ahnve *et al.*, 1979).

Some discrepancies between surveys may reflect problems with self-administered questionnaire techniques, but Keith *et al.* (1965) also had poor results with the interview method. Coronary patients, healthy controls and men with peptic ulcers were assessed blindly and classified as A or B. Only 47 per cent of cardiac patients were considered to be Type A, while 32 per cent of controls fell into the same category. On the other hand, a number of cross-sectional investigations support the coronary-prone behaviour concept, albeit with important cultural and socioeconomic variations (Shekelle *et al.*, 1976; Cohen, 1978). Significant associations between ischaemic heart disease and Type A ratings were found in both men and women at Framingham in cross-sectional surveys, although the differences in prevalence were not large (Haynes *et al.*, 1978a, b).

Type A behaviour seems to show many of the properties of conventional cardiac risks identified in epidemiological surveys. It has been evaluated both prospectively and retrospectively, and may contribute independently to the incidence of ischaemic heart disease. As with high blood pressure and other established factors, a large number of people considered to be Type A remain symptom-free. Yet despite this empirical robustness, a number of discrepant results have been reported. It is possible that the behaviour pattern is not associated with ischaemia in all cultures and populations, but only when certain demands prevail. Additionally, unreliabilities in assessment may contribute to the variability of links with heart disease.

Assessment of coronary-prone behaviour

Amongst the methods used to distinguish Type As, the interview technique piloted by Friedman and Rosenman (1959) predicts ischaemic heart disease most accurately. The interview is a semi-structured conversation of varying length, in which as much weight is placed on the patient's manner as on replies to the questions themselves. Restlessness, impatience and explosive speech all contribute to the final rating. The procedure is used not only to distinguish broad categories of Type A and B, but to identify sub-divisions of more or less developed "behavioural styles". Different divisions have been proposed, but commonly either A_1, A_2, B_1 and B_2, or else A_1, A_2, B and an intermediate category X have proved useful.

The precise criteria are not explicitly described in the literature, since they rely a good deal on broad impressions. Impressions of course can differ — thus some have claimed rarely to encounter Type A characteristics in their clinical practice (Russek and Russek, 1977). But the measurement and labelling is not made in a neutral setting, as the interview is specifically designed to elicit Type A behaviours. Examiners are trained by the original investigators or their colleagues, both in assessment and in the administration of the interview itself. The procedure even requires some acting skills; for example, on occasions the interviewer hesitates over questions, to see whether the client will show impatience, interrupt or try to hurry things along. Consequently, the training procedure is time consuming, involves the development of intuitive as well as objective skills, and does not succeed in making all candidates proficient (Jenkins *et al.*, 1968; Rowland and Sokol, 1977).

When examiners have been adequately trained, a reliability of 70–80 per cent in categorising people as A or B is common. Caffrey (1969) reported inter-rater reliabilities of 76 per cent, whilst reassessment of taped interviews previously analysed produced agreement on 74–80 per cent of occasions (Keith *et al.*, 1965; Friedman, M., *et al.*, 1968). Similarly, when an individual was re-examined after an interval of months or years, he was assigned to his original category in 80 per cent of cases (Rosenman *et al.*, 1964).

However, these levels of reliability are maintained only with the binary split into A and B; with the four-point scale, agreement drops to 54–60 per cent (Jenkins *et al.*, 1968). This is particularly disturbing in view of the fact that many differences between Type As and others are only apparent when the behaviour pattern is "fully developed" (Friedman and Rosenman, 1959; Rosenman and Friedman, 1974). The variability may be a reflection of imprecise measurement criteria. Attempts have been made to determine what aspects of behaviour actually contribute to interview ratings. Schucker and Jacobs (1977) analysed the vocal characteristics of interviewees; the most important features were the speed and volume of speech, which together correlated 0·69 with judgements of coronary-prone behaviour. Other facets of speech, such as interruptions, uneven talking and pauses, were involved to a lesser degree. Broadly similar effects were observed in a student sample, where emphasis, speed and delays in responding were all important (Scherwitz *et al.*, 1977). Interestingly, these vocal stylistics were not consistently related to each other. They seemed to have been judged independently and connected only by the conceptual scheme developed during interview training. The patients' replies are relatively unimportant in distinguishing types. But since deportment and non-verbal behaviours are not categorised formally, the subjective component in assessment is large.

In view of these shortcomings, standardised tests or questionnaires would appear to have advantages. However, such procedures assume that reactive characteristics will be displayed in the absence of the conducive atmosphere generated in the interview. Furthermore, self-report measures rely on people having insight into their behaviour, and being able to identify their own habitual actions. This may not be justified, since Type A individuals are said to be especially poor at self-appraisal (Rosenman, 1978). The JAS has been developed with great industry, but correlations with interview assessments are not high; misclassifications of up to one third of patients have been calculated. The inconsistency is underlined by the relatively poor predictive power of the JAS in distinguishing patients with ischaemic heart disease (Jenkins *et al.*, 1971). Jenkins *et al.* (1974) concluded that the scale was insufficiently precise to warrant general clinical application.

Assessment procedures remain amongst the weakest components of coronary-prone behaviour research, and are in urgent need of refinement. The method with the greatest predictive power is the most subjective, whilst the systematically scored questionnaires are weaker. However, the latter are used extensively in epidemiological and laboratory studies. A student version of the JAS has been devised, but its relationship with ischaemic heart disease is unknown. Correlations between the student JAS and interview ratings have been low or insignificant (Scherwitz *et al.*, 1977; Matthews and Saal, 1978). Mac-Dougall *et al.* (1979) found that agreement between the procedures exceeded modest levels only when extreme questionnaire scores were used.

Nevertheless, imperfections in measurement are not likely to account for all discrepancies between studies relating Type As with ischaemic heart disease. There may also be genuine variations, contingent on the cultural and personal demands to which an individual is exposed.

The nature of the behaviour pattern

One way of understanding coronary-prone behaviour is as a fixed trait or attribute, developing under the influence of constitutional factors or early environment. The Type A characterisation is similar to other descriptions of personality, such as McClelland's (1978) "need for power", and correlates with ratings of dominance, impulsiveness and sociability (Glass, 1977). Attempts have been made to examine the underlying properties through factor analysis of the JAS. Items on the scale cluster into three independent dimensions, labelled by the investigators as "hard driving", "job involvement" and "speed and impatience". Yet although these factors are robust statistically, their significance is less clear. None of the sub-scales have been consistently associated with ischaemic heart disease incidence or recurrent infarction, and some negative correlations have been recorded (Jenkins *et al.*, 1971; 1974; 1976). More recently, new sub-scales have been derived from statistical manipulations of questionnaire answer clusters (Jenkins *et al.*, 1978).

It may be more fruitful to consider coronary-prone behaviour as a response style, and not a reflection of fixed traits. This is implicit in the use of a challenging rather than neutral assessment interview; it is assumed that Type A characteristics are not always observable, but have to be provoked by suitable conditions. The poor showing of some questionnaire measures may be attributable to the relatively neutral settings in which they are administered. A comparison of interview and questionnaire techniques in Belgium bears out this explanation (Kittel *et al.*, 1978). Broadly equal numbers of Types A and B were found on interview, with a fifth of the population falling into an intermediate category. However, JAS scores were predominantly negative (in the Type B direction), with an overall mean of $-3 \cdot 0$.

The incidence of Type A behaviour differs between populations, suggesting that not all environments and cultures elicit the response pattern. Even if some people display the behaviours on assessment, they may not habitually respond in this fashion, due to the absence of appropriate eliciting stimuli in their normal lives. It is possible to specify more precisely the environments that do foster coronary-prone behaviour. The pattern was first described amongst middle-aged men in California, the majority of whom belonged to middle income groups. It may therefore be closely related to the individual occupational ambitions of Western urban culture. Shekelle *et al.* (1976) reported consistent positive correlations with socioeconomic status, and associations with educational achievement have also been identified (Waldron *et al.*, 1977). Amongst supermarket employees in Georgia, the average Type A scores varied directly with job levels, from $6 \cdot 22$ in administrators down to $-8 \cdot 47$ in labourers and drivers (Zyzanski, 1978). Black people in the USA tend to score lower than whites, and ratings may also decline in late middle age, when occupational goals have been achieved. There are indications that fewer children in rural schools display Type A behaviours than those from urban backgrounds, although the values fostered by different religious traditions may also contribute to this pattern (Butensky *et al.*, 1976). The coronary-prone behaviour pattern is more common amongst employed than unemployed women, but only in higher educated groups.

The distribution of Type A scores in different groups sheds further light on eliciting conditions (Zyzanski, 1978). The average JAS scores for European groups have been consistently negative, in comparison with the Californian WCGS mean of 0. On the other hand, US physicians, business administration graduates and NASA executives average very high, at 5·4, 4·2 and 5·3 respectively. Thus the behaviour pattern seems to be embedded within the social context of competitive occupational careers in the United States and similar cultures. Within this setting, it may be a highly adaptive response style, leading to the desired material goals. Van Dijl (1977) showed positive associations with self ratings of "aggressivity", ambition and a positive attitude to work. Significant correlations between Type A behaviour, and promotion or income change have also been identified (Mettlin, 1976). The behaviour pattern is a strikingly successful strategy, in terms of material gains. The high scores of employed women may reflect their involvement in competitive roles. These data also indicate the difficulties that are likely to encounter widespread intervention programmes.

The urban environment of developed countries may encourage rapid aggressive performance, and foster these response patterns. Yet it would be wrong to ascribe all blame to contemporary mores. Substantial proportions of the population, even in Western cities, do not display Type A behaviour, and only a fraction sustain ischaemic heart disease. Conversely, it would appear that even monasteries can have their share of "Type A atmosphere" (Caffrey, 1969). So it is essential to delineate the type of challenge that provokes coronary-prone behaviour. This aim has been pursued in recent years through experimental studies.

Type As tend to strive ceaselessly, working hard to achieve goals even in the absence of external pressures. This has been documented in the laboratory, in students divided by median split of JAS scores into Types A and B (Burnam *et al.*, 1975). All were administered a series of mental arithmetic problems, but while half were given a 5-minute deadline, the remainder had no time limit. Type A and B students attempted the same number of problems in the deadline condition; yet in the absence of any time limit, the former worked harder, trying to complete more arithmetic problems. The work rate of Type As did not in fact differ between deadline and no deadline conditions. Other studies have focused on the chronic sense of time urgency displayed by the coronary-prone (Glass, 1977); unfortunately, although some differences from Type Bs have been seen, many results have been of marginal statistical significance, implicating situational factors as major determinants of experimental outcome.

While Type As do apparently have a large capacity for work, it is not certain whether they strive actively under all circumstances. Glass (1977) has suggested that in the face of uncontrollable aversive stimulation, the coronary-prone initially struggle hard to cope with harassment. But with prolonged exposure, they give up, and manifest greater degrees of helplessness than Type Bs. Their behaviour will then mirror learned helplessness patterns (Seligman, 1975).

The conclusion that Type A individuals show greater helplessness when confronted with taxing environments is surprising, since the group is said to go to considerable lengths to exert and maintain control in their lives. In these learned helplessness experiments, participants have typically been exposed in the first instance to unpleasant stimuli such as loud noise. All subjects believe that there is some response they can make with a lever or button to terminate the noise. But this is true for only half the participants (escape condition); the other half experience failure and uncontrollable noise. The groups are matched so that the level of stimulation is the same, and only the control–escape variable distinguishes them. Those in inescapable conditions commonly show a series of behavioural deficits, and fail to perform efficiently on subsequent soluble tasks.

In a series of interrelated studies, Glass (1977) found that after brief exposure to uncontrollable noise, Type As made more efforts to solve or master subsequent tasks than Type Bs. The second hypothesis, that the coronary-prone become more helpless after prolonged uncontrollable stimulation, was less secure. Krantz *et al.* (1974) did not record greater ratings of helplessness in Type A students, nor were larger performance deficits seen. In fact, under some circumstances, Type Bs were the more disturbed group. Glass (1977) reported similar effects in a second study.

These experiments tend to show greater efforts at active behavioural coping from Type As, and attempts to master the environment persist even when such responses are inappropriate. Yet conclusions must be extremely tentative; these laboratory psychological investigations do not bear the weight of some interpretations that have been proposed (e.g. Glass, 1978; Williams *et al.*, 1978). Many results have been of only borderline significance, depending strongly on unpredicted changes in the comparison Type B groups. The bulk of studies have been performed on students rather than mature Type As, classified according to the modified JAS. The reliability of this categorisation is doubtful, particularly when groups are divided by median split, as is the case in many studies (Krantz *et al.*, 1974; Glass, 1977). It was noted on p. 178 that there may be considerable unreliability in assignment to Types A and B when distinctions are made on the population median (Mac-Dougall *et al.*, 1979).

Psychological studies of the coronary-prone have yet to define precisely either the nature of the behavioural characteristics, or the eliciting environments. It may be inappropriate, however, to consider the response patterns only on the behavioural level, since much can be gained from exploring the biological components of reactivity.

Physiological mechanisms underlying Type A responses

A number of studies indicate that coronary-prone behaviour may be associated not only with manifest ischaemic heart disease, but also with the degree of coronary stenosis. If this is the case, it provides the firmest evidence available that behavioural factors have an impact on atherogenesis in man. The first report of such a link was from an autopsy survey of coronary atheroma in patients who died during the first years of the WCGS (Friedman, M., *et al.*, 1968). Fifty-one were examined, of whom 25 had died of ischaemic heart disease. Although the ratings of occlusion were higher in the Type A than Type B groups, this was primarily due to the high proportion of cardiac deaths amongst the former. When the men who died from heart disease were excluded, the evidence for greater stenosis in the coronary-prone was slight overall, and altogether absent in the younger cohort, so the connection was spurious.

Yet subsequent coronary angiography studies have revealed more substantial associations. A series of over 90 men was examined in Boston (Zyzanski *et al.*, 1976). The patients were suffering from a variety of complaints, including congestive heart failure, aortic stenosis and ischaemic heart disease. All completed the JAS before surgery, and their coronary angiograms were rated blindly for degree of obstruction. Patients with greater levels of stenosis scored significantly higher on the Type A scale and its three sub-scales. The difference could not be accounted for by severity of symptoms or number of previous hospitalisations, and so was not due to high rating men simply being more ill. The men with severe atherosclerosis also admitted to more social insecurity and self consciousness — an interesting fact in view of the associations between myocardial ischaemia and social incongruity discussed in Chapter 9 (Jenkins *et al.*, 1977).

These findings were confirmed by Blumenthal and associates (1978), although in this case only interview assessments and not JAS scores correlated with ratings of stenosis. Table 10.2 summarises data from the series of consecutive angiographies examined by Frank *et al.* (1978). Patients were classified into four categories by interview, and the mean number of coronary arteries with 50 per cent or more occlusion increased with grade of coronary-prone behaviour. Disease severity was also correlated with serum cholesterol, sex and age; however, even when these factors, together with blood pressure and smoking were entered into a multiple regression analysis, the relation of stenosis to Type A rating persisted. Thus the association was not due to the presence of other risks. The high proportion of Type As included in Table 10.2 is not unexpected, since the bulk of patients undergoing coronary angiography have suspected ischaemic heart disease.

TABLE 10.2
Type A behaviour and severity of coronary artery stenosis (Frank *et al.*, 1978)

Behaviour type	Number of cases	Mean number of coronary arteries with 50% or more stenosis
A_1	75	2·13
A_2	33	2·07
B_3	32	1·35
B_4	7	0·84

The coronary-prone behaviour pattern may actually show closer connections with atheroma than with some clinical manifestations of ischaemic heart disease; it was striking, for example, that in the WCGS, the mean JAS score of sudden cardiac death victims was $-2·15$, well within the Type B range for this population (Zyzanski, 1978). The data are not entirely consistent however, since Dimsdale *et al.* (1979) failed to identify associations between the extent of stenosis revealed through angiography, and coronary-prone characteristics. Negative results were also recorded by Krantz and colleagues (1979) in a study of men who underwent repeat angiography. The group was divided into those who showed progression of disease between the two examinations, with increased stenosis, or no progression. There were so significant differences between the two cohorts in Type A scores derived from the structured interview assessment, or in the JAS ratings of progression and no progression groups.

The mechanisms translating behavioural aspects must presumably operate through the autonomic or neuroendocrine pathways described in Chapter 2, unless some unknown process is operating. A series of studies by Friedman, Rosenman and their colleagues (1960; 1963; 1964) suggested that Type A individuals showed relatively high catecholamine excretion, serum cholesterol, rate of blood clotting and fasting triglyceride level. But methodological deficiencies cast doubt on these observations. The groups were small, the same pool of men being used in part for each comparison, leading to mixtures of experienced and naive subjects. Apart from interview behaviour, additional selection procedures were involved, while differences between groups in smoking habits and weight were also present. Subsequent studies also employed auxiliary selection methods, such as the questioning of business associates (Friedman *et al.*, 1970).

The data relating to coronary-prone behaviour to other cardiovascular risks are conflicting. Jenkins (1966) reported that extreme A and B scorers differed in serum cholesterol levels, but this was not confirmed either in cardiac patients or healthy groups (Keith *et al.*, 1965; Friedman, E. *et al.*, 1968). There are few indications of excessive tonic adrenocortical activity in the coronary-prone (Friedman *et al.*, 1970; 1972). Howard and his associates (1976) scrutinised over 200 men of managerial rank in Canadian companies. Those rated as Type A had elevated levels of blood pressure, serum cholesterol and triglycerides, while a greater percentage smoked. This would implicate Type A as one component of a high risk physical and behavioural profile. On the other hand, it should be recalled that coronary-prone behaviour emerged as an independent factor in the WCGS; elsewhere too, few associations with biological vulnerabilities have been uncovered (Shekelle *et al.*, 1976).

However, if Type A behaviour is a reaction pattern, rather than a fixed trait, then neuroendocrine correlates might only be manifest under conditions of challenge. This is consistent with the study of adrenomedullary reactivity performed by Friedman *et al.* (1975). Fifteen pairs of middle-aged Type A and B males were classified on interview assessments, and recruited into a competitive experiment. They were required to work against each other on mental puzzles for 15 minutes, and the prize for the winner was a bottle of wine. The puzzles were actually insoluble, so neither member of the pair could win. Figure 10.2 summarises the noradrenaline responses of the two

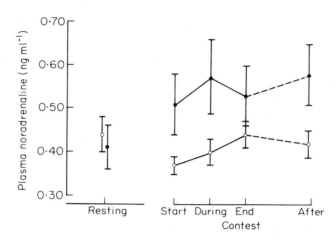

Fig. 10.2. Plasma noradrenaline concentrations in Type A and B men, during performance of a challenging cognitive task. Means ± s.d. over test period, and for resting control values sampled one week later. ●——●, Type A; ○——○, Type B. (Friedman *et al.*, 1975.)

groups. There was no difference at the start of the test, or in the control values taken one week later. However, the increase during the task period was significantly greater amongst Type A men, remaining high after the end of the test. Plasma adrenaline did not change.

The pattern suggests a heightened sympathetic nervous system response amongst Type As, when confronted with actively challenging conditions. The coronary-prone were more involved behaviourally with the task as well; they concentrated intensely, and even afterwards were restless and agitated. In contrast, resting sympathetic nervous function is not disturbed amongst Type A individuals.

Additional studies have explored the possibility that young people likely to develop into fully fledged Type A subjects show exaggerated autonomic reactivity. Dembroski and his associates (1977; 1978; 1979) have assessed cardiovascular adjustments to cognitive and psychomotor tests, principally in students, but also in mature patients. Some of the results, classified on the bases of the student JAS, are listed in Table 10.3; a high score on the scale indicates greater tendencies to coronary-prone behaviour. No differences were recorded on basal systolic or diastolic pressure, or in heart rate. But reactive increases were more substantial in the Type A students, the pressure changes in those scoring 6 or above being significantly larger than responses of the low rating group. The correlations between changes in systolic

TABLE 10.3
Cardiovascular reactions in students classified on JAS A–B scores
(Dembroski *et al.*, 1978)

| | JAS score | | |
	12+	11 − 6	5 −
Systolic pressure change (mmHg)	16·8	13·2	8·6
Diastolic pressure change (mmHg)	8·2	7·0	4·1
Heart rate change (bpm)	9·5	5·3	5·4

pressure and heart rate were reliable, a pattern of adjustment similar to that described in conditions of active coping (see Chapter 6).

It has been argued in Chapters 6 and 8 that this type of reaction predisposes individuals to essential hypertension. If it is also displayed by the coronary-prone, it is surprising that high blood pressure is not characteristic of Type A people. However, the haemodynamic adjustments reported by Dembroski have not been consistently confirmed. Scherwitz *et al.* (1978) failed to find any important differences in reactivity between student A and B groups during mental arithmetic, maze learning or the imagining of distressing scenes, although cardiovascular responses were unusually small throughout this study. A series of investigations by Manuck *et al.* (1978b, 1979) identified differences in systolic pressure increase on performance of complex cognitive tasks, but only amongst male Type As; there was no distinction in heart rate reactions, or in female participants. Similarly, a study of cardiovascular reactions, elicited by mental arithmetic tasks administered in the presence of unpleasant noise, showed no differences between Type A and B female students (Weidner and Matthews, 1978).

All these experiments have employed discontinuous techniques of blood pressure monitoring, and brief tasks. Consequently, very few systolic and diastolic readings were available. Steptoe and Ross (1980a) assessed cardiovascular function continuously with pulse transit time and interbeat interval, during performance of three actively engaging mental tasks. No reliable differences in reactivity were present amongst extreme scorers on a student JAS, selected from the total sample of 36 men and women. Figure 10.3 illustrates the reactivity of high and low scoring men—a high score on the 21-item scale indicates extreme Type A responses. Contrary to prediction, low scoring men were more reactive in heart rate and transit time. More-

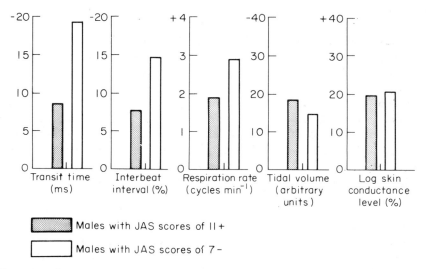

Males with JAS scores of II +

Males with JAS scores of 7 –

FIG. 10.3. Pattern of psychophysiological reactions during three mental task trials, plotted as changes from average baseline. Six subjects per group. (Steptoe and Ross, 1980a.)

over, the baseline heart rate of low scorers was 78·2 bpm, compared with 68·8 in high raters, further emphasising the heightened arousal of the former. These results are again contradictory to the hypothesis that Type As show heightened haemodynamic reactivity.

The psychophysiological investigations of students present a confused picture. A number of laboratories have failed to identify differential haemodynamic or catecholamine responses to tasks that provide little mental challenge, such as the cold pressor (Simpson *et al.*, 1974; Lott and Gatchel, 1978). But even in actively demanding conditions. hyper-reactivity is uncommon. Lundberg and Forsman (1979) found no differences between Type A and B students in their catecholamine or cortisol excretion during challenging tasks, while Simpson's (1974) assessment of platelet aggregation was unfortunately compromised by differences in resting characteristics. It is possible that the behaviour patterns assessed in students have little in common with mature coronary-prone activities, since examination and course requirements may impose certain forms of coping. Friedman's (1975) data on middle-aged Type As suggest that these individuals engage in vigorous attempts to master their environments, and that their responses have neurohumoral concomitants. Whether the latter are instrumental in mediating the risk of ischaemic heart disease remains to be determined.

Summary and conclusions

Despite disagreements about the precise characteristics of the behaviour pattern, there is sound evidence relating Type A activities and ischaemic heart disease. The behaviours, including restlessness, a chronic sense of urgency and hard drive, seem common amongst coronary patients, and those predisposed to later clinical disease. Coronary-prone behaviour is not the only aspect of emotion or interaction with the social environment important in ischaemic heart disease, as the arguments outlined in Chapter 9 indicate. Nor may it be specific to heart disease; although few other forms of pathology have been studied systematically, the behaviour pattern may put people at risk for varied physical and social morbidity.

Type A behaviour is not a universal characteristic of coronary patients, but may be fostered in the context of Western materialistc culture. In a society based on individual achievement and ambition, reactions are frequently channelled into occupational roles. Parents generate motivation for advancement in this sphere of life, through developing high expectations and aspirations in their children, encouraging and reinforcing appropriate behaviours (Matthews, 1978). But under different circumstances, this behavioural coping style will be elicited by other aspects of the social environment. Hence, it is not surprising that Type A behaviour is less significant outside the Western middle-class ambience. For instance, the challenges that confront Japanese Americans trying to emancipate themselves from traditional culture (see p. 161) may be very different from those evoking active striving in other groups.

The mechanisms translating Type A behaviours into cardiovascular risk remain unresolved. It seems probable that differences lie in reactive components rather than tonic levels of haemodynamic or endocrine function, and further laboratory experiments may identify the salient pathways. A catecholaminergic process, operating through lipid metabolism or platelet aggregation, is attractive, but undocumented. Type A behaviour may have a long-term impact on atherogenesis, rather than triggering clinical symptoms in people with advanced stenosis. This latter role may be filled by acute life events, as will be seen in the next chapter.

11
Psychosocial Factors as Acute Precursors of Cardiovascular Events

It has been argued in previous sections that emotional and behavioural factors may operate at a number of different stages in the cardiovascular disease process. The last two chapters have been concerned with the impact of chronic harassments and patterns of behaviour on ischaemic heart disease. Here the emphasis is shifted to acute precipitants of clinical symptoms, usually acting in individuals already at risk with severe atheroma. The psychosocial features involved at this late triggering state may differ from those implicated in long-term aetiology. It is interesting that many of the parameters associated chronically with ischaemic heart disease, such as coronary-prone behaviour, are not closely linked to sudden cardiac death (Zyzanski, 1978). Acute emotional disturbances may be particularly significant in this condition; similarly, research into the precursors of stroke has also focused on emotional traumas in the period immediately preceding the event.

Life crises and acute coronary events

An association between extreme emotion or distress and sudden death can be traced from the earliest medical literature. The range of circumstances thought to precipitate fatal attacks is bewilderingly wide. Thus in the seventeenth century, Bonetus wrote that "not a few have experienced the harm of terror. The fear of an evil is often worse than the evil itself, and how many die before their time from a dread of death." (East, 1958.) A nineteenth-century physician observed that sudden cardiac death might follow "playing Hamlet, or holding the breath during a military flogging". Many famous cases can be cited: the Danish sculptor Thorwaldsen, for example, died in 1844 at a Copenhagen theatre, during the performance of one of Wagner's "new" operas. The surgeon John Hunter collapsed and died after a heated meeting at the Medical School from which I am now writing.

The link between emotional trauma and sudden death can be explored systematically by examining individuals who have undergone severe life crises. Bereavement through loss of a spouse or close friend is one of the most harrowing experiences faced by many people in their lives. The connection between bereavement and subsequent ill-health or death has been frequently documented (Rowland, 1977). Only a proportion of the bereaved are likely to be at risk for sudden cardiac death of course, and many factors may contribute to the raised mortality rate. Grieving relatives may fail to eat properly or maintain adequate hygiene, and the dead and their families may have shared similar unfavourable environments. Yet when Parkes *et al.* (1969) followed up a large cohort of middle-aged widowers, the prime cause of the 40 per cent elevation in death rate was heart disease and arteriosclerosis. Thus deaths from these disorders accounted for 60 per cent of the increased mortality during the first 6 months of bereavement.

A raised cardiovascular death rate may follow general disasters, as well as personal traumas. Mackay (1974) was able to study the effects of the 1971 Civil War in Bangladesh on a community of 40 000 tea workers. The population was well documented, having previously been provided with a good health service. The war interrupted medical treatments, supplies and programmes of malaria eradication. Consequently, the major result was a massive increase in death due to anaemia, malnutrition, and dysentery. Infants and young children were the most vulnerable, but the death rate also rose 65·2 per cent amongst adult workers. When children were excluded from the statistics, the rise in cardiovascular death rate was 54 per cent. So although cardiac deaths were masked by high mortality from other causes, they still responded to these dreadful events. Again, mortality was elevated after the sudden but brief Bristol flood of 1968 (Bennet, 1970). Death rates increased more than 50 per cent in the year following the flood, compared with the previous 12 months. It is likely that cardiovascular disorders made a substantial contribution to this rise.

Studies of this type are based on the grossest of traumas that occur in people's lives, and it is possible that the influence of acute emotional responses extends beyond such crises. Life Event methodology has been applied to investigate the effects of a broader range of experiences. The Schedule of Recent Events (SRE), developed by Holmes and Rahe (1967), is a checklist of incidents thought to require personal or social adjustment. The subject simply endorses whether or not these have been experienced over a specified measurement period. The events, from divorce to a vacation, clearly differ in their salience, so a weighting system was devised in which items were rated against an arbitrary score of 50 for marriage. Weightings were judged by a number of population samples, so as to establish the relative importance of different occurrences. Experiences likely to require more adjustment than marriage were given values over 50, while minor incidents have lower scores. The rank ordering of items is said to be relatively uniform over different populations (Holmes and Masuda, 1974). By adding the weighted values of events actually experienced, a total score in Life Change Units (LCU) can be calculated for each time period. Thus for example, a scaling survey of Finnish adults gave the items "new home improvements" and "unpaid bills leading to threat of legal action" 26 LCU each, compared with 64 for "going to gaol" (Rahe *et al.*, 1974b).

The method has been used extensively in studies of the events preceding non-fatal cardiac crises, yet no consistent build-up of incidents has generally been recorded. Its application to heart disease is complicated by the fact that recently ill people will score high, irrespective of the nature of their problem. This is because illness itself is included in the SRE, together with items such as "change in working conditions" that are likely to be influenced by poor health (Rahe and Arthur, 1967). Consequently, those with a history of angina or undefined pain will have large LCU totals and no build-up may be seen. Rahe and Passikivi (1971) studied 30 coronary patients, for whom an acute infarct was the first sign of ischaemia or ill-health. They completed the SRE for the previous four years retrospectively. No reliable increases of LCU were found, since levels during the months immediately surrounding the attack were not significantly different from those of earlier periods. Theorell and Rahe (1971) administered the SRE to 54 male survivors of infarction, and to a smaller matched control group. Although weighted LCU increased between the third year and the year preceding the coronary crisis, the pattern did not differ significantly from that in controls. In a comparison of twins, one of whom only had died with ischaemic heart disease, no differential trends in LCU were recorded, except in the small sample of monozygotic pairs (De Faire, 1975).

One reason for this failure to uncover reliable associations may lie in the use of LCU scores. It is assumed that life crises simply accumulate in an additive fashion. Although weighting systems have been assessed on several different groups, there are marked variations in the importance placed on particular experiences (Holmes and Masuda, 1974; Chiriboga, 1977). Women rate events more severely than men, while lower scores are produced by people aged over 60 (Horowitz *et al.*,

1977; Masuda and Holmes, 1978). The well educated, and those who have actually experienced the events they are asked to judge, also allot higher LCU. Many questions are related to marriage and the family, and so are not appropriate for all groups. An individual may attach particular importance to occurrences that are not generally considered distressing. Thus Lundberg *et al.* (1975) failed to show a difference between victims of myocardial infarction and controls in LCU; but when participants were allowed to use their own weightings of "upsettingness", patients scored above average. The impact of events may of course be modified by a number of factors, such as social support, that are not assessed by the SRE.

Brown (1974) has criticised the SRE because questions are vague and open ended, and the events to be judged are imprecisely defined. The burden of interpretation is put upon patients, but their perceptions may be influenced by their state of health. Brown and his colleagues (1973) devised an alternative interview method for life event assessment, through which the incidents that are relevant to the individual could be specified. Connolly (1976) used this technique with 91 patients in a coronary care unit, comparing them with an equal number of healthy controls. No assumption was made that the impact of events summated, so analysis was confined to the numbers reporting events, rather than cumulative scores. Significantly more patients than controls confirmed that they had experienced disturbing life events in the three weeks prior to the cardiac crisis. When the patients were divided into angina and acute onset groups, the association with life events was only reliable in the latter. Moreover the differences across the whole 12-week study period in numbers experiencing events was statistically significant.

This result is interesting, since events possibly related to illness were eliminated from analysis. For instance, redundancies following poor work that might have been secondary to chest pain were excluded. The data suggest that when assessments are geared towards the individual patient, firmer associations may be uncovered. Yet the proportion of patients reporting important events was still low. Thus in the three weeks preceding admission only 18 of the 91 cardiac patients experienced events, compared with 6 controls. So it would appear that the number of cases in which acute life disturbances do precipitate nonfatal clinical attacks is not large.

The evidence relating emotional traumas with sudden cardiac death is somewhat firmer. A large study in Finland compared 279 survivors of myocardial infarction with 226 fatalities. Both groups were divided into subsets of victims with or without prior illness (Rahe *et al.*, 1974b).

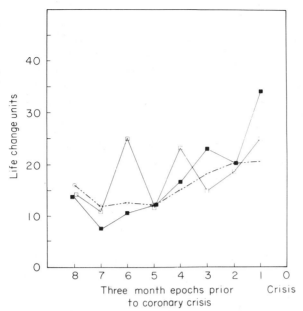

F_IG_. 11.1. Mean life change units (LCU) for each three-month epoch in the two years preceding coronary crises for three groups who had experienced no recent illness. O—–·–·—–O, Myocardial infarction survivors; ■———■, sudden cardiac deaths; □———□, delayed cardiac deaths. (Rahe *et al.*, 1974b.)

LCU increased during the months immediately preceding myocardial infarction, but the rise was greater in the sudden death group. Figure 11.1 summarises data from patients without prior illness. There are seasonal fluctuations in LCU because some items relate to work and vacations, so it is proper to compare levels over the parallel periods of each year. A 69 per cent increase was recorded from survivors during the six months prior to onset, while LCU rose by 143 per cent in the sudden death group.

Unfortunately two difficulties hamper simple interpretations. The low score for more distant periods might simply reflect forgetfulness, since there are clear recency effects in reporting (Masuda and Holmes, 1978). Additionally, data on the sudden death group were solicited from spouses, and their reports are not always reliable. Rahe *et al.* (1974b) tested accuracy by comparing LCU ratings from survivors and their spouses; for this cohort correlations were variable, and did not reach statistical significance for one subgroup. Hence, the differential increase of LCU may be artefactual.

Reporting problems in life event research are minimised by study designs in which incidents are scored as they occur. Theorell and Rahe (1975) used this concurrent method in a case note survey. Patients with previous myocardial infarctions were examined every three months, and during these interviews psychosocial information was gathered informally. The case notes of 18 patients who subsequently died abruptly were compared with those of age and sex matched survivors, and all were rated blind for life events. The LCU totals over the two years that ended in death for half the patients are plotted in Fig. 11.2. The mean value was significantly higher amongst fatalities for the period 7–12 months before death. These differences were unlikely to be biased by

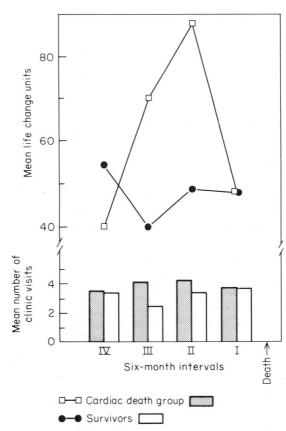

FIG. 11.2. Mean life change units (LCU) and number of clinic visits for each six months of the two years prior to coronary death (Theorell and Rahe, 1975).

forgetting or reporting inaccuracy. However, patients were not inter-
rogated systematically, so events were identified only after unstandard-
ised questionning by physicians. It can be seen in Fig. 11.2 that patients
who subsequently died also had higher consulting rates, and may
therefore have been provided with greater opportunities for revealing
their problems and experiences. Only a prospective assessment of
sudden cardiac death, with events recorded soon after they occur, will
determine whether the relationship is robust.

It may be significant that in Theorell and Rahe's survey, the high
rates of life disturbance did not occur immediately before death, but
sometime earlier. Kuller *et al.* (1975) determined the frequency of acute
precipitating events by interviewing next of kin. Clear triggers could
be identified in only 14 per cent of 484 sudden cardiac death cases, and
the rate amongst infarct survivors was identical. Longer prodromal
periods may have to be scrutinised in order to establish an association
between life events and cardiac death.

The identification of links between severe but relatively common life
experiences and cardiac mortality, raises a question that has already
been considered in earlier chapters; whether emotional or psychosocial
disturbances are specifically connected with cardiovascular disease, or
have more general consequences. Bereavement and life events may be
significant in a range of medical disorders, including psychiatric and
physical complaints (Parkes and Brown, 1972; Brown *et al.*, 1975).
Conversely, women who died suddenly were characterised by a variety
of social morbidity, including alcoholism and marital instability
(Talbott *et al.*, 1977). Since cardiac crises generally occur only in
people with moderate or severe coronary stenosis, the interaction between physical vulnerability and life experience may be crucial.

An association of this type was identified by Rahe and his associates
(1976) in Finland. The inhabitants of Karelia in East Finland have a
much higher incidence of ischaemic heart disease than those living in
the south western part of the country. Both groups are primarily rural,
living in subarctic conditions, and many efforts have gone into un-
covering the causes of the difference. Rahe *et al.* (1976) found that
East Finns not only had higher systolic pressure, serum cholesterol and
smoking rates, but also experienced greater numbers of life events. The
eastern section is poor, so the inhabitants suffer more redundancy,
financial and familial problems. Thus life experience may contribute,
along with other factors, in the construction of the risk profile of the
Karelian population. The interaction of behaviour, environment and
pathology can be further clarified by considering the processes operating in sudden cardiac death.

Behaviour and the mechanisms of sudden cardiac death

Psychological factors may be involved in the precipitation of sudden cardiac death through influences on the electrical stability of the heart. The interaction between autonomic discharge and coronary stenosis in modifying the fragility of the myocardium was described in Chapter 2 (pp. 31–33). Animal research has concentrated on the effects of two integrated behavioural–autonomic activity patterns on cardiac vulnerability (see pp. 91–95). The same aspects can be considered in clinical cases.

The first approach stems from the hypothesis that sudden death is due to extreme bradycardia following severe vagal overstimulation. It has been suggested that such activity is associated with depression, helplessness, and "giving up" on the part of the patient (Richter, 1957; Wolf, 1967; Engel, 1971). Vagal discharge, leading to ventricular failure and standstill, has been implicated as a mechanism of sudden death in the absence of myocardial infarction (Hellerstein and Turell, 1964).

This theory has drawn support from two areas of experimental research, although neither is entirely consistent. The work on swimming death in rats was interpreted in terms of helplessness, since sinking and death apparently followed the termination of attempts to escape (Richter, 1957). Yet as has been argued in Chapter 5, the evidence is weak both for death following on helplessness, and for a neurogenic arrest. Nevertheless, other studies do suggest that parasympathetic tone may be augmented during unavoidable or severe stimulation from the environment. Laboratory research in humans was drawn in at the suggestion of Wolf (1967) who argued that the "diving reflex", the vagally induced bradycardia observed on face immersion, may parallel the changes seen in sudden cardiac death. With extreme emotional harassment, a profound vagal bradycardia might precipitate complete cessation of the cardiac contractions. However mental stimulation appears not to exaggerate, but attenuate the reduction of heart rate seen on face immersion (Fig. 2.4, p. 29). Severe vagal overactivity, leading to bradycardia of sufficient size to be clinically disturbing, has not been documented extensively in humans (Wolf et al., 1978).

The hypothesis predicts that sudden cardiac death will be preceded by depression or a sense of hopelessness and giving up. Unfortunately, most surveys to date have been concerned with establishing the presence of a psychological trigger, rather than analysing the nature of the precursors. The single cases smattered in the literature emphasise overwhelming anger or fright, although several other emotions were also described (Engel, 1971). Engel's own survey was based on the unsystematic review of newspaper items, few of which were backed by medical information; there is no evidence that the circumstances described in these extracts are at all representative of sudden death in general. Greene *et al.* (1972) explored the conditions surrounding 26 sudden deaths amongst employees of a large commercial concern. Almost all victims had histories of ischaemic heart disease, and 80 per cent apparently showed recent signs of depression. However, these data were solicited from the victims' wives rather than physicians, and the primary contact with these widows was a telephone interview. In none of the case notes was there any indication of proneness to vasovagal syncope. The lethargy and reduced activity may have resulted from cardiac insufficiency, being effects rather than causes of dysfunction.

The most dramatic parallels to experimental observations of helplessness are the cases of "voodoo" death. Previously healthy victims are said to decline and die rapidly following the realisation that they are in the clutches of malignant powers (Cannon, 1957). Although poisoning may sometimes be involved, on other occasions there have been no signs of physical interference. Yet again, these may not be vagally induced effects; Cannon himself concluded that fear-related sympathatic "nervous" activation might provoke dehydration and reductions in blood volume. It may be significant that taboo victims usually refuse food and water, exacerbating the deficits.

Glass (1977) attempted a more systematic analysis of events preceding non-fatal infarctions by comparing patients in a coronary care unit with groups of non-cardiac hospitalised, and healthy controls. A modified SRE was administered, items being separated into uncontrollable losses (such as the death of a relative) and others. Uncontrollable losses are thought likely to induce a state of helplessness (Seligman, 1975). Although some difference in the proportion of each group experiencing a loss over the previous 12 months was uncovered, methodological drawbacks make the study difficult to interpret. Of the cardiac patients 40 per cent refused to participate, so it is uncertain whether the sample was representative. The hospitalised controls were predominantly psychiatric patients, including a number of alcoholics; reporting abilities may not therefore have been comparable in the different groups. Furthermore, the samples varied on a number of characteristics, including age, class and racial distribution that are known to influence life event measurement.

A final problem with the vagal hypothesis is the significance of this parasympathetic mechanism in cardiac disturbances. As was seen in Chapter 1, the sinus bradycardias recorded at the time of myocardial infarction may be benign. Moreover, vagal stimulation protects against ventricular fibrillation, the process that commonly leads to death.

The alternative conceptualisation of psychological influence relates to the mechanisms affecting vulnerability to ventricular fibrillation. Physiological research, discussed in Chapter 2, suggests that ventricular fibrillation may follow intense activity in the cardiac sympathetic fibres, notably in people already suffering from coronary stenosis. Data from laboratory studies of animals indicates that behavioural stimuli can likewise provoke traffic of sufficient magnitude in the autonomic pathways.

The same process may operate in man. A series of investigations by Lynch and his associates demonstrate that psychological or emotional stimuli may result in modifications of cardiac rhythm and stability in patients with ischaemic heart disease (Lynch *et al.*, 1974; 1977). Patients were studied in a coronary care unit, and the apparently innocuous pulse palpation procedure, or the presence of a nurse beside the bed, altered the pattern of arrhythmias dramatically. In formal testing, the frequency of ectopic beats increased significantly during pulse palpation, in comparison with control periods. When the generally younger and non-ischaemic admissions to emergency accident units were examined, arrhythmias were less frequent; but tachycardia was recorded during bedside discussions by doctors, even when the patients were curarised to prevent seizure movements.

The importance of cardiac sympathetic tone in the initiation of ventricular arrhythmias may also account for the changes in ectopic activity during sleep. Lown *et al.* (1973b) undertook 24-hour ECG monitoring of cardiac patients with ectopic activity. The frequency of premature ventricular contractions fell during sleep in 78 per cent of participants, often to a dramatic degree. It is significant that these changes occur despite heart rate slowing, since arrhythmias are generally more frequent at slow rates. But as was noted on p. 50, β blockers exert their major antihypertensive effects in the daytime, suggesting that cardiac sympathetic traffic is reduced at night (Millar-Craig *et al.*, 1979).

The significance of asymptomatic disturbance of ventricular rhythm has not been entirely established, since associations with subsequent cardiac vulnerability are inconsistent (Hinkle *et al.*, 1969; Fisher and Tyroler, 1973). However the frequency and pattern of arrhythmias must be considered. Using 24-hour ambulatory ECG monitoring,

Calvert *et al.* (1977) found 67 per cent of people with normal coronary arteries manifest some ectopic activity. But premature ventricular beats appeared with greater regularity and persisted for longer periods in patients with stenosis. Prevalence was higher amongst those with multiple rather than single vessel disease. The circumstances under which arrhythmias occurred in this study were unfortunately not recorded. When Rose (1974) recorded ECGs telemetrically from cardiac patients while they were attending football games, half the cases showed abnormal electrical activity. Premature ventricular contractions and ST segment changes were particularly frequent at exciting moments of the game. The cardiac sympathetic innervation is further implicated by the reduction in sudden death incidence amongst survivors of infarction treated with β blockade (Wilhelmsson *et al.*, 1974).

These data are important for behavioural investigations of sudden cardiac death, since the conditions that elicit cardiac sympathetic arousal are very different from those associated with vagal stimulation. The pathway is generally provoked by novel or very severe excitatory stimuli, or else by conditions that demand active behavioural coping. This contrasts with the depression and withdrawal apparently responsible for augmented parasympathetic tone. Nevertheless, a number of case studies are consistent with this emphasis. Levine (1963) described a patient who had displayed a benign atrial fibrillation for more than 40 years. His blood pressure was normal, and no other cardiovascular disturbances were observed in regular checkups throughout this period. At the age of 63 he was walking in some woods when he came across a fawn which had been wounded by a poacher. While talking to the gamewarden about the incident, he became extremely agitated and distressed, and died suddenly. No extensive atheroma or infarction were revealed on autopsy, and death seems to have followed intense electrical cardiac disturbance. A sudden death with ventricular fibrillation occurred in a hypertensive man after he rode a large and frightening corkscrew rollercoaster at an amusement park (Glasser *et al.*, 1978), while Nakamoto (1965) documented several cases in which paroxysmal arrhythmias apparently followed life traumas or crises. In an early series examined by Stevenson and associates (1949), excitement and anxiety were the commonest emotional concomitants of extrasystolic activity.

In most of these examples, electrical instability was superimposed on a background of ischaemia and atheroma. Yet on occasion, behavioural factors may be sufficiently powerful to provoke disturbance in the absence of stenosis. Such an explanation was proposed for a 39-year-old patient who displayed ventricular fibrillation without any evidence of hypertension, ST segment depression or blood chemical abnormalities (Lown *et al.*, 1976). The man was living under considerable strain, having experienced a major career setback, while his wife was depressed over a bereavement. Another interesting phenomenon was identified during exercise stress tests of firefighters in Los Angeles (Barnard *et al.*, 1976). Coronary risks are generally low amongst these men, since only very fit people are admitted to the service. However, 10 per cent of the sample showed ischaemic ECG responses to exercise. Subsequent coronary angiography of 6 men revealed severe stenosis in two; the other 4 exhibited myocardial instability in the absence of coronary occlusion. They may have succumbed to the repeated alerting required in this occupation.

Despite such case studies, there is little systematic evidence about the contrasting psychological profiles proposed in sudden death. In part the solution must depend on clarification of the physiopathology of the condition, and the frequency of different prodromata. The behaviours and environmental conditions that place people at risk may then be distinguished more conclusively.

Psychological precipitants of stroke

A further area in which psychosocial factors may predispose towards clinical crises is in the case of cerebrovascular accidents. Unfortunately, well-controlled data are sparse. For although interest in stroke patients has been intense, it has focused on a narrow range of phenomena. Disturbances of cognition, perception and other consequences have received considerable attention, to the neglect of psychosocial precursors. Descriptive information on sex or urban–rural differences in stroke incidence is incomplete, and many variations in prevalence between populations have not been explained in a satisfactory manner (Abu-Zeid *et al.*, 1975; Kagan *et al.*, 1976b). Since few studies have explored emotional or behavioural factors, the uncontrolled, retrospective reports in the literature must be interpreted cautiously.

One popular notion is that strokes are triggered by extreme emotional excitement. In Storey's (1968) large cohort of subarachnoid haemorrhage cases, four patients spontaneously described acute precipitating incidents. One patient had a stroke on being told that her best friend had just hung herself, while another collapsed on learning of her son's motor cycle accident. A third heard that the aeroplane, on which she believed her son was travelling, had blown up, and the fourth had a stroke on discovering that her husband was seeking a divorce, on the grounds of her supposedly secret adultery. In each case, the emotional trauma immediately presaged the stroke.

However, such clear associations are rarely identified, and may be very uncommon; these four were the only convincing cases from amongst more than 250 studied by Storey. In a series of 32 mixed stroke patients, Adler *et al.* (1971) found acute precursors in only two. Other information was collected in open-ended interviews, which suggested that certain behavioural characteristics were common to their group. Many displayed chronically pressured, energetic behaviour, were vigorous and determined, and saw themselves as very hard working. A substantial number were also thought to have difficulties with controlling anger. The strokes themselves were frequently preceded by personal failures, excessive environmental demands and threat of loss. This pattern implies that objectively defined life events may be associated with stroke, but data were unfortunately not collected in a standardised form, nor was a control group included. Moreover, most of the patients could be interviewed within three days of the crisis, so the cerebrovascular events must in many cases have been relatively small. Other investigations have claimed to identify emotional precursors in a much higher proportion of patients during uncontrolled studies (Ecker, 1954).

The position is further complicated by the possibility that psychosocial factors are more important in some types of stroke than others. Storey (1968) hypothesised that emotional disturbances were linked with subarachnoid haemorrhage in a greater proportion of cases when angiograms revealed no cerebral berry aneurysms. Penrose (1972) recorded life events in 44 patients with subarachnoid haemorrhage using the Brown interview technique. Systematic enquiries were pursued about events in the previous three months, with relatives rather than patients being interviewed, since the latter were too ill. Seventeen patients had no berry aneurysms, and of these 48 per cent had experienced a significant life event in the three weeks preceding the stroke. This compared with 28 per cent of patients with berry aneurysms, and 19 per cent of controls abstracted from an earlier investigation (Brown and Birley, 1968). The difference from control was reliable only for patients without aneurysms.

This life event survey suggests that emotional factors may be associated with particular forms of stroke. But general conclusions are unwarranted. A chain of physiopathology linking emotion to cerebrovascular accident cannot be described with confidence. Autonomic discharge might provoke the acute changes in cerebral blood flow, and hypertensive episodes are thought to underlie some strokes. Yet this area of psychosocial experience has not been researched in depth.

Summary and conclusions

Psychosocial factors may be involved at different stages of the cardio-vascular disease process. The salient features vary at each phase, and with the diverse clinical manifestations of disease; consequently, the elements discussed in Chapters 9 and 10 in relation to long-term aetiology may not be significant in the acute phase.

Life event methodologies have been applied to the analysis of acute influences. Many techniques have distinct weaknesses, while poor controls and other features confound some studies. Reactions to disturbing events are modified by social supports and other chronic factors, and these have rarely been taken into account (Cobb, 1976). Thus only the grossest connections between life events and ischaemic heart disease have been confirmed to date. The association appears firmest in cases of sudden death, since the correlation with non-fatal cardiac crises is inconsistent. The latter may be related to chronic perturbations, rather than chronically distressing events. There are no indications that life events can provoke heart attacks in the absence of severe atheroma.

The types of behaviour or experience that are most significant for sudden cardiac death are not yet known. However, connections are beginning to be formed between the pathological endpoint, the neural mechanisms involved, and the psychological conditions likely to pro-mote activity in these pathways. Ventricular fibrillation tends to be linked with intense excitement and behavioural activation. The con-trasting relationship between vagal overstimulation and depression or helplessness has yet to be substantiated. Greater understanding of the physiopathological mechanisms underlying sudden cardiac death will clarify these issues.

In comparison with ischaemic heart disease, the prodromata of stroke have been largely neglected. Acute emotional triggers are present in only a few cases, while chronic distress is evident in rather more. However, the uncontrolled nature of most investigations pro-hibits any generalisations.

These data further underline the argument that the endpoints of cardiovascular disease cannot be grouped together in psychosocial research. Nor do "psychological stressors" act in a uniform way on circulatory dysfunctions. A greater sophistication in both psychological and clinical analysis must be exercised if the relationships are to be established with any precision.

12
Psychological Aspects of Prevention and Management

The last decade has witnessed a rapid expansion of research and practice in behavioural medicine. Much of this work has been directed at cardiovascular disorders, as books devoted to acute coronary care (Gentry and Williams, 1975; Cromwell *et al.*, 1977), rehabilitation (Stocksmeier, 1976; Wenger and Hellerstein, 1978), and recovery from myocardial infarction (Croog and Levine, 1977; Finlayson and McEwen, 1977) indicate. A detailed discussion of these aspects would occupy more space than can be given here. Nevertheless, it is important to consider the implications of the arguments put forward in previous chapters. Psychological factors are involved at several different stages in the development of cardiovascular disorders, at each of which modifications of behaviour may prove valuable.

Figure 12.1 summarises the sequence of events salient in ischaemic heart disease, indicating the areas in which behavioural factors figure prominently. Interventions fall into two broad groups. Firstly, attempts have been made to change overt behaviours that are likely to increase the individual's cardiovascular vulnerability. These include risk behaviours such as lack of exercise and smoking, and actions secondary to medical intervention, amongst which failures to adhere to treatment and drug regimens are most important. These activities are viewed as problem behaviours, and considered as analogous to other behavioural difficulties; thus counselling, self-monitoring, operant techniques and other procedures may be employed as appropriate.

Secondly, direct modifications of the autonomic and endocrine components of cardiovascular dysfunction have been studied. Recent developments in biofeedback and relaxation techniques offer patients the opportunity of being directly responsible for the management of their own problems, and may provide valuable adjuncts to conventional medical procedures. As can be seen in Fig. 12.1, psychophysiological

Target problem	Primary prevention		Symptoms of myocardial ischaemia	Coronary care and rehabilitation	
	Physical and psychological risk factors	Essential hypertension	Angina pectoris Cardiac arrhythmias	Acute coronary care	Recovery and return to home and work environment
Psychological and behavioural contributions	Modification of risk behaviours: Smoking reduction Diet and weight control Exercise training Alteration of coronary-prone behaviour	Biofeedback and relaxation Improving adherence to medication Weight control Reduction of salt intake	Exercise training Biofeedback	Patient education, support	Improving transmission of information to patients and families Relaxation training Improving compliance Secondary reduction of risk behaviours

Fig. 12.1. Summary of behavioural interventions in cardiac disorders.

methods are applied at several stages in cardiovascular morbidity, from primary modifications of risk factors to the restoration of haemo-dynamic patency in the post-infarction period.

The emphasis here will fall on this second class of interventions, since many of the preceding chapters have been concerned with psycho-social factors in aetiology, and their mediation through autonomic pathways. Nevertheless, modifications in attitudes and overt behaviour must also be considered.

Risk behaviour intervention

The energies of health agencies have increasingly been directed towards modifications of risk factors, in an effort to prevent the spread of serious cardiovascular disorders. Even in the absence of identifiable pathology, the occurrence of heavy smoking, high serum lipid levels and elevated blood pressure in otherwise healthy individuals is cause for concern. Some risk factors are themselves behaviours, and can be treated as such; in other cases, modifications of voluntary actions may prove the most accessible pathway to prevention.

Occasionally, simple warnings about the danger of particular habits, and instructions to change them, prove sufficient to induce alterations in behaviour. For example, some success in arterial pressure control has emerged from encouraging patients to reduce salt intake. A cohort of 75 Japanese hypertensive women was divided into three groups (Shibata and Hatano, 1979). The first was given a $2\frac{1}{2}$-hour lecture on diet, blood pressure and salt, and was instructed to lower salt usage. The second group was mobilised one week later, while the third set acted as controls. Systolic and diastolic pressures fell immediately and significantly within the first week in Group 1, and a similar decrease was recorded after instructing Group 2. The systolic reduction of some 10 mmHg was associated with lower 24-hour sodium excretion rates. These short-term modifications were equivalent to those produced by conventional drugs. Similarly, Morgan *et al.* (1978) found that the pressure change following administration of detailed dietary instructions about salt restriction compared favourably with drug interventions, even at two year follow-up.

More commonly however, high risk behaviours are difficult to modify. Thus although short-term reductions in smoking and body weight may be achieved by a variety of techniques, there is considerable recidivism (Ley, 1977; Raw, 1977). When control procedures are incorporated to account for non-specific effects of attention and therapeutic expectations, little difference is observed between treatment groups. The high relapse rates may reflect failures to promote long-term maintenance following active intervention, and neglect of the part played by the individual's family and personal circle in the enterprise.

A major problem may lie in widespread scepticism about the dangerous consequences of risk behaviours. A useful conceptualisation of health-related behaviour is furnished by the Health Belief Model, which suggests that action depends on several aspects of belief and experience (Becker and Maiman, 1975). These include the perception of susceptibility to the disorder, realisation of the seriousness of the dysfunction, and perception of the benefits of the proposed remedial action. Thus smokers may not accept that their behaviour is putting them at risk, they may consider the risk worth taking, or may believe that it is too late to reverse any medical complications. In this respect, it is notable that smokers' motivation for change is greatly increased after they have suffered a myocardial infarction, presumably because the threat becomes more tangible (Acker, 1976; Finlayson and McEwan, 1977). Similarly, health beliefs influence responses to weight control programmes. Becker and associates (1977) assessed attitudes in mothers of obese children from a predominantly black, low income population. Weight loss in children was not related to sex, size of family, income or education. However, it was associated with the mother's general concern about her child's health, her belief in her child's vulnerability to illness, and her perception of the dangers of being overweight.

Another important component is the personal cost to individuals of altering habits. Behaviour change may have ramifications throughout a person's life, from the initial effort of participating in an intervention programme, to lasting effects on social activities. Weight reduction, for example, may involve modifications in shopping, cooking and eating habits, interfere with social life, and require changes in daily routines so that exercise can be included. This amounts to a formidable price that the client may not be prepared to pay.

Risk behaviour modification shares a further drawback with other forms of intervention: the maintenance of compliance or adherence to regimes. Many of the factors related to compliance are common to different clinical procedures. For convenience therefore, the matter will be considered with specific reference to antihypertensive treatment.

Treatment of high blood pressure

The problem of high blood pressure attracts vast therapeutic resources, and the limits that should be placed on the application of drugs remain controversial (Perry and Smith, 1978). Yet a significant proportion of patients prescribed antihypertensive medication continue to show elevated pressure levels. For example, Langfield (1973) surveyed 185 patients whose blood pressures were recorded by anaesthesiologists prior to surgery for non-cardiovascular problems. Fifty-one were considered hypertensive, and of these 50 per cent were under treatment. Many other failures to lower arterial pressure have been reported (Taguchi and Fries, 1974). Deficiencies in medication may account for some pressure instability, but in a proportion of patients, adherence to treatment is poor. Compliance with chronic medication is generally low, and the problems are compounded in the case of asymptomatic disorders. Unfortunately, there are major difficulties in determining adherence to antihypertensive treatment (Sackett *et al.*, 1979). Blood pressure itself is a poor criterion, since changes depend on dosage — the absence of desired reductions may reflect low compliance, or incorrect prescription. Pill counts, when the number of pills removed from the container is compared with the prescription, are based on the assumption that all missing tablets are actually taken by the patient. Using this method, McKenney and co-workers (1973) estimated that some 80 per cent of hypertensive outpatients were non-compliant, while other investigators have put the rate at about 50 per cent (Sackett *et al.*, 1975). An even simpler expedient for assessing compliance is to ask patients whether they are adhering to treatment; although the people who lie will be missed, those who admit being lax are generally telling the truth. Furthermore, uncontrolled blood pressure is more prevalent amongst those who confess that their compliance is poor (Nelson *et al.*, 1978).

A number of factors influence the likelihood of compliance with antihypertensive medication. Nelson *et al.* (1978) studied patients after 2 years of treatment, and noted more faithful adherence in the older patients, those who considered the problem severe, and amongst people who were prescribed chronic medications for other complaints. This suggests that health beliefs are relevant; however, Sackett *et al.* (1979) found that attitudes to health, assessed at the beginning of treatment, were generally not predictive of subsequent compliance. Other aspects of medical care are significant. Complex medication regimes are followed less reliably, both because of memory problems and lack of comprehension. All treatments have a behavioural cost, reflected in the amount of effort that must go into compliance. In addition, adherence depends on the patient's satisfaction with medical consultations and procedures. Those who are dissatisfied with their doctor's communications, who are not given sufficient information about their problem and its management, and whose expectations are not met, tend to show low levels of treatment compliance (Ley, 1977).

Methods of improving patient compliance

Faced with this recalcitrance on the part of patients, efforts are being made to increase adherence with treatment. Some methods concern the ways in which health information and advice is presented. Thus training physicians in communication skills, and providing information to patients in readily comprehensible and memorable forms, may improve compliance behaviours (Ley, 1977). For example, Ley compared two versions of a booklet written to encourage women to follow a low carbohydrate diet. Although the contents were identical, one leaflet presented material in the standard form, while the other was laid out in an especially simple manner, with explicit categorisation of advice and deliberate repetition. The obese subjects who received the easy version produced significantly more weight loss than the ordinary leaflet group, with an average reduction of 15·4 lb at 16 weeks, compared with 8·2 lb.

In the case of blood pressure, specific procedures have been developed to increase the efficiency of control through antihypertensive drugs (Sackett *et al.*, 1979). Teaching patients to measure their own pressures may be valuable. Carnahan and Nugent (1975) provided half the patients in a cohort of newly diagnosed hypertensives with sphygmomanometers, and they were instructed to measure pressure twice daily. The results of this 6-month intervention are summarised in Table 12.1. Although both groups showed similar reductions of diastolic pressure, the systolic change was significantly greater in the self-monitoring condition.

Self-monitoring was also included in a package of special attention procedures administered to a group of non-compliant hypertensive steelmen (Haynes *et al.*, 1976). The men were seen fortnightly by a research worker who encouraged self-monitoring and the charting of pill takings, and helped patients to solve compliance problems by working out convenient occasions for drug administration. Diastolic pressures fell consistently in this group by an average of 5·6 mmHg on

6 months reassessment, while levels in the drug treated, no intervention controls remained unchanged.

These studies have unfortunately confounded self-monitoring with extra medical attention, and it is possible that the latter is very important. When self-monitoring is introduced without increasing contact and attention, its effects on compliance are modest (Johnson *et al.*, 1978). Moreover, vigorous efforts to improve patient supervision have effects in the absence of blood pressure self-monitoring. Thus in another experiment, hypertensive outpatients were interviewed every month by a pharmacist, who discussed drug reactions, complications and therapeutic responses, provided information and monitored treatment (McKenney *et al.*, 1973). During the 5-month intervention period, compliance rates (assessed by pill counts) rose to 70 per cent in experimental subjects, compared with less than 20 per cent in controls. Diastolic pressures were better regulated, so that 19 out of 25 patients were stabilised below 90 mmHg, while only 5 of the 25 controls reached this state. Even though the pharmacist spent an average of only 6 minutes with each patient every month, the therapeutic gains were substantial.

The changes in patient behaviour fostered by these interventions are not simply products of non-specific interest, but follow from attempts to tailor treatment to the individual. No substantial changes in compliance result when extra attention is not directed at these goals (Johnson *et al.*, 1978). Furthermore, the effects of increased supervision may not endure, and there is rapid reversion to baseline once special attention is withdrawn — only 25 per cent of McKenney's patients, for example, remained compliant during follow-up. Therefore, if improvements in adherence are to prove valuable, the problem of maintaining the behaviour without expending vast clinical resources will have to be solved.

TABLE 12.1
The effects of self-monitoring on the control of hypertension
(Carnahan and Nugent, 1975)

	Initial levels (mmHg)		Final levels (mmHg)	
	Systolic	Diastolic	Systolic	Diastolic
Experimental group	152·7	101·7	134·7	91·3
Control group	156·6	103·6	146·1	93·3

Voluntary control of blood pressure

Poor compliance is one of several problems with conventional anti-hypertensive treatments. Complaints about side effects are widespread amongst recipients of medication, although they do not appear to constitute a major cause of failure to take drugs (Bulpitt and Dollery, 1973; Sackett *et al.*, 1979). Nevertheless, the agents available do not suit everybody, and pressure control is not always adequate even when regimens are fulfilled (Hanssen and Henning, 1978). Significant proportions of patients have negative attitudes towards drug-taking and dependence on medicines. This difficulty is compounded by the nature of the risk from hypertension. Serious consideration is being given to active management at lower and lower levels of arterial pressure; yet only a minority of those with moderately elevated pressure progress to higher values, while still fewer actually succumb to cardiovascular disorders (Miall and Brennan, 1979). Consequently, growing numbers of people are faced with the prospect of medication beginning in early middle age and continuing indefinitely, in order to avoid an illness that may not ever develop.

There has been increasing interest over recent years in the development of alternative management procedures, based on voluntary control with biofeedback and relaxation. Yet although many methods have been devised, there are major difficulties in assessing their efficacy with essential hypertensives. The condition is notoriously sensitive to placebos and therapeutic expectations, so that quite ineffective techniques can provoke dramatic responses (Goldring *et al.*, 1956). Thus experiments have to be rigorously controlled, so that effects are not attributed to the wrong elements. Several studies of biofeedback and relaxation in hypertension have been methodologically deficient in these respects (Steptoe, 1977a, 1978a).

However, some controlled investigations of psychological techniques have demonstrated valuable pressure reductions. Patel and North (1975) recruited hypertensive outpatients from a general practice list, allocating them to treatment and control groups at random. The treatment patients received educational material, and then carried out twelve 30 minute sessions of instructed relaxation and meditation. During these periods, patients were seen individually, and taught to relax using instructions focusing progressively on different parts of the body. Feedback of skin conductance or muscle tension was also included as an aid to relaxation. Controls attended for the same number of sessions, but were asked to relax without being given specific assistance.

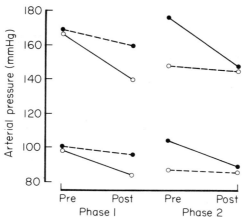

Fig. 12.2. Average changes in blood pressure in two groups of hypertensive patients. Phase 1: O——O, behavioural treatment group ($n = 17$); ●----●, control group ($n = 17$). Phase 2: O----O, former experimental group given no further treatment; ●——●, former control group given behavioural treatment. Each phase lasted 6 weeks. Post-treatment values are averaged across readings taken fortnightly for a three-month follow-up. (Patel and North, 1975.)

The results plotted in Fig. 12.2 indicate that pressure fell in both conditions. But reductions in systolic and diastolic pressure were significantly greater after the relaxation programme. The modification amongst controls may have been due to adaptation, treatment expectations and non-specific attentional factors. Two months later, the controls were switched to active therapy, and they too showed large falls in arterial pressure, while the former treatment group maintained gains. Although parts of the study remain difficult to interpret, the results appear robust, and encourage this approach to high blood pressure.

Other explorations of relaxation confirm that changes cannot be attributed merely to attentional factors. Taylor and associates (1977) observed greater pressure control in relaxation than in patients given standard medical treatment, or non-specific supportive counselling. The same team reported a further comparison of relaxation, learned either from a therapist or from audio tapes, and psychotherapy (Brauer *et al.*, 1979). A series of medicated outpatients attended for 10 sessions, and those in the psychotherapy condition were counselled on the stresses of life, and ways of coping with them. No differences between groups were apparent at the end of treatment, as can be seen in Table 12.2. Yet the therapist conducted relaxation group continued to show gains at six months follow-up, with a mean reduction of 17·8/9·70 mmHg; in contrast, pressure reverted towards basal levels in other conditions. Some alterations in medication were recorded, but these did not differ between conditions. The pattern of results suggests that patients in all groups responded transiently to vigorous treatment, and the non-specific elements of therapeutic interaction. However, arterial pressure decreases were only sustained by those taught relaxation on a personal basis.

The mechanism of pressure change may involve the sympathetic branch of the autonomic nervous system. Stone and DeLeo (1976) showed that the decreases in arterial pressure produced by a cohort of young unmedicated patients were correlated with reductions in plasma $D\beta H$ (see p. 18 for the use of this measure). Moreover, plasma renin activity also fell in the treatment group, while Davidson *et al.* (1979) found plasma noradrenaline was lowered in relaxing coronary patients.

In comparison with these data, the effects of training subjects with direct feedback of blood pressure have been disappointing. Although small decreases are regularly recorded within treatment sessions, they are often not translated into useful effects. Some of the greatest changes were generated in a series of outpatients given intensive systolic pressure feedback training (Benson *et al.*, 1971). Decreases of 30 mmHg were observed in some cases, while a number failed to respond. Other carefully designed comparisons of blood pressure feedback with alternative psychological techniques have yielded predominantly negative results (Frankel *et al.*, 1978; Surwit *et al.*, 1978; Blanchard *et al.*, 1979). The difficulty of maintaining large changes is mirrored in studies on normotensive volunteers, where again feedback effects are slight. When treatments are compared with appropriate control conditions, the decreases produced with biofeedback do exceed those of instructed sub-

TABLE 12.2
Relaxation therapy in the control of high blood pressure (Brauer *et al.*, 1979)

	Baseline mmHg	Post-treatment mmHg	Six-month follow-up mmHg
Relaxation, live therapist	153/92·7	142·8/86·6	136/83
Relaxation, taped instructions	150/94·8	144·7/93·8	150·7/90·2
Non-specific therapy	145·2/93·1	136·4/88·6	143·6/92

jects (Steptoe, 1977c; Elder *et al.*, 1979). However, the alterations are generally no greater than those produced with simple relaxation procedures (Steptoe, 1978b; Fey and Lindholm, 1978).

Two factors may account for the relatively poor results with blood pressure feedback techniques. The first problem lies in methods of measurement. Voluntary control is thought to depend on the quality of the feedback, and will improve as the amount of information available to the subject increases (Steptoe, 1979a). Conventional indirect blood pressure recording devices are not sufficient, since they have discontinuous outputs. Furthermore, repeated squeezing of a limb with an occlusion cuff may itself be distracting, and handicap attempts to lower arterial pressure. Dynamic measures of cardiovascular function may be more appropriate tools in feedback treatment (Steptoe, 1980a).

The second difficulty concerns the manner in which psychological training procedures are applied. Skills are generally taught in undistracting, resting conditions, but these may not be the most suitable, as will be seen in the next section.

Control of cardiovascular reactivity

Psychological factors may play a role in the initiation of hypertension through stimulation of traffic in the cardiac sympathetic fibres. These pathways are activated most strongly when people attempt to cope actively with sources of threat or disturbance. In the resting state, their contribution to haemodynamic regulation is less pronounced. Consequently, voluntary control techniques might be more useful in overcoming pressor reactions, than in modifying tonic levels of cardiovascular activity (Steptoe, 1979b). Biofeedback and relaxation procedures have usually been administered in undisturbing conditions, in the hope that the skills acquired might generalise to more taxing environments. However, the voluntary control of reactions may utilise resources that are not tapped in the resting state.

Over a number of years, the author and his colleagues have developed laboratory analogues of stressful conditions in order to assess the value of biofeedback and relaxation in this context. The initial studies indicated that while feedback and relaxation instructions produced equivalent modifications in cardiovascular activity at rest, feedback allowed greater control of reactions to mental tasks (Steptoe, 1978b). The feedback group was provided with a visual analogue display of pulse transit time, an index that varies with arterial pressure, while also being sensitive to cardiac sympathetic influences (Steptoe *et al.*,

1976; Newlin and Levenson, 1979). Groups trained with feedback apparently showed more rapid control over circulatory reactions to mental arithmetic and other demanding tests than volunteers performing relaxation exercises. However, recent investigations suggest that both methods are useful. Fig. 12.3 summarises data from a further comparison, in which cardiovascular reactions were assessed in three groups of normotensives (Steptoe and Ross, 1980b). Transit time feedback was again used, while relaxation subjects followed a sequence of instructions designed to help them achieve muscular and autonomic calm. A third set performed the same laboratory tasks as the other

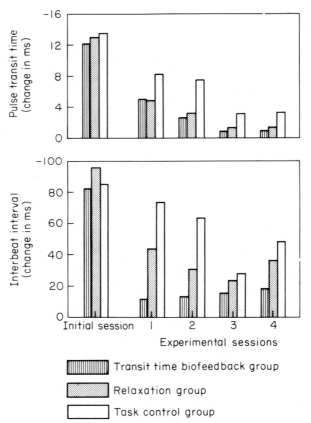

FIG. 12.3. Mean transit time (top) and interbeat interval (bottom) reactions in three groups of volunteers ($n = 10$ per group). Initial session reactions were monitored during task performance when no voluntary control was attempted. In subsequent sessions, biofeedback and relaxation subjects attempted to control cardiovascular activity during task performance. (Steptoe and Ross, 1980b.)

groups, but were not asked to control blood pressure. The results indicate that substantial cardiovascular reactions were produced by all groups before training; however, during later treatment sessions, significantly smaller tachycardias and pressor responses were shown in the feedback and relaxation conditions. Differences between these treatment groups were modest, although biofeedback may again have permitted more rapid control over reactions.

These short-term laboratory experiments confirm the feasibility of training subjects to overcome cardiovascular reactions. They are based on consideration of the physiopathology of high arterial pressure, and the contribution of psychological elements. They indicate ways through which the efficacy of voluntary control techniques may be improved. Other investigators have demonstrated reactivity control using procedures such as heart rate biofeedback and meditation (Patel, 1975; DeGood and Adams, 1976). It must be emphasised that these psychological methods require a fundamental reorientation of patients and medical professionals. Instead of physicians taking the major role in deciding on treatment and administering medication, the behavioural approach challenges the patient to active involvement in management. Blood pressure regulation thus becomes a joint venture, in which the motivation and application of the patient is as important as the physician's ability to train appropriate voluntary control skills.

Type A coronary-prone behaviour

Since Type A behaviour has been recognised as a risk factor, at least in some cultures, it may be a legitimate target for modification. However, the agent who attempts to change such a wide-ranging behavioural style faces grave responsibilities. The logic of prevention implies that healthy Type A individuals may be encouraged to alter their way of life, ambitions, gratifications and goals, for the sake of a potential threat to wellbeing in the future. Evidence discussed in Chapter 10 suggests that modification of the behaviour may even have economic repercussions for the client. On the other hand, since Type A characteristics have been formulated so vaguely, it is not certain that all the behaviours associated with the pattern would have to be altered in order to reduce cardiac risk (Friedman, 1979).

An additional problem is the choice of outcome variables in the assessment of interventions. Once patients recognise the elements considered to be undesirable, they may conceal these facets during evaluation. Both interview and questionnaire measures can be defrauded, leading to spurious changes in behaviour⌊An alternative is to monitor modifications in other factors such as serum cholesterol or blood pressure; yet since Type A behaviour is regarded as an independent risk, the significance of fluctuations in these variables is uncertain⌋ It may be useful to develop techniques of assessment by independent parties including relatives or colleagues, who could identify changes outside the treatment setting. Such procedures are only likely to be reliable if assessors are required to measure specific actions, rather than vague generalities about behavioural style. Ideally intervention should be followed by analysis of long term cardiovascular morbidity, as in the case of other attempts at primary prevention.

The published reports on altering Type A behaviour reflect these special methodological difficulties.⌊Suinn and Bloom (1978) for example, hypothesised that the link between coronary-prone behaviour and ischaemic heart disease is mediated by "stress"⌋ Accordingly, they adapted the methods of Anxiety Management Training (AMT) for a group of seven middle-class males, recruited by advertisements describing the Type A behaviour pattern. AMT involves relaxation, followed by the evocation of anxiety through imagery, so that the physical cues associated with arousal can be identified. Finally, relaxation is incorporated as a method of coping with the arousal. The treatment group was compared with a matched series of waiting list controls.

Following six training sessions, those who had undergone AMT reported lower anxiety on the State–Trait inventory, but there were no reliable differences in modifications of blood pressure or serum cholesterol. The Type A scores on the JAS did not change significantly, although there was an alteration on one subscale of the questionnaire. Thus the fluctuations in anxiety were not accompanied by adjustments in Type A characteristics. Similarly, training based on Suinn's technique failed to modify Type A behaviour in a study conducted by Jenni and Wollersheim (1979). These investigators compared AMT with a cognitive restructuring programme, which involved the identification of thoughts associated with tension cues or threats. Clients were taught to evaluate these cognitions, and replace them with more reasonable self-statements. A third group acted as waiting-list controls. Only the cognitive therapy group reduced their Type A profiles, as assessed with a self-rated questionnaire. Few reliable changes were measured in physiological variables, although the AMT group showed a small rise in serum cholesterol.

Both these interventions utilised procedures designed for the management of psychological stress and anxiety. However, unless the coronary-prone are noted for their anxiety, such techniques may not be appropriate. Roskies *et al.* (1978; 1979) took a different approach, comparing brief psychotherapy and behavioural methods. Psychotherapy was centred on the hypothesis that coronary-prone characteristics originate in specific patterns of family dynamics early in life, while the behavioural group were taught relaxation and self-monitoring of tension. After 14 sessions of treatment, both groups exhibited significant decreases in systolic pressure and serum cholesterol. There were no important differences between the modifications, although the effects of the behavioural therapy were more enduring on 6-month follow-up.

It is certain that many efforts will be made to modify Type A behaviour over future years. These attempts will be helped by an identification of the precise activities considered dangerous, so that specific proposals about management can be put forward. Bids to change global features of personality or behaviour are rarely successful, and may result in unnecessary distress. The environmental conditions that promote Type A activities must also be explored, since the behaviour pattern does not exist in isolation. Unless the social context in which the individual operates is brought into consideration, lasting changes in behaviour are unlikely to emerge.

Multiple risk factor intervention

The value of preventive techniques would be greatly enhanced if a single procedure led to changes in several cardiovascular risks. Mass media and community programmes of counselling and education about heart disease are progressing in several centres, although changes in risk factor prevalence are not invariably found (Aronow *et al.*, 1975). The Belgian Heart Disease Prevention Project has had some success with these methods however (Kornitzer *et al.*, 1980). Over 1500 blue collar workers were categorised as high risk on the basis of arterial pressure, job activity level, smoking and serum cholesterol. They were allocated to the intervention group, and given individual counselling twice yearly. During these sessions, they were advised about fat intake, smoking and activity, and were encouraged to consult their physicians about high blood pressure. High risk control subjects were also screened, but given no counselling. At 2-year follow-up, serum cholesterol had fallen by an average of 3·9 per cent in the high risk intervention cohort, compared with an increase of 0·4 per cent in the high risk controls. Systolic pressure was down by 7·8 per cent, while controls showed a 3·4 per cent change. The number of cigarette smokers declined in both groups, but the change in daily cigarette consumption was less in the control condition. In combination it was estimated that these modifications had reduced the risk of heart disease by 20 per cent in the intervention group, contrasting with an increase of 12·5 per cent in the vulnerability of high risk controls.

The Belgian study has not utilised systematic behavioural techniques for altering cardiovascular risks, but relies on more traditional medical advisory consultation. The same is true of several other community based primary prevention programmes (MRFIT, 1976; Puska *et al.*, 1979). However, experimental psychological research suggests that behavioural change may be enhanced by procedures such as modelling, self-monitoring and contingency management. Combinations of mass education and propaganda with individual instructions may also prove valuable. Such approaches have been pioneered in the Stanford Heart Disease Prevention Program. Meyer and Henderson (1974) compared a number of individually based techniques, assessing their applicability in primary prevention. Subjects identified as high risk during screening were allocated to three groups. Those in the behaviour modification condition ($N=12$) concentrated on altering activities thought to promote risk. Overweight and high cholesterol diets, for example, were considered to be dependent on shopping habits, the type and quality of food consumed, the frequency of eating and other aspects. Educational, self-monitoring, modelling and reward techniques were all mobilised to alter these behaviours. A second group ($N=10$) had individual counselling, in which information and encouragement were supplied without specific behavioural instructions. A third, control group had just one session with a physician, in which advice was given about risks.

Members of all groups reduced weight where this was appropriate, but the changes were significantly greater in the two treatment conditions. Alterations in diet and physical activity were also recorded. Although behaviour modification and counselling strategies showed effects of a similar order, improvements were sustained more consistently by the former. For instance, the average serum cholesterol level fell by 18·1 per cent across the treatment phase in the behaviour modification group, and by 16·4 per cent in the counselling condition. But at 3-months follow-up, the counselled subjects had regressed to 10·3 per cent while the behaviour modification group maintained a 16·3 per cent decrease; the corresponding change in controls was 6·90 per cent.

A programme based on the behaviour modification package was incorporated into the full-scale project (Farquhar *et al.*, 1977; Meyer *et al.*, 1980). Three Californian towns were selected for the study. One

(Tracy) acted as control, while the second (Gilroy) was subject to an extensive mass media campaign for two years. Television, radio, newspaper and advertising drives against cardiac risks were accompanied by information designed to increase knowledge of heart disease. In the third town (Watsonville), the media campaigns were augmented by intensive instruction in two-thirds of high-risk subjects.

The results over the three study years suggest that both mass and individually based interventions have an effect on cardiovascular risks. Table 12.3 illustrates the changes on risk, estimated from multiple logistic formulae. The small reduction of risk in the mass media groups after one year had extended to 25 per cent by the second follow-up. This contrasts with the relatively small changes of risk in the control (Tracy) sample. The modifications in the intensive instruction group were larger, and sustained throughout the study. Knowledge of risk behaviours and heart disease complimented the reduced vulnerability of the intervention groups.

The breakdown of factors contributing to the multiple risk adjustments reveal some interesting patterns. Systolic blood pressure fell in both mass and intensive instruction groups. Since there were no significant differences in body weight, this may have been a consequence of improved drug treatment or increased compliance. Surprisingly little change was recorded in physical exercise measures, while all treatment groups modified dietary intake of cholesterol and saturated fats. The alterations in diet tended to be larger in the intensive instruction condition, but the greatest advantage of this procedure lay in smoking modifications. The reported number of cigarettes consumed per day was down by more than 45 per cent in the second and third

TABLE 12.3
Percentage change in risk in the Stanford Heart Disease Prevention Program
(Meyer *et al.*, 1980)

	Follow-up years		
	1	2	3
Intensive instruction (Watsonville)	− 27·8	− 30·1	− 29·0
Mass media (Watsonville)	− 11·6	− 25·6	− 23·1
Mass media (Gilroy)	− 8·1	− 25·5	− 16·1
Control (Tracy)	5·7	− 2·3	− 8·0

year follow-ups, compared with less than 20 per cent in the mass media groups.

None of the procedures described thus far have attempted to alter activity in the autonomic nervous pathways directly. However the relaxation and biofeedback techniques applied to essential hypertension may also be valuable in a broader context. Patel (1976) found that the patients participating in her treatment programme also showed decreases in cholesterol. The mean pretrial concentration of 241·6 mg/100 ml (6·24 mmol l^{-1}) fell an average of 24·5 mg/100 ml (0·63 mmol l^{-1}) after six weekly treatment sessions. Weight and medication were constant, although some individuals showed decreases of more than 50 mg/100 ml (1·29 mmol l^{-1}). This uncontrolled series was subsequently extended in a multiple risk intervention study (Patel *et al.*, note 1). Over 1100 middle-aged industrial employees were screened, and those not already under treatment who fulfilled blood pressure, serum cholesterol and cigarette smoking criteria were recalled. Blood pressures were reassessed to exclude cases where readings fell below 140/90 mmHg. Consequently, 230 subjects remained at risk on two or three of the factors: pressure over 140/90 mmHg, cholesterol more than 243·8 mg/100 ml (6·3 mmol l^{-1}), and 10 or more cigarettes per day. The 240 who consented to participate were allocated to two groups, matched on age, sex, and risk factors. Treatment subjects attended 8 group sessions of one hour, in which they learned the biofeedback and meditation procedures described earlier (p. 211). They also had access to health education material, while controls had only a short counselling session plus health literature.

Some of the principle results are summarised in Table 12.4. Amongst those individuals with high blood pressure, significant decreases were measured in both groups, but the effects of active treatment were greater. This pattern persisted at 6 months, confirming the observations of Patel and North (Fig. 12.2). Serum cholesterol also fell, with biofeedback subjects producing larger changes post treatment, but not on follow-up. Nearly 68 per cent of smokers in the therapy condition had restricted their usage by the end of treatment, compared with 39 per cent of controls, and modest changes were seen in the number of cigarettes consumed each day. Reductions of noradrenaline, plasma renin activity and aldosterone were also recorded in biofeedback subjects, suggesting some of the mechanisms by which the treatment may operate.

Psychological procedures may therefore be useful in the modification of risk factors on a large scale, even in populations that are not especially attuned to prevention. Patel and her colleagues have calculated that

TABLE 12.4
Modification of cardiovascular risk factors. (Patel *et al.* Reference Note 1.)

Variable	% of group at risk Biofeedback (n=99)	% of group at risk Control (n=93)	Reduction: Pre-post treatment Mean ± s.e. Biofeedback	Reduction: Pre-post treatment Mean ± s.e. Control	Reduction: Pre-6 months follow-up Mean ± s.e. Biofeedback	Reduction: Pre-6 months follow-up Mean ± s.e. Control
Blood pressure						
Systolic (mmHg)	64	62	18·0 ± 1·72[a]	8·8 ± 1·42	20·2 ± 1·99[a]	11·2 ± 1·70
Diastolic (mmHg)			10·6 ± 1·37[a]	3·8 ± 1·04	11·5 ± 1·43[a]	3·2 ± 1·32
Serum cholesterol mg per 100 ml plasma (mmol l^{-1})	82	87	34·8 ± 4·64[b] (0·90 ± 0·12)	20·1 ± 4·64 (0·52 ± 0·12)	29·8 ± 3·87 (0·77 ± 0·10)	21·7 ± 4·26 (0·56 ± 0·11)
Cigarette smoking (average number of cigarettes per day)	82	70	5·8 ± 0·73[a]	2·6 ± 0·75	4·8 ± 0·77	2·3 ± 0·74

[a] Significant difference between groups (t test), $p < 0.01$–0.001.
[b] Significant differences between groups (t test), $p < 0.05$.

these adjustments would lessen the likelihood of death from heart disease by some 20 per cent; such benefits cannot be ignored.

Exercise, biofeedback and myocardial function

Behavioural methods do not lose their importance once ischaemic heart disease has been identified. They may be particularly valuable in helping to expand the functional capacity of the circulatory system. The effects of physical exercise have been explored in both animals and man. Froelicher (1978) reviewed studies of swimming and treadmill exercise in rodents, and concluded that changes typically included increased cardiac performance and coronary artery calibre, myocardial hypertrophy and a raised capillary-to-fibre ratio in myocardial tissue. Modifications of cardiac ultrastructure, with enlargement of mitochondria, have also been observed.

[Carefully graded systematic programmes of physical conditioning are recommended both for prevention, and the rehabilitation of patients following infarction (Naughton and Hellerstein, 1973; Wenger, 1978). Cardiovascular function is not improved by all forms of exercise; isometrics, and training in violent but brief anaerobic work (e.g. sprinting), are not beneficial (Froelicher, 1973). Similarly gentle, casual exercise, such as walking or golf, is thought to be ineffective (Cureton, 1966). Three to four sessions weekly of 30 minutes work at 60 per cent of maximal oxygen consumption will generally promote cardiovascular adaptation (Scheuer and Tipton, 1977). However, exercise programmes for cardiac patients have to be carefully managed, since overwork may be dangerous (Hellerstein and Franklin, 1978).

A low resting heart rate is regularly observed after physical training, being typical of athletes, and those who have exercised consistently for a few months (Froelicher, 1973). The mechanism remains obscure, although both increases in vagal tone, and reductions of cardiac sympathetic traffic, may be involved. Heart rate responses to submaximal exercise are also attenuated, and this permits the maximal workload to rise. Although resting arterial pressure may not alter, responses during exercise are again less marked.

These adjustments of haemodynamic response have clear implications for the management of angina pectoris. Patients with stable angina develop pain at a relatively constant workload, after correction for heart rate. A critical value of cardiovascular function can be established, by multiplying heart rate by arterial pressure; this rate–

pressure product predicts when pain will develop in exercise-induced angina (Robinson, 1967). Physical training allows work to be performed at a smaller cardiovascular cost; consequently, the amount of activity that can be produced before the rate–pressure product is reached will be larger. Direct benefits to ischaemic patients might also result from improvements in myocardial vascularity, and the opening up of collateral vessels — but unfortunately, such effects have not been demonstrated angiographically in man (Conner *et al.*, 1976). Changes in the peripheral circulation appear to combine with cardiac modifications in augmenting haemodynamic efficiency.

Despite current enthusiasm for physical conditioning, positive effects for cardiac morbidity and mortality have yet to be established. Epidemiological studies have uncovered prevalence differences between the sedentary and fit, but have not evaluated exercise training *per se*. The prospective assessment of long-term consequences for healthy subjects would be a formidable undertaking; efforts have therefore been concentrated on high risk post-infarction groups thus far. Yet neither of the randomised trials of training, in Scandinavia and in the USA, showed significant differences between exercising patients and controls (Wilhelmsen *et al.*, 1975; Froelicher, 1978). Moreover, physical conditioning programmes are subject to drop-outs and non-compliance, in the same way as other interventions. Reported rates of adherence vary from 13 to 81 per cent at 12 months follow-up, but may be inflated in many cases by the use of volunteer groups. Oldridge *et al.* (1978) found that only 57 per cent of the post-infarction patients randomly assigned to different training groups were still in programmes after one year. Of the non-compliers 46 per cent dropped out within one month, and these people appeared to belong to the subsection of the group at greatest risk. They were more likely to have suffered recurrent infarcts, show Type A characteristics, and be inactive smokers. It is unfortunate, but haemodynamic improvements are only maintained with persistent training; as in animals, effects are reversed after a few weeks of inactivity (Scheuer and Tipton, 1977).

An additional behavioural technique has recently been explored that may also be valuable in helping angina sufferers to perform more work at lower cardiovascular cost. This involves the introduction of biofeedback of heart rate or blood pressure in exercising individuals Clemens and Shattock (1979) demonstrated that healthy volunteers can modify their heart rate responses to static muscular effort, and studies of heart rate control during dynamic (treadmill) work have also been reported (Goldstein *et al.*, 1977). In Fig. 12.4, the results collected by Perski and Engel (1980) are illustrated, showing the haemodynamic

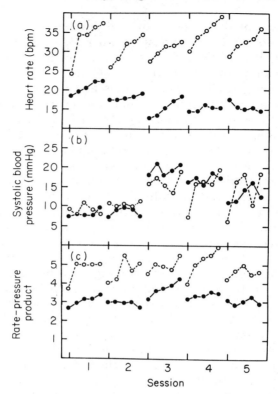

Fig. 12.4. Changes in heart rate (a), systolic blood pressure (b) and rate–pressure product (c) during the five trials of five successive experimental sessions. ●——●, Exercise + feedback; ○----○, exercise without feedback. (Perski and Engel, 1980.)

responses of two groups exercising on bicycle ergonometers at rates of 370–380 kg m min^{-1}. The feedback group watched visual displays of their heart rates, and were instructed to lower rate while exercising. The overall difference in heart rate response was significant, and emerged consistently in all five sessions. Systolic pressure increases were not attenuated, but the decrease in tachycardia was sufficiently great to reduce the rate–pressure product for this level of physical work. If these modifications are duplicated in patients with angina, and can be extended outside the laboratory, they will constitute a useful addition to the armoury of behavioural techniques for assisting the patient with coronary stenosis.

Biofeedback in the regulation of cardiac arrhythmias

The application of voluntary control procedures to the management of cardiac arrhythmias has also been pioneered by Engel. A series of eight patients with premature ventricular contractions was studied in 1971; although the therapeutic effects were compromised by the brevity of pretraining baselines and the lack of a control group, the results remain interesting (Weiss and Engel, 1971). Patients were trained with heart rate feedback, being taught both to raise and lower rate, and finally to retain the rhythm within a narrow range. After very extended treatment programmes many patients showed reductions in frequency of premature ventricular contractions, and these were maintained at follow-up over a year later. Pretreatment extrasystole incidences of up to 20 per minute, were attenuated to 0–1 per minute on follow-up. The single cases studied by Pickering and his associates also indicate some success with this technique (Pickering and Miller, 1977). Pickering and Graham's (1975) patient initially displayed a ventricular parasystolic rhythm whenever heart rate exceeded 72 bpm. After 12 biofeedback sessions, the arrhythmia did not emerge until heart rates were more than 106 bpm. Engel and Bleeker (1974) showed modifications in patients with a variety of other arrhythmias, including atrial fibrillation and supraventricular tachycardia. In several cases, voluntary control produced improvements where drug treatments had been ineffective.

None of these investigations have included control groups, so feedback effects cannot be distinguished from changes due to treatment expectation, clinical attention and laboratory habituation. Moreover, it appears that the acquisition of voluntary skills requires extensive training with relatively sophisticated monitoring techniques; the bulk of Weiss and Engel's (1971) successes, for example, participated in more than 45 sessions of treatment. Thus unless robust and stable responses can be generated in a greatly abbreviated treatment time, it is unlikely that biofeedback will be recommended as an alternative, or even an adjunct, to pharmacological interventions with the problem.

Acute coronary care and rehabilitation

The medical literature is well stocked with admonishments on the failure of staff to treat cardiac patients as complete people, but as inanimate objects with mechanical problems. Recommendations about social and psychological counselling are common, yet few have been evaluated systematically. Uncontrolled assessments of psychologically orientated management programmes are of limited value, since patients vary considerably in recovery rates and severity of illness. Furthermore, opinions about patterns of medical care are divided, and methods of treatment, such as early or late mobilisation, can differ widely between centres (Lindvall *et al.*, 1979); consequently, trends in psychosocial rehabilitation may be confounded with other factors.

There is, however, general agreement that one of the problems most frequently encountered by patients and their relatives is a lack of information. Patients often have little understanding of their illness or its treatment, and complain that they have been told even less (Mayou *et al.*, 1976). They also tend to be dissatisfied about the advice given on discharge, and remain uncertain about what activities are permitted, what food may be eaten, and what relatives can do about care. Misconceptions about heart attacks are rife — Hackett and Cassem (1978) have listed several common errors, including the beliefs that mild exercise, sex and motorcar driving are all forbidden, that heart attacks will recur on anniversaries, and that patients will die at the same age as their parents. Many sufferers think a myocardial infarction means that a hole has been punctured through the heart.

Special efforts at communication and education have been introduced in some clinics, and these do seem to have an impact on the patients' knowledge (Bracken *et al.*, 1977). Acker (1976) compared patients given routine coronary care and hospital rehabilitation with a special care group. The latter were provided with a special patient area, with activity and educational schemes, psychological support and a vigorous orientation towards recovery. The average number of days spent in hospital was significantly shorter in the special care group (19·3 compared with 22·7), while convalescence time was also reduced (78·9 and 100·9 days). The differences in rate of returning to work or re-employment were most marked amongst the younger (< 50 year), lower class patients. Another trial, with random allocation of infarct survivors to psychological rehabilitation and control groups, also found effects on speed of returning to work, but little impact on ratings of emotional stability (Naismith *et al.*, 1979).

The patterns observed in these studies may have been due to the amount of attention and interest shown in patients, rather than specific effects of the procedures themselves. A more detailed evaluation of different forms of attention was provided by Cromwell and associates (1977) in a comparison of coronary care regimens. Three factors were manipulated:

a. Level of information — half the patients were provided with detailed information about heart conditions and the Coronary Care Unit (CCU), together with advice on recovery, diet, work and risk behaviours. The low information group was given the conventional description of the CCU and hospital procedures.

b. Level of diversion — the high group had television, windows near their beds, reading material and relaxed visiting hours, while these sources of diversion were more restricted in the low condition.

c. Level of participation — the high participation group were encouraged to involve themselves in the recovery process. They could switch on their ECGs when they experienced symptoms, and were given systematic exercise schedules in the CCU. By contrast, low participation patients were treated with complete bedrest, and little movement.

The factors were combined in all permutations in a factorial design for a large number of infarction victims. Patients allocated to low information, low diversion, low participation were not deprived, but were in the position common in most CCU. All received the same intensive nursing.

Unfortunately, the obvious differences in treatment format prevented a blind assessment of recovery, and subtle fluctuations in medical care may have been present. Nevertheless, the length of stay in the CCU and hospital was longest amongst patients who received information, but no diversion or opportunity to participate (mean 28·0 days); by contrast, high information plus high levels on one of the other factors was associated with a short stay (19·5 days for information plus diversion, and 20·9 for information plus participation). Those exposed to high levels on all three factors recovered at an intermediate rate. This pattern was reflected in some of the other outcome variables, although reinfarction and re-employment were unrelated to the interventions. The study suggests that information alone is not sufficient to promote change. Information is helpful, provided that it is coupled with some practical action. However, too much stimulation may not be beneficial.

The role of psychosocial factors in rehabilitation is well established. Clinical impressions and correlational surveys suggest that recovery and return to former activities are dependent on psychic wellbeing and the social context. The reasons for failures to resume work at an early date are predominantly social and personal, rather than medical (Mulcahy, 1976; Pancheri *et al.*, 1978). The depressed are especially vulnerable, and may be at greater risk for readmission (Stern *et al.*, 1977). However, socioeconomic factors cannot be ignored. The rate of re-employment is greater in professional and executive circles, and lowest amongst manual workers (Croog and Levine, 1977; Finlayson and McEwen, 1977).

Nagle *et al.* (1976) introduced a special education scheme, involving general practitioners, patients and hospital staff, in order to encourage the social rehabilitation of infarction survivors. The proportion of cases classified as mild on clinical criteria, who returned to work, increased from 55 to 69 per cent. Another strategy that has been exploited is relaxation training. Short-term studies of patients with organic heart disease indicate that relaxation is associated with falls in plasma noradrenaline and cardiac contractility, suggesting that sympathetic tone to the heart is reduced (Davidson *et al.*, 1979). Fielding (1979) provided group counselling and relaxation training, demonstrating positive effects in terms of recovery and relapse rate, in comparison with minimally treated controls. Compliance with rehabilitation programmes may also be a problem; some patients have unrealistic expectations of future work capacity, refuse to slow down, and may even doubt the reality of their illness. Baile and Engel (1978) encouraged such patients to become involved in the structuring of rehabilitation, monitoring pulse rate during exercises and systematically scheduling their progress. These procedures appeared to enhance compliance in a small group of recalcitrant subjects, confirming that adherence to treatment may be increased by engaging patients directly, and giving them responsibility.

Several methods of aiding social recovery, and helping patients come to terms with their problem, are thus being explored. Their value and general applicability cannot be gauged at present, but as more behavioural scientists are attracted to the field, the advantages of a multidiscplinary approach may become more apparent.

Summary and conclusions

This chapter reflects the recent changes of emphasis in psychosocial studies of cardiovascular morbidity. More and more behavioural scientists have moved from description to action, and have become involved in attempts to reduce risk and aid recovery. Much interesting descriptive material on acute cardiovascular disease has unfortunately been omitted. For example, the reasons why patients delay seeking help after their first experience of symptoms have received much attention. These delays appear due primarily to misinterpretation of symptoms and the time taken to reach decisions about appropriate action, rather than transportation and other physical hindrances (Gentry, 1975). Similarly, the impact of acute crises on patients and their families, and analyses of the social context of rehabilitation, have been passed over (Croog and Levine, 1977; Finlayson and McEwen, 1977).

Many of the interventions discussed have derived from the psycho-physiological laboratory, and their application to patients is still at a preliminary stage. Biofeedback, relaxation and other techniques for the voluntary control of cardiovascular function may be relevant at all phases of coronary morbidity from primary risk to rehabilitation. The use of these methods in regulating high arterial pressure may be facilitated by procedures aimed at overcoming hyper-reactivity, and lability in the presence of psychosocial threats. Similarly, the extension of self control to angina involves training patients to modify cardiac responses during physical exercise.

Behavioural interventions are establishing their importance in the armoury of preventive techniques. Many primary risks are themselves behaviours, while others may be reduced most economically by altering habits and actions. Risk intervention programmes have been administered both on a population basis, disseminating health education and advice, and to individuals or small groups. The individual approach may be more costly in the short term, but ultimately more powerful, since methods can be tailored to idiosyncratic problems. Attention has to be paid as much to maintenance of change, as to the initial intervention. Behaviour change is in many ways more appealing than pharmacological regimens in primary prevention.

It is difficult to predict the ultimate status of psychological procedures in the battery of clinical methods. Enthusiasm for a treatment does not depend simply on its efficacy, but on a whole constellation of secondary factors, including expense, ease of administration and professional training requirements. Thus even if psychological interventions are fruitful, they may not be favoured over pharmacological or surgical procedures. However, a number of behavioural strategies are efficient and economic, in that they can be administered by auxiliary personnel, and may repay initial efforts with long-term benefits. Some may be preferred on humanitarian as well as medical grounds, in giving patients greater control over their own fate. Many individuals like a share in responsibility for their own care, rather than complete dependence on external aids.

References

ABILDSKOV, J. A. and VINCENT, G. M. (1977). The autonomic nervous system in relation to electrocardiographic waveform and cardiac rhythm. *In* "Neural Regulation of the Heart" (W. C. Randall, Ed.), pp. 409–424. Oxford University Press, Oxford.

ABU-ZEID, H., CHOI, N. W. and NELSON, N. A. (1975). Epidemiologic features of cerebrovascular disease in Manitoba; Incidence by age, sex and residence, with etiologic implications. *Can. med. Ass. J.* **113**, 379–384.

ACKER, J. E. (1976). Socio-economic factors affected by an in-hospital cardiac rehabilitation program. *In* "Psychological Approach to the Rehabilitation of Coronary Patients" (U. Stocksmeier, Ed.), pp. 96–100. Springer-Verlag, New York.

ADAMS, D. B., BACCELLI, G., MANCIA, G. and ZANCHETTI, A. (1969). Cardiovascular changes during naturally elicited behaviour in the cat. *Am. J. Physiol.* **216**, 1226–1235.

ADLER, R., MACRITCHIE, K. and ENGEL, G. L. (1971). Psychologic process and ischaemic stroke (occlusive cerebrovascular disease). 1. Observations on 32 men with 35 strokes. *Psychosom. Med.* **33**, 1–30.

ADSETT, C. A., SCHOTTSTAEDT, W. W. and WOLF, S. G. (1962). Changes in coronary blood flow and other haemodynamic indicators induced by stressful interviews. *Psychosom. Med.* **24**, 331–336.

AHNVE, S., DE FAIRE, U., ORTH-GOMÉR, K. and THEORELL, T. (1979). Type-A behaviour in patients with non-coronary chest pain admitted to a CCU. *J. psychosom. Res.* **23**, 219–223.

AGNOLI, A. and FAZIO, C. (Eds) (1977). "Platelet aggregation in the pathogenesis of cerebrovascular disorders". Springer-Verlag, New York.

ALEXANDER, F. (1952). "Psychosomatic Medicine". Allen and Unwin, London.

ALEKSANDROW, D. (1967). Studies on the epidemiology of hypertension in Poland. *In* "The Epidemiology of Hypertension" (J. Stamler, R. Stamler and T. N. Pullman, Eds), pp. 82–96. Grune and Stratton, New York.

ANDERSON, D. E. and BRADY, J. V. (1973). Prolonged preavoidance effects on blood pressure and heart rate in the dog. *Psychosom. Med.* **35**, 4–12.

ANDERSON, D. E. and BRADY, J. V. (1976). Cardiovascular responses to avoidance conditioning in the dog: effects of beta-adrenergic blockade. *Psychosom. Med.* **38**, 181–189.

ANDERSON, D. E. and TOSHEFF, J. G. (1973). Cardiac output and total peripheral resistance changes during preavoidance periods in dogs. *J. appl. Physiol.* **34**, 650–654.

ARDLIE, N. G., GLEW, G. and SCHWARTZ, C. J. (1966). Influence of catecholamines on nucleotide-induced platelet aggregation. *Nature, Lond.* **212**, 415–417.

ARKEL, Y. S. (1976). Evaluation of platelet aggregation in disorders of hemostasis. *Med. Clins. N. Am.* **60**, 881–911.

ARKEL, Y. S., HAFT, J. I., KREUTNER, W., SHERWOOD, J. and WILLIAMS, R. (1977). Alteration in second phase platelet aggregation associated with an emotionally stressful activity. *Thromb. Haemost.* **38**, 552–561.

ARMITAGE, P. and ROSE, G. A. (1966). The variability of measurements of casual blood pressure. 1. Laboratory study. *Clin. Sci. molec. Med.* **30**, 325–335.

ARONOW, W. S., ALLEM, W. H., DE CHRISTOFARO, D. and UNGERMANN, S. (1975). Follow-up of mass screening for coronary risk factors in 1817 adults. *Circulation*, **51**, 1038–1045.

AVERILL, J. R. (1973). Personal control over aversive stimuli and its relationship to stress. *Psychol. Bull.* **80**, 286–303.

AX, A. (1953). The physiological differentiation between fear and anger in humans. *Psychosom. Med.* **15**, 433–442.

AXELROD, J. (1965). The metabolism, storage and release of catecholamines. *Recent Prog. Horm. Res.* **21**, 597–622.

AXELROD, J. (1976). Catecholamines and hypertension. *Clin. Sci. molec. Med.* **51**, 415S–421S.

BAILE, W. F. and ENGEL, B. T. (1978). A behavioral strategy for promoting treatment compliance following myocardial infarction. *Psychosom Med.* **40**, 413–419.

BALTER, M. and LEVINE, J. (1977). Psychiatric aspects of hypertension. *In* "Stress and the Heart" (D. Wheatley, Ed.). pp. 157–173. Raven Press, New York.

BANAHAN, B. F., SHARPE, T. R., BAKER, J. A., LIAO, W. C. and SMITH, M. C. (1979). Hypertension and stress: a preventative approach. *J. psychosom. Res.* **23**, 69–75.

BARD, P. (1960). Anatomical organisation of the central nervous system in relation to control of the heart and blood vessels. *Physiol. Rev. Suppl.* **4**, 3–26.

BARNARD, R. J., GARDNER, G. W. and DIACO, N. V. (1976). "Ischaemic" heart disease in firefighters with normal coronary arteries. *J. occup. Med.* **18**, 818–820.

BAROLDI, G. (1969). Lack of correlation between coronary thrombosis and myocardial infarction or sudden "coronary" heart death. *Ann. N.Y. Acad. Sci.* **156**, 504–525.

BAUMANN, R., ZIPRIAN, H., GODICKE, W., HARTRODT, W., NAUMANN, E. and
LAUTER, J. (1973). The influence of acute psychic stress situations on biochemical and vegetative parameters of essential hypertensives at the early
stages of the disease. *Psychother. Psychosom.* **22**, 131–140.

BEAGLEHOLE, R., SALMOND, C. E., HOOPER, A., HUNTSMAN, J., STANHOPE,
J. M., CASSEL, J. C. and PRIOR, I. A. M. (1977). Blood pressure and social
interaction in Tokelauan migrants in New Zealand. *J. chron. Dis.* **30**,
803–812.

BEAGLEHOLE, R., EYLES, E., SALMOND, C. and PRIOR, I. A. M. (1978). Blood
pressure in Tokelauan children in two contrasting environments. *Am. J.
Epid.* **108**, 283–286.

BEAMER, V. and SHAPIRO, A. P. (1973). Comparison of pressor and adrenergic
responses derived from direct and indirect methods of cardiovascular
testing. *Psychosom. Med.* **35**, 112–120.

BECKER, M. H. and MAIMAN, L. A. (1975). Sociobehavioural determinants of
compliance with health and medical care recommendations. *Med. Care.*
13, 10–24.

BECKER, M. H., MAIMAN, L. A., KIRSCHT, J. P., HAEFNER, D. P. and DRACH-
MAN, R. H. (1977). The health belief model and prediction of dietary
compliance: a field experiment. *J. Hlth soc. Behav.* **18**, 348–368.

BEECHER, H. K. (1966). Pain: one mystery solved. *Science*, **151**, 840–841.

BELL, B. A. and SYMON, L. (1979). Smoking and subarachnoid haemorrhage.
Br. med. J. **I**, 577–578.

BELLET, S., RONAN, L. and KOSTIS, J. (1969). The effect of automobile driving
on catecholamine and adrenocortical excretion. *Am. J. Cardiol.* **24**,
365–368.

BELLO, C. T., SEVY, R. W. and HARAKAL, C. (1967). Relationship between
severity of disease and haemodynamic patterns in essential hypertension.
Am. J. med. Sci. **256**, 194–208.

BENDITT, E. P. (1976). Implications of the monoclonal character of human
atherosclerotic plaques. *Beitr. Path. Verdan Org.* **158**, 405–416.

BENGTSSON, C., HÄLLSTRÖM, T. and TIBBLIN, G. (1973). Social factors, stress
experience, and personality traits in women with ischaemic heart disease,
compared to a population sample of women. *Acta med. scand., Suppl.* **549**,
82–92.

BENNET, G. (1970). Bristol floods 1968, controlled survey of effects on health of
local community disaster. *Br. med. J.* **III**, 454–458.

BENSON, H., COSTAS, R., GARCIA-PALMIERI, M. R., FELIBERTI, M., AIXALA, R.,
BLANTON, J. H. and COLON, A. A. (1966). Coronary heart disease risk
factors: a comparison of two Puerto Rican populations. *Am. J. publ. Hlth*,
56, 1057–1060.

BENSON, H., HERD, J. A., MORSE, W. H. and KELLEHER, R. T. (1969).
Behavioral induction of hypertension and its reversal. *Am. J. Physiol.* **217**,
30–34.

BENSON, H., SHAPIRO, D., TURSKY, B. and SCHWARTZ, G. E. (1971). Decreased systolic blood pressure through operant conditioning techniques in patients with essential hypertension. *Science,* **173**, 740–742.

BERDINA, N. A., KOLENKO, O. L., KOTZ, I. M., KUZNETZOV, A., RODIONOV, I., SAUTCHENKO, A. and THOREVSKY, V. I. (1972). Increases in skeletal muscle performance during emotional stress in man. *Circulation Res.* **30**, 642–650.

BERGLUND, G., WILHELMSEN, L., SANNERSTEDT, R., HANSSON, L., ANDERSSON, O., SIVERTSSON, R., WEDEL, H. and WIKSTRAND, J. (1978). Coronary heart disease after treatment of hypertension. *Lancet,* **I**, 1–5.

BERGMAN, L. R. and MAGNUSSON, D. (1979). Overachievement and catecholamine excretion in an achievement-demanding situation. *Psychosom. Med.* **41**, 181–188.

BEVAN, A. T., HONOUR, J. and STOTT, F. H. (1969). Direct arterial pressure recording in unrestricted man. *Clin. Sci.* **36**, 329–344.

BIGLIERI, E. G. (1978). An approach to mineralocorticoid hormone hypertension. *In* "Hypertension: Mechanisms, Diagnosis and Treatment" (G. Onesti and A. N. Brest, Eds), pp. 91–97. F. A. Davis, Philadelphia.

BINIK, Y. M., THERIAULT, G. and SHUSTACK, B. (1977). Sudden death in the laboratory rat: cardiac function, sensory and experiential factors in swimming deaths. *Psychosom. Med.* **39**, 82–92.

BINIK, Y. M., DEIKEL, S. M., THERIAULT, G., SHUSTACK, B. and BALTHAZARD, C. (1979). Sudden swimming deaths: cardiac function, experimental anoxia and learned helplessness. *Psychophysiology,* **16**, 381–391.

BIRKENHÄGER, W. H. and SCHALEKAMP, M. A. D. H. (1976). "Control Mechanisms in Essential Hypertension". Elsevier, Amsterdam.

BLAIR, M. L., FEIGL, E. O. and SMITH, O. A. (1976). Elevation of plasma renin activity during avoidance performance in baboons. *Am. J. Physiol.* **231**, 772–776.

BLALOCK, H. M. (1967). Status inconsistency, social mobility, status integration and structural effects. *Am. Soc. Rev.* **32**, 790–800.

BLANCHARD, E. B., MILLER, S. T., ABEL, G. G., HAYNES, M. R. and WICKER, M. R. (1979). Evaluation of biofeedback in the treatment of borderline essential hypertension. *J. appl. Behav. Anal.* **12**, 99–109.

BLATT, C. M., VERRIER. R. L. and LOWN, B. (1977). Acute blood pressure elevation and ventricular fibrillation threshold during coronary occlusion and reperfusion in the dog. *Am. J. Cardiol.* **39**, 513–518.

BLISS, E. L., MIGEON, C. J., BRANCH, C. H. and SAMUELS, L. T. (1956). Reaction of the adrenal cortex to emotional stress. *Psychosom. Med.* **18**, 56–76.

BLIX, A. S., STRØMME, S. B. and URSIN, H. (1974). Additional heart rate – an indicator of psychological activation. *Aerospace Med.* **45**, 1219–1222.

BLOOM, D. S., STEIN, M. G. and ROSENDORFF, C. (1976). Effects of hypertensive plasma on responses of a isolated artery preparation to nor-adrenaline. *Cardiovasc. Res.* **10**, 268–274.

BLOOM, G., VON EULER, U. S. and FRANKENHAEUSER, M. (1963). Catecholamine excretion and personality traits in paratroop trainees. *Acta physiol. scand.* **58**, 77–89.

BLUMENTHAL, J. A., WILLIAMS, R. B., KONG, Y., SCHANBERG, S. M. and THOMPSON, L. W. (1978). Type A behavior pattern and coronary atherosclerosis. *Circulation*, **58**, 634–639.

BLUMENTHAL, J. A., THOMPSON, L. W., WILLIAMS, R. B. and KONG, Y. (1979). Anxiety-proneness and coronary heart disease. *J. Psychosom. Res.* **23**, 17–21.

BOHR, D. F. and BERECEK, K. H. (1976). Relevance of vascular structural and smooth muscle sensitivity changes in hypertension. *Aust. N.Z. J. Med.* **6**, Suppl. 2, 26–34.

BORN, G. V. R. (1977). Platelet aggregation in the pathogenesis of cerebro-vascular disorders. *In* "Platelet Aggregation in the Pathogenesis of Cerebrovascular Disorders" (A. Agnoli and C. Fazio, Eds), pp. 8–16. Springer-Verlag, New York.

BOURNE, P. G., ROSE, R. M. and MASON, J. W. (1967). Urinary 17-OHCS levels—data on seven helicopter medics in combat. *Archs gen. Psychiat.* **17**, 104–110.

BOURNE, P. G. (1970). "Man, Stress and Vietnam". Little, Brown and Co., Boston.

BRACKEN, M. B., BRACKEN, M. and LANDRY, A. B. (1977). Patient education by videotape after myocardial infarction: An empirical evaluation. *Archs phys. Med. Rehabil.* **58**, 213–219.

BRADY, J. V. (1965). Experimental Studies on psychophysiological responses to stressful situations. *In* "Symposium on Medical Aspects of Stress in the Military Climate". Walter Reed Army Institute of Research, Government Printing Office, Washington, D.C.

BRAND, R. J. (1978). Coronary-prone behavior as an independent risk factor for coronary heart disease. *In* "Coronary-prone Behavior" (T. M. Dembroski, S. M. Weiss, J. L. Shields, S. G. Haynes and M. Feinleib, Eds), pp. 11–24. Springer-Verlag, New York.

BRAND, R. J., ROSENMAN, R. H., SHOLTZ, R. I. and FRIEDMAN, M. (1976). Multivariate prediction of coronary heart disease in the Western Collaborative Group Study compared to the findings of the Framingham Study. *Circulation*, **53**, 348–355.

BRAND, R. J., PAFFENBARGER, R. S., SCHOLTZ, R. I. and KAMPERT, J. B. (1979). Work activity and fatal heart attack studied by multiple logistic risk analysis. *Am. J. Epidemiol.* **110**, 52–62.

BRAUER, A. P., HORLICK, L., NELSON, E., FARQUHAR, J. W. and AGRAS, W. S. (1979). Relaxation therapy for essential hypertension: A VA outpatient study. *J. behav. Med.* **2**, 21–29.

BRENER, J., PHILLIPS, K. and CONNALLY, S. R. (1977). Oxygen consumption and ambulation during operant conditioning of heart rate increases and decreases in rats. *Psychophysiology*, **14**, 483–491.

BRENER, J., PHILLIPS, K. and CONNALLY, S. (1980). Energy expenditure, heart rate and ambulation during shock-avoidance conditioning of heart rate increases and ambulation in freely-moving rats. *Psychophysiology*, **17**, 64–74.

BRITTON, J., HAWKEY, C., WOOD, W. G. and PEELE, M. (1974). Stress—a significant factor in venous thrombosis. *Br. J. Surg.* **61**, 814–820.

BROD, J., FENCL, V., HEJL, Z. and JIRKA, J. (1959). Circulatory changes underlying blood pressure elevation during acute emotional stress in normotensive and hypertensive subjects. *Clin. Sci.* **18**, 269–279.

BROOKS, D., FOX, P., LOPEZ, R. and SLEIGHT, P. (1978). The effect of mental arithmetic on blood pressure variability and baroreflex sensitivity. *J. Physiol.* **276**, 75P–76P.

BROWN, D. F., KINCH, S. and DOYLE, J. (1965). Serum triglycerides in health and ischaemic heart disease. *New Engl. J. Med.* **273**, 947–952.

BROWN, G. W. (1974). Meaning, measurement and stress of life events. *In* "Stressful Life Events: Their Nature and Effects" (B. S. Dohrenwend and B. P. Dohrenwend, Eds), pp. 217–243. Wiley, Chichester.

BROWN, G. W. and BIRLEY, J. L. T. (1968). Crises and life changes and the onset of schizophrenia. *J. Hlth soc. Behav.* **9**, 203–214.

BROWN, G. W., SKLAIR, F., HARRIS, T. O. and BIRLEY, J. L. T. (1973). Life events and psychiatric disorder: 1. Some methodological issues. *Psychol. Med.* **3**, 74–87.

BROWN, G. W., BHROLCHAIN, M. N. and HARRIS, T. (1975). Social class and psychiatric disturbance among women in an urban population. *Sociology*, **9**, 225–254.

BROWN, R. G., DAVIDSON, L. A. G., MCKEOWN, T. and WHITEFIELD, A. G. W. (1957). Coronary-artery disease: Influence affecting its incidence in the seventh decade. *Lancet*, **2**, 1073–1077.

BRUHN, J. C., WOLF, S., LYNN, T., BIRD, H. and CHANDLER, B. (1968). Social aspects of coronary-heart disease in a Pennsylvannia German community. *Soc. Sci. Med.* **2**, 201–212.

BRUHN, J. C., CHANDLER, B. and WOLF, S. (1969). A psychological study of survivors and nonsurvivors of myocardial infarction. *Psychosom. Med.* **31**, 8–19.

BRUNSWICK, A. F. and COLLETTE, P. (1977). Psychophysical correlates of elevated blood pressure: A study of urban black adolescents. *J. Human Stress*, **3** (4), 19–31.

BRUYNEEL, K. and OPIE, L. (1974). The baboon as an experimental animal for the production of myocardial infarction: Comparison with the mongrel dog. *In* "Effect of Acute Ischaemia on Myocardial Function" (M. F. Oliver, Ed.), pp. 18–23. Williams and Wilkins, Baltimore.

BUCHWALD, H., MOORE, R. B. and VARCO, R. L. (1977). Maximum lipid reduction by partial ideal bypass: A test of the lipid–atherosclerosis hypothesis. *Lipids*, **12**, 53–58.

BÜHLER, F. R., LARAGH, J. H., BAER, L., VAUGHAN, D. and BRUNNER, H. R. (1972). Propranolol inhibition of renin release. *New Engl. J. Med.* **287**, 1209–1214.

BUHLER, H. V., DA PRADA, M., HAEFELY, W. and PICOTTI, G. B. (1978).

Plasma adrenaline, noradrenaline and dopamine in man and different animal species. *J. Physiol,* **276**, 311–320.

BULPITT, C. J. and DOLLERY, C. T. (1973). Side effects of hypotensive agents evaluated by a self-administered questionnaire. *Br. med. J.* **III**, 485–490.

BURNAM, M. A., PENNEBAKER, J. W. and GLASS, D. C. (1975). Time consciousness, achievement striving and the type A coronary-prone behavior pattern. *J. abnorm. Psychol.* **84**, 76–79.

BUTENSKY, A., FARALLI, V., HEEBNER, D. and WALDRON, I. (1976). Elements of the coronary-prone behavior pattern in children and teenagers. *J. psychosom. Res.* **20**, 439–444.

CAFFREY, B. (1969). Behavior patterns and personality characteristics related to prevalence of coronary heart disease in American monks. *J. chron. Dis.* **22**, 93–103.

CAIRNCROSS, K. and BASSETT, J. R. (1975). Changes in myocardial function as a consequence of prolonged emotional stress. *Prog. Brain Res.* **42**, 313–318.

CALVERT, A., LOWN, B. and GORLIN, R. (1977). Ventricular premature beats and anatomically defined coronary heart disease. *Am. J. Cardiol.* **39**, 627–634.

CANNON, W. B. (1915). "Bodily Changes in Pain, Hunger, Fear and Rage". Routledge and Kegan Paul, London.

CANNON, W. B. (1957). "Voodoo" death. *Psychosom. Med.* **19**, 182–190.

CAPLAN, R. D., COBB, S., FRENCH, J. R. P., HARRISON, R. V. and PINNEAU, S. R. (1975). Job demands and worker health. NIOSH Report, DHEW Publication 75–160, Washington, D.C.

CARLSON, L., LEVI, L. and ORÖ, L. (1968). Plasma lipids and urinary excretion of catecholamines in man during experimentally induced emotional stress, and their modification by nicotinic acid. *J. clin. Invest.* **47**, 1795–1805.

CARNAHAN, J. E. and NUGENT, C. A. (1975). The effects of self-monitoring by patients on the control of hypertension. *Am. J. med. Sci.* **269**, 69–73.

CARROLL, D. and ANASTASIADES, P. (1978). The behavioural significance of heart rate: The Laceys' hypothesis. *Biol. Psychol.* **7**, 249–275.

CARRUTHERS, M. and TAGGART, P. (1973). Vagotonicity of violence: Biochemical and cardiac responses to violent films and television programmes. *Br. med. J.* **III**, 384–389.

CARRUTHERS, M., ARGUELLES, A. F. and MOSOVICH, A. (1976). Man in transit: Biochemical and physiological changes during intercontinental flights. *Lancet,* **I**, 977–981.

CHAMOVE, A. S. and BOWMAN, R. E. (1978). Rhesus plasma cortisol response at four dominance positions. *Aggress. Behav.* **4**, 43–55.

CHANDLER, A. B. and POPE, J. T. (1975). Arterial thrombosis in atherogenesis. *In* "Blood and Arterial Wall in Atherogenesis and Arterial Thrombosis" (J. G. A. J. Hautvast, R. J. J. Hermus and F. Van Der Haar, Eds), pp. 111–118. E. J. Brill, Leiden.

CHAPMAN, W. P., LIVINGSTON, R., LIVINGSTON, K. and SWEET, W. (1950).

Possible cortical areas involved in arterial hypertension. *Res. Publ. Assoc. Res. Nerv. Ment. Dis.* **29**, 775–798.

CHAU, N. P., SAFAR, M. E., WEISS, Y. A., LONDON, G. M., SIMON, A. and MILLIEZ, P. L. (1978). Relationships between cardiac output, heart rate and blood volume in essential hypertension. *Clin. Sci. molec. Med.* **54**, 175–180.

CHIRIBOGA, D. A. (1977). Life events weighting systems: A comparative analysis. *J. psychosom. Res.* **21**, 415–422.

CHOBANIAN, A. V., GAVRAS, H., GAVRAS, I., BRESNAHAN, M., SULLIVAN, P. and MELBY, J. C. (1978). Studies on the activity of the sympathetic nervous system in essential hypertension. *J. Human Stress*, **4** (3), 22–28.

CHRISTIAN, J. J. (1970). Social subordination, population density, and mammalian evolution. *Science*, **168**, 84–90.

CIARANELLO, R., WOOTON. G. F. and AXELROD, J. (1976). Regulation of rat adrenal dopamine-beta-hydroxylase II. Receptor interaction in the regulation of enzyme synthesis and degradation. *Brain Res.* **113**, 349–362.

CLAMAGE, D. M., VANDER, A. J. and MOUW, D. R. (1977). Psychosocial stimuli and human plasma renin activity. *Psychosom. Med.* **30**, 393–401.

CLARK, D. A., ARNOLD, E., FOULDS, E., BROWN, D., EASTMEAD, D. and PARRY, E. (1975). Serum urate and cholesterol levels in Air Force Academy cadets. *Aviat. Space Environ. Med.* **46**, 1044–1048.

CLARKE, N. P., SMITH, O. A. and SHEARN, D. W. (1968). Topographical representation of vascular smooth muscle of limbs in primate motor cortex. *Am. J. Physiol.* **214**, 122–129.

CLEMENS, W. J. and SHATTOCK, J. R. (1979). Voluntary heart rate control during static muscular effort. *Psychophysiology*, **16**, 327–323.

COBB, L. A., BAUM, R. S., ALVAREZ, H. and SHAFFER, W. (1975). Resuscitation from out of hospital ventricular fibrillation. 4 year follow-up. *Circulation*, **51–52**, *Suppl.* 111, 223.

COBB, S. (1974). Physiologic changes in men whose jobs were abolished. *J. psychosom. Res.* **18**, 245–258.

COBB, S. (1976). Social support as a moderator of life stress. *Psychosom. Med.* **38**, 300–314.

COBB, S. and ROSE, R. M. (1973). Hypertension, peptic ulcer and diabetes in air traffic controllers. *J. Am. med. Ass.* **224**, 489–492.

COBB, S. and KASL, S. V. (1977). Termination: The consequences of job loss. NIOSH Research Report, DHEW Publication, 77–224.

COCHRANE, R. (1973). Hostility and neuroticism among unselected essential hypertensives. *J. psychosom. Res.* **17**, 215–218.

COHEN, J. B. (1978). The influence of culture on coronary-prone behavior. *In* "Coronary-prone Behavior" (T. Dembroski, S. Weiss, J. Shields, S. Haynes and M. Feinleib, Eds), pp. 191–198. Springer-Verlag, New York.

Cole, F. M. and Yates, P. O. (1967). The occurence and significance of intra-cerebral microaneurysms. *J. Path. Bact.* **93**, 393–411.

COLERIDGE, H. M., COLERIDGE, J. C. G. and ROSENTHAL, F. (1976). Prolonged inactivation of cortical pyramidal tract neurones in cats by distension of the carotid sinus. *J. Physiol.* **256**, 635–649.

CONNER, J., LACAMERA, F., SWANICK, E. (1976). Effects of exercise on coronary collateralization—angiographic studies of six patients in a supervised exercise program. *Med. Sci. Sports*, **8**, 145–151.

CONNER, R. L., VERNIKOS-DANELLIS, J. and LEVINE, S. (1971). Stress, fighting and neuroendocrine function. *Nature, Lond.* **234**, 564–566.

CONNOLLY, J. (1976). Life events before myocardial infarction. *J. Human Stress*, **2** (4), 3–17.

CONNOR, W. E. and CONNOR, S. L. (1977). Dietary treatment of hyper-lipidemia. *In* "Hyperlipidemia—Diagnosis and Therapy" (B. M. Rofkind and R. I. Levy, Eds), pp. 79–93. Grune and Stratton, New York.

CONWAY, J. (1978). Beta blocking drug therapy in hypertension. *In* "Hypertension: Mechanisms, Diagnosis and Treatment" (G. Onesti and A. N. Brest, Eds), pp. 253–261. F. A. Davis, Philadelphia.

COOVER, G. D., URSIN, H. and LEVINE, S. (1973). Plasma-corticosterone levels during active avoidance learning in rats. *J. comp. physiol. Psychol.* **82**, 170–174.

CORBALAN, R., VERRIER, R. and LOWN, B. (1974). Psychological stress and ventricular arrhythmias during myocardial infarction in the conscious dog. *Am. J. Cardiol.* **34**, 692–696.

CORLEY, K. C., MAUCK, H. P. and SHIEL, F. O'M. (1975). Cardiac responses associated with yoked chair shock avoidance. *Psychophysiology*, **12**, 439–444.

CORLEY, K. C., SHIEL, F. O'M., MAUCK, H. P. and BARBER, J. H. (1977). Myocardial degeneration and cardiac arrest in squirrel monkey: Physiological and psychological correlates. *Psychophysiology*, **14**, 322–328.

CORLEY, K. C., MAUCK, H. P., SHIEL, F. O'M., BARBER, J. H., CLARK, L. S. and BLOCHER, C. R. (1979). Myocardial dysfunction and pathology associated with environmental stress in squirrel monkey: Effect of vagotomy and propranolol. *Psychophysiology*, **16**, 554–560.

Coronary Drug Project Group (1975). Clofibrate and niacin and coronary heart disease. *J. Am. med. Ass.* **231**, 360–381.

CORUM, C. R. and THURMOND, J. B. (1977). Effects of acute exposure to stress on subsequent aggression and locomotor performance. *Psychosom. Med.* **39**, 436–443.

COUSINEAU, D., LAPOINTE, L. and DE CHAMPLAIN, J. (1978). Circulating catecholamines and systolic time intervals in normotensive and hypertensive patients with and without left ventricular hypertrophy. *Am. Heart J.* **96**, 227–234.

COWLEY, A. W., LIARD, J. F. and GUYTON, A. C. (1973). Role of baroreceptor reflex in daily control of arterial blood pressure and other variables in dogs. *Circulation Res.* **32**, 564–576.

CRAMPTON, R. S. and SCHWARTZ, P. J. (1978). Some aspects of sudden cardiac death. *In* "Neural Mechanisms in Cardiac Arrhythmias" (P. J. Schwartz,

A. M. Brown, A. Malliani and A. Zanchetti, Eds), pp. 1–6. Raven Press, New York.

CRANEFIELD, P. F., WIT, A. L. and HOFFMAN, B. F. (1973). Genesis of cardiac arrhythmias. *Circulation*, **47**, 190–204.

CROMWELL, R., BUTTERFIELD, E. C., BRAYFIELD, F. M. and CURRY, J. J. (1977). "Acute Myocardial Infarction – Reaction and Recovery". C. V. Mosby, St Louis.

CROOG, S. H. and LEVINE, S. (1969). Social status and subjective perceptions of 250 men after myocardial infarction. *Publ. Hlth Rep., Wash.* **84**, 989–997.

CROOG, S. M. and LEVINE, S. (1977). "The Heart Patient Recovers". Human Sciences Press, New York.

CRUZ-COKE, R. (1960). Environmental influences on arterial blood pressure. *Lancet*, **II**, 885–886.

CRUZ-COKE, R., DONOSO, H. and BARRERA, R. (1973). Genetic ecology of hypertension. *Clin. Sci.* **45**, *Suppl.* 1, 55–65.

CURETON, T. K. (1966). The relative value of various exercise programs to protect adult human subjects from degenerative heart disease. *In* "The Prevention of Ischaemic Heart Disease" (W. Raab, Ed.), pp. 321–330. Charles Thomas, Springfield.

DAHL, H. and SPENCE, D. P. (1971). Heart rate and task characteristics. *Psychophysiology*, **7**, 369–375.

DAHL, L. K. (1961). Possible role of chronic excess salt consumption in the pathogenesis of essential hypertension. *Am. J. Cardiol.* **8**, 571–575.

DAHL, L. K. and LOVE, R. A. (1957). Etiological role of sodium chloride intake in essential hypertension in humans. *J. Am. med. Ass.* **164**, 397–400.

DAHL, L. K., KNUDSON, K. D., HEINE, M. and LEITL, G. (1968). Hypertension and stress. *Nature, Lond.* **219**, 735–736.

DANEV, S. G., DE WINTER, C. R. and WARTNA, G. F. (1972). Information processing and psychophysiological functions in a task with and without time stress. *Acta Nerv. Super.* **14**, 8–12.

D'ATRI, D. A. (1975). Psychophysiological responses to crowding. *Envir. Behav.* **7**, 237–252.

DAVIDSON, D. M., WINCHESTER, M. A., TAYLOR, C. B., ALDERMAN, F. A. and INGELS, N. B. (1979). Effects of relaxation therapy on cardiac performance and sympathetic activity in patients with organic heart disease. *Psychosom. Med.* **41**, 363–369.

DAVIES, M. H. (1971). Is high blood pressure a psychosomatic disorder? *J. chron. Dis.* **24**, 239–258.

DAVIES, M. J. (1977). The pathology of myocardial ischaemia. *J. clin. Path.* **30**, Suppl. 11, 45–52.

DAVIES, M. J., WOOLF, N. and ROBERTSON, W. B. (1976). Pathology of acute myocardial infarction with particular reference to occlusive coronary thrombosis. *Br. Heart J.* **38**, 659–664.

DAVIS, J. O. and FREEMAN, R. H. (1976). Mechanisms regulating renin release. *Physiol. Rev.* **56**, 1–56.

DAWBER, T. R., KANNEL, W. B., KAGAN, A., DONADEBIAN, R. K., McNAMARA, P. M. and PEARSON, G. (1967). Environmental factors in hypertension. *In* "The Epidemiology of Hypertension" (J. Stamler, R. Stamler and T. N. Pullman, Eds), pp. 255–283. Grune and Stratton, New York.

DE CHAMPLAIN, J. and VON AMERINGEN, M. (1973). Role of sympathetic fibres and adrenal medulla in the maintenance of cardiovascular homeostasis in normotensive and hypertensive rats. *In* "Frontiers in Catecholamine Research" (E. Usdin and S. H. Snyder, Eds), pp. 860–868. Pergamon Press, Oxford.

DE CHAMPLAIN, J., KRAKOFF, L. R. and AXELROD, J. (1968). Relationship between sodium intake and norepinephrine storage during the development of essential hypertension. *Circulation Res.* **23**, 479–491.

DE FAIRE, U. (1975). Life change patterns prior to death in ischaemic heart disease: A study on death-discordant twins. *J. psychosom. Res.* **19**, 273–278.

DE JONG, W., PROVOOST, A. P. and SHAPIRO, A. P. (Eds) (1977). The nervous system in arterial hypertension. *Prog. Brain Res.* **47**. Elsevier, Amsterdam.

DE JONG, W., ZANDBERG, P., PALKOVITS, M. and BOHUS, B. (1977). Acute and chronic hypertension after lesions and transection of the rat brainstem. *Prog. Brain Res.* **47**, 189–197.

DE QUATTRO, V. and CHAN, S. (1972). Raised plasma catecholamines in some patients with primary hypertension. *Lancet*, **I**, 806–809.

DE QUATTRO, V., MIURA, Y., LURVEY, A., COSGROVE, M. and MENDEZ, R. (1975). Increased plasma catecholamine concentrations and vas deferens norepinephrine biosynthesis in men with elevated blood pressure. *Circulation Res.* **36**, 118–126.

DE QUATTRO, V., BARBOUR, B. H., CAMPESE, V., FINK, E. J., MIAND, L. and ESLER, M. (1977). Sympathetic nervous hyperactivity in high-renin hypertension. *Mayo Clinic Proc.* **52**, 369–373.

DE SILVA, R. A., VERRIER, R. L. and LOWN, B. (1978). The effects of psychological stress and vagal stimulation with morphine on vulnerability to ventricular fibrillation in the conscious dog. *Am. Heart J.* **95**, 197–203.

DE WIED, D. (1974). Pituitary–adrenal system hormones and behaviour. *In* "Neurosciences Third Study Program" (F. O. Schmitt and F. G. Warden, Eds), pp. 653–666. M.I.T. Press, Cambridge, Massachusetts.

DeGOOD, D. E. (1975). Cognitive control factors in vascular stress responses. *Psychophysiology*, **12**, 399–401.

DeGOOD, D. E. and ADAMS, A. S. (1976). Control of cardiac responses under aversive stimulation. *Biofeedback self-regulation*, **1**, 373–385.

DELGADO, J. M. R. (1960). Circulatory effects of cortical stimulation. *Physiol. Rev.* **40**, *Suppl.* 4, 146–178.

DEMBROSKI, T. M., MacDOUGALL, J. M. and SHIELDS, J. L. (1977). Physiologic reactions to social challenge in persons evidencing the Type A coronary-prone behavior pattern. *J. Human Stress*, **3** (3), 2–10.

DEMBROSKI, T. M., MACDOUGALL, J. M., SHIELDS, J. L., PETITTO, J. and LUSHENE, R. (1978). Components of the coronary-prone behavior pattern and cardiovascular responses to psychomotor performance challenge. *J. Behav. Med.* **1**, 159–176.

DEMBROSKI, T. M., MACDOUGALL, J. M. and LUSHENE, R. (1979). Interpersonal interaction and cardiovascular response in Type A subjects and coronary patients. *J. Human Stress*, **5** (4), 28–36.

DHSS (1976). "On the State of the Public Health for the Year 1975". HMSO, London.

DIMSDALE, J. E., HACKETT, T. P., CATANZANO, D. M. and WHITE, P. J. (1979). The relationship between diverse measures of Type A personality and coronary angiographic findings. *J. psychosom. Res.* **23**, 289–294.

DINSDALE, H. B., ROBERTSON, D. M., HAAS, R. A. and DAVIS, P. E. (1976). Acute hypertension, blood–brain damage and the role of adrenal steroids. *In* "Cerebral Vessel Wall" (J. Cervós-Navarro, E. Betz, F. Matakas and R. Wullenweber, Eds), pp. 253–260. Raven Press, New York.

DINTENFASS, L. and ZADER, I. (1975). Effect of stress and anxiety on thrombus formation and blood viscosity factors. *Biblthca haemat.* **41**, 133–139.

DOLL, R. and HILL, A. B. (1964). Mortality in relation to smoking: 10 year's observations of British doctors. *Br. med. J.* **I**, 1399–1410.

DREW, G. M. and LEACH, G. D. H. (1971). Corticosteroids and their effects on cardiovascular sensitivity in the pithed adrenalectomised rat. *Archs int. Pharmacodyn. Thér.* **191**, 255–260.

DUNNE, J. F. (1969). Variation of blood pressure in untreated hypertensive outpatients. *Lancet*, **I**, 391–392.

DYKMAN, R. A. and GANTT, W. A. (1960). Experimental psychogenic hypertension: blood pressure changes conditioned to painful stimuli. *Bull. Johns Hopkins Hosp.* **107**, 72–89.

EAST, T. (1958). "The Story of Heart Disease". W. Dawson, London.

ECKER, A. (1954). Emotional stress before strokes: A preliminary report of 20 cases. *Annls int. Med.* **40**, 49–56.

EHRSTRÖM, M. C. (1945). Psychogene Blutdruckssteigerung – Kriegshypertonien. *Acta med. scand.* **122**, 546–570.

EICH, R. H., CUDDY, R. P., SMULYAN, H. and LYONS, R. H. (1966). Hemodynamics in labile hypertension: A followup study. *Circulation*, **34**, 299–307.

ELDER, S. T., GAMBLE, E. H., MCAFEE, R. D. and VAN VEEN, W. J. (1979). Conditioned diastolic pressure. *Physiol. Behav.* **23**, 875–880.

ELIOT, R. S., CLAYTON, F. C., PIEPER, G. M. and TODD, G. L. (1977). Influence of environmental stress on pathogenesis of sudden cardiac death. *Fed. Proc.* **36**, 1719–1724.

ELLIOTT, R. (1969). Tonic heart rate: Experiments on the effects of collative variables lead to a hypothesis about its motivational significance. *J. Person. soc. Psychol.* **12**, 211–228.

ELLIOTT, R. (1974). The motivational significance of heart rate. *In* "Cardiovascular Psychophysiology" (P. A. Obrist, A. H. Black, J. Brener and L. V. DiCara, Eds), pp. 505–537. Aldine, Chicago.

ELMADJIAN, F., HOPE, J. M. and LANSON, E. T. (1957). Excretion of epinephrine and norepinephrine in various emotional states. *J. clin. Endocr. Metab.* **17**, 608–620.

ENGEL, B. T. and BLEECKER, E. R. (1974). Application of operant conditioning techniques to the control of the cardiac arrhythmias. *In* "Cardiovascular Psychophysiology" (P. A. Obrist, A. H. Black, J. Brener and L. V. DiCara, Eds), pp. 456–476. Aldine, Chicago.

ENGEL, G. L. (1971). Sudden and rapid death during psychological stress. Folklore or folk wisdom? *Annls int. Med.* **74**, 771–782.

ENGEL, R. R., MÜLLER, F., MÜNCH, V. and ACKENHEIL, M. M. (1980). Plasma catecholamine response and autonomic functions during short-term psychological stress. *In* "Catecholamines and Stress: Recent Progress" (E. Usdin, R. Kvetňanský and I. J. Kopin, Eds). Elsevier, New York.

ESLER, M. D. and NESTEL, P. J. (1973a). Sympathetic responsiveness to head-up tilt in essential hypertension. *Clin. Sci.* **44**, 213–226.

ESLER, M. D. and NESTEL, P. J. (1973b). Renin and sympathetic nervous system responsiveness to adrenergic stimulation in essential hypertension. *Am. J. Cardiol.* **32**, 643–649.

ESLER, M. D., JULIUS, S., ZWEIFLER, A., RANDALL, O., HARBURG, E., GARDINER, H. and DE QUATTRO, V. (1977). Mild high-renin essential hypertension: A neurogenic human hypertension? *New Engl. J. Med.* **296**, 405–411.

ETTEMA, J. H. and ZIELHUIS, R. L. (1971). Physiological parameters of mental load. *Ergonomics*, **14**, 137–144.

FARQUHAR, J. W., MACCOBY, N., WOOD, P. D., ALEXANDER, J. K., BREITROSE, H., BROWN, B. W., HASKELL, W. L., MCALISTER, A. L., MEYER, A. J., NASH, J. D. and STERN, M. P. (1977). Community education for cardiovascular health. *Lancet*, **I**, 1192–1195.

FEJFAR, Z. (1975). Prevention against ischaemic heart disease: A critical review. *In* "Modern Trends in Cardiology – III" (M. Oliver, Ed.), pp. 465–499. Butterworths, London.

FEJFAR, Z. and WIDIMSKY, J. (1962). Juvenile hypertension. *In* "The Pathogenesis of Essential Hypertension. Proceedings of a Joint WHO-Czech Cardiological Society Symposium" (J. H. Cort, V. Fencl, Z. Hejl and J. Jirka, Eds), pp. 33–42. Pergamon Press, Oxford.

FELDMAN, J. and BROWN, G. (1976). Endocrine responses to electric shock and avoidance conditioning in the rhesus monkey: cortisol and growth hormone. *Psychoneuroendocrinology*, **1**, 231–242.

FELDMAN, S., CONFORTI, N., CHOWERS, I. and DAVIDSON, J. (1970). Pituitary–adrenal activation in rats with medial basal hypothalamic islands. *Acta Endocr.* **63**, 405–414.

FENZ, W. D. (1975). Strategies for coping with stress. *In* "Stress and Anxiety" (I. Sarason and C. Spielberger, Eds), vol. 2, pp. 305–336. Wiley, Chichester.

FENZ, W. D. and EPSTEIN, S. (1967). Changes in gradients of skin conductance, heart rate and respiration rate as a function of experience. *Psychosom. Med.* **29**, 33–51.

FERRARIO, C. M. and PAGE, I. H. (1978). Current views concerning cardiac output in the genesis of experimental hypertension. *Circulation Res.* **43**, 821–831.

FERRARIO, C. M., GILDENBERG, P. and McCUBBIN, J. W. (1972). Cardiovascular effects of angiotensin mediated by the central nervous system. *Circulation Res.* **30**, 257–262.

FEY, S. G. and LINDHOLM, E. (1978). Biofeedback and progressive relaxation: Effects on systolic and diastolic blood pressure and heart rate. *Psychophysiology*, **15**, 239–247.

FIELDING, R. (1979). Behavioural treatment in the rehabilitation of myocardial infarction. *In* "Research in Psychology and Medicine" (D. J. Oborne, M. M. Gruneberg and J. R. Eiser, Eds), vol. 1, pp. 176–182. Academic Press, London.

FINDLEY, J. D., BRADY, J. V., ROBINSON, W. W. and GILLIAM, W. J. (1971). Continuous cardiovascular monitoring in the baboon during long term behavioral performance. *Communs behav. Biol.* **6**, 49–58.

FINLAYSON, A. and McEWEN, J. (1977). "Coronary Heart Disease and Patterns of Living". Croom Helm, London.

FINN, F., MULCAHY, R. and HICKEY, N. (1974). The psychological profiles of coronary and cancer patients. *Ir. J. med. Sci.* **143**, 176–178.

FISHER, F. D. and TYROLER, H. A. (1973). Relationship between ventricular premature contractions on routine electrocardiography and subsequent sudden death from coronary heart disease. *Circulation*, **47**, 712–719.

FLEISCHMAN, A. I., BIERENBAUM, M. L. and STIER, A. (1976). Effects of stress due to anticipated minor surgery upon *in vivo* platelet aggreggation in humans. *J. Human Stress*, **2** (1), 33–37.

FLODERUS, B. (1974). Psychosocial factors in relation to coronary heart disease and associated risk factors. *Nord. Hyg. Tidskr.*, Suppl. 6.

FLOREY, C. Du V. and CUADRADO, R. R. (1968). Blood pressure in native Cape Verdeans and in Cape Verdean immigrants and their descendants living in New England. *Human Biol.* **40**, 189–211.

FOLKOW, B. (1976). Structural changes in heart and vessels during hypertension with aspects of their reversibility. *Aust. N.Z. J. Med.* **6**, *Suppl.* 2, 35–39.

FOLKOW, B., and VON EULER, U. S. (1954). Selective activation of noradrenaline and adrenaline producing cells in cat's adrenal gland by hypothalamic stimulation. *Circulation Res.* **2**, 191–195.

FOLKOW, B. and RUBINSTEIN, E. H. (1966). Cardiovascular effects of acute and chronic stimulation of the hypothalamus defence area in the rat. *Acta physiol. scand.* **68**, 48–57.

FOLKOW, B. and NEIL, E. (1971). "Circulation". Oxford University Press, Oxford.

FOLKOW, B., HALLBÄCK, M., LUNDGREN, H. and WEISS, L. (1970). Background of increased flow resistance and vascular reactivity in spontaneously hypertensive rats. *Acta physiol. scand.* **80**, 93–106.

FORSYTH, R. P. (1968). Blood pressure and avoidance conditioning. *Psychosom. Med.* **30**, 125–133.

FORSYTH, R. P. (1969). Blood pressure responses to long term avoidance schedules. *Psychosom. Med.* **31**, 300–309.

FORSYTH, R. P. (1971). Regional blood flow changes during 72 hour avoidance. *Science*, **173**, 546–548.

FORSYTH, R. P., HOFFBRAND, B. I. and MELMON, K. L. (1971). Hemodynamic effects of angiotensin in normal and environmentally stressed monkeys. *Circulation*, **44**, 119–129.

FOUAD, F. M., TARAZI, R. C., DUSTAN, H. P. and BRAVO, E. L. (1978). Hemodynamics of essential hypertension in young subjects. *Am. Heart J.* **96**, 646–654.

FRANCO-MORSELLI, R., ELGHOZI, J., JOLY, E., DIGIULIO, S. and MEYER, P. (1977). Increased plasma adrenaline concentration in benign essential hypertension. *Br. med. J.* **II**, 1251–1254.

FRANK, K. A., HELLER, S. S., KORNFELD, D. S., SPORN, A. A. and WEISS, M. B. (1978). Type A behavior pattern and coronary angiographic findings. *J. Am. med. Ass.* **240**, 761–763.

FRANKEL, B. L., PATEL, D. J., HOROWITZ, D., FRIEDEWALD, W. T. and GAARDER, T. R. (1978). Treatment of hypertension with biofeedback and relaxation training. *Psychosom. Med.* **40**, 276–293.

FRANKENHAEUSER, M. (1975). Sympathetic-adrenomedullary activity, behaviour and the psychosocial environment. *In* "Research in Psychophysiology" (P. Venables and M. J. Christie, Eds), pp. 71–97. Wiley, Chichester.

FRANKENHAEUSER, M. and GARDELL, G. (1976). Underload and overload in working life: Outline of a multidisciplinary approach. *J. Human Stress*, **2** (2), 35–46.

FRANKENHAEUSER, M. and JOHANSSON, G. (1976). Task demand as reflected in catecholamine excretion and heart rate. *J. Human Stress*, **2** (1), 15–23.

FRANKENHAEUSER, M. and LUNDBERG, U. (1977). The influence of cognitive set on performance and arousal under different noise loads. *Motiv. Emot.* **1**, 139–149.

FRANKENHAEUSER, M. and RISSLER, A. (1970). Effects of punishment on catecholamine release and efficiency of performance. *Psychopharmacologia*, **17**, 378–390.

FRANKENHAEUSER, M., POST, B., NORDHEDEN, B. and SJOBERG, H. (1969). Physiological and subjective reactions to different physical work loads. *Perc. mot. Skills*, **28**, 343–349.

FRANKENHAEUSER, M., NORDHEDEN, B., MYRSTEN, A. L. and POST, B. (1971).

Psychophysiological reactions to understimulation and overstimulation. *Acta psychol. scand.* **35**, 298–308.

FRANKENHAEUSER, M., DUNNE, E. and LUNDBERG, U. (1976). Sex differences in sympathetic-adrenal medullary responses induced by different stressors. *Psychopharmacologia*, **47**, 1–5.

FRIEDMAN, E. H., HELLERSTEIN, H. K., EASTWOOD, G. L. and JONES, S. E. (1968). Behavior patterns and serum cholesterol in two groups of normal males. *Am. J. med. Sci.* **255**, 237–244.

FRIEDMAN, G. D., URY, H. K., KLATSKY, A. L. and SIEGELAUB, A. B. (1974). A psychological questionnaire predictive of myocardial infarction: Results from the Kaiser–Permanente epidemiologic study of myocardial infarction. *Psychosom. Med.* **36**, 327–343.

FRIEDMAN, M. and KASANIN, J. S. (1943). Hypertension in only one of identical twins. *Archs intern. Med.* **72**, 767–774.

FRIEDMAN, M. and ROSENMAN, R. H. (1959). Association of specific overt behavior pattern with blood and cardiovascular findings. *J. Am. med. Ass.* **169**, 1085–1096.

FRIEDMAN, M., ROSENMAN, R. H. and CARROLL, V. (1958). Changes in serum cholesterol and blood clotting time in men subjected to cyclic variations of occupational stress. *Circulation*, **17**, 852–861.

FRIEDMAN, M., ST GEORGE, S. and BYERS, S. O. (1960). Excretion of cate-cholamines, 17-ketosteroids, 17-hydroxy-corticoids and 6-hydroxy-indole in men exhibiting a particular behavior pattern (A) associated with high incidence of clinical coronary artery disease. *J. clin. Invest.* **39**, 758–764.

FRIEDMAN, M., ROSENMAN, R. H. and BROAN, F. (1963). The continuous heart rate in men exhibiting an overt behavior pattern associated with increased incidence of clinical coronary artery disease. *Circulation*, **28**, 861–866.

FRIEDMAN, M., ROSENMAN, R. H. and BYERS, S. (1964). Serum lipids and conjunctival circulation after fat ingestion in men exhibiting Type A behavior pattern. *Circulation*, **29**, 874–886.

FRIEDMAN, M., ROSENMAN, R. H., STRAUS, R., WURM, M. and KOSITCHEK, R. (1968). The relationship of behavior pattern A to the state of the coronary vasculature. *Am. J. Med.* **44**, 525–537.

FRIEDMAN, M., BYERS, S., ROSENMAN, R. H. and ELEVITCH, F. R. (1970). Coronary-prone individuals (Type A behavior pattern). Some bio-chemical characteristics. *J. Am. med. Ass.* **212**, 1030–1038.

FRIEDMAN, M., BYERS, S. and ROSENMAN, R. H. (1972). Plasma ACTH and cortisol concentration of coronary-prone subjects. *Proc. Soc. exp. Biol. Med.* **140**, 681–684.

FRIEDMAN, M., BYERS, S., DIAMANT, J. and ROSENMAN, R. H. (1975). Plasma catecholamine response of coronary-prone subjects (Type A) to a specific challenge. *Metabolism*, **24**, 205–210.

FRIEDMAN, M. J. and BENNET, P. L. (1977). Depression and hypertension. *Psychosom. Med.* **39**, 134–142.

FRIEDMAN, R. and DAHL, L. K. (1975). Effect of chronic conflict on the blood pressure of rats with a genetic susceptibility to experimental hypertension. *Psychosom. Med.* **37**, 402–416.

FRIEDMAN, R. and IWAI, T. (1976). Genetic predisposition and stress-induced hypertension. *Science*, **193**, 161–162.

FRIEDMAN, S. B., MASON, J. W. and HAMBURG, D. A. (1963). Urinary 17-hydroxycorticosteroid levels in parents of children with neoplastic disease. *Psychosom. Med.* **25**, 364–376.

FRIES, E. D. (1967). Effects of treatment on morbidity in hypertension. Results in patients with diastolic pressures averaging 115 through 129 mmHg. *J. Am. med. Ass.* **202**, 1028–1034.

FRIES, E. D. (1970). Effects of treatment on morbidity in hypertension II. Results in patients with diastolic pressures averaging 90 through 114 mmHg. *J. Am. med. Ass.* **213**, 1143–1152.

FRIES, E. D. (1976). Salt, volume and the prevention of hypertension. *Circulation*, **53**, 589–595.

FRIESINGER, G. C., PAGE, E. E. and ROSS, R. (1970). Prognostic significance of coronary arteriography. *Trans. Ass. Am. Physns*, **93**, 78–92.

FROELICHER, V. F. (1973). The haemodynamic effects of physical conditioning in healthy young and middle aged individuals, and in coronary heart disease patients. *In* "Exercise Testing and Exercise Training" (J. Naughton and H. K. Hellerstein, Eds), pp. 63–78. Academic Press, London.

FROELICHER, V. F. (1978). Exercise and the prevention of coronary atherosclerotic heart disease. *In* "Exercise and the Heart" (N. K. Wenger, Ed.), pp. 13–23. F. A. Davis, Philadelphia.

FROHLICH, E. D., KOZUL, V. J., TARAZI, R. C. and DUSTAN, H. P. (1970). Physiological comparison of labile and essential hypertension. *Circulation Res.* **27**, Suppl. 1, 55–63.

FRY, D. L. (1973). Responses of the arterial wall to certain physical factors. *In* "Atherogenesis: Initiating Factors". CIBA Foundation Symp. 12. pp. 93–120. Elsevier, Amsterdam.

FULTON, R. M. and DUCKETT, K. (1976). Plasma-fibrinogen and thromboembolism after myocardial infarction. *Lancet*, **II**, 1161–1164.

FUNKENSTEIN, D. (1956). Norepinephrine-like and epinephrine-like substances in relation to human behavior. *J. nerv. ment. Dis.* **124**, 58–68.

FUREDY, J. and BIEDERMAN, G. (1976). The preference for signalled shock phenomenon: A taxonomy of signal type and signal content. *Aust. J. Psychol.* **28**, 167–179.

GALOSY, R. A. and GAEBELEIN, C. J. (1977). Cardiovascular adaptations to environmental stress: Its role in the development of hypertension, responsible mechanisms and hypotheses. *Biobehav. Rev.* **1**, 165–175.

GALOSY, R. A., CLARKE, L. K. and MITCHELL, J. H. (1979). Cardiac changes during behavioural stress in dogs. *Am. J. Physiol.* **236**, H750–H758.

GANONG, W. F. (1974). Brain mechanisms regulating the secretion of the pituitary gland. *In* "The Neurosciences Third Study Program" (F. O.

Schmidt and F. G. Warden, Eds), pp. 549–563. M.I.T. Press, Cambridge, Massachusetts.

GANTT, W. H., NEWTON, J. E. O., ROYER, F. L. and STEPHENS, J. H. (1966). Effect of person. *Cond. Reflex*, **1**, 18–35.

GEBBER, G. L. and SNYDER, D. W. (1970). Hypothalamic control of baroreceptor reflexes. *Am. J. Physiol.* **218**, 124–131.

GEBBER, G. L. and KLEVANS, L. R. (1972). Central nervous system modulation of cardiovascular reflexes. *Fed. Proc.* **31**, 1245–1252.

GEER, J. H., DAVISON, G. C. and GATCHEL, R. I. (1970). Stress effects of perceived control of aversive stimulation. *J. Person. soc. Psychol.* **16**, 731–738.

GENTRY, W. D. (1975). Preadmission behaviour. *In* "Psychological Aspects of Myocardial Infarction and Coronary Care" (W. D. Gentry and R. B. Williams, Eds), pp. 53–62. C. V. Mosby, St. Louis.

GENTRY, W. D. and WILLIAMS, R. B. (Eds) (1975). "Psychological Aspects of Myocardial Infarction and Coronary Care". C. V. Mosby, St. Louis.

GILLUM, R. F. and PAFFENBARGER, R. S. (1978). Chronic disease in former college students XVII. Sociocultural mobility as a precursor of coronary heart disease and hypertension. *Am. J. Epidemiol.* **108**, 289–298.

GITTLEMAN, B., SHATIN, L., BIERENBAUM, M. L., FLEISCHMAN, A. and HAYTON, T. (1968). Effects of quantified stressful stimuli on blood lipids in man. *J. nerv. ment. Dis.* **147**, 196–201.

GLASS, D. C. (1977). Behavior patterns, stress and coronary disease. LEA, Hillsdale.

GLASS, D. C. and SINGER, J. E. (1972). "Urban Stress". Academic Press, London and New York.

GLASS, D. C., SINGER, J. E., LEONARD, H. S., KRANTZ, D., COHEN, S. and CUMMINGS, H. (1973). Perceived control of aversive stimulation and the reduction of stress responses. *J. Personal.* **41**, 577–595.

GLASSER, S. P., CLARK, P. I. and SPOTO, E. (1978). Heart rate response to "fright stress". *Heart Lung*, **7**, 1006–1010.

GLINER, J. A., BROWE, A. C. and HORVATH, S. M. (1977). Haemodynamic changes as a function of classical aversive conditioning in humans. *Psychophysiology*, **14**, 281–286.

GLINER, J. A., BEDI, J. F., and HORVATH, S. M. (1979). Somatic and nonsomatic influences on the heart: Haemodynamic changes. *Psychophysiology*, **16**, 358–362.

GOLDBOURT, V., MEDALIE, J. H. and NEUFELD, H. N. (1975). Clinical myocardial infarction over a 5 year period III. A multivariate analysis of incidence, the Israel ischaemic heart disease study. *J. chron. Dis.* **28**, 217–237.

GOLDRING, W., CHASIS, H., SCHREINER, G. E. and SMITH, H. W. (1956). Reassurance in the management of benign hypertensive disease. *Circulation*, **14**, 260–264.

GOLDSTEIN, D. S., ROSS, R. S. and BRADY, J. V. (1977). Biofeedback heart rate training during exercise. *Biofeedback and Self-regulation*, **2**, 107–126.

GOLDSTEIN, K. (1942). "The After Effects of Brain Injuries in War". Grune and Stratton, New York.

GOODWIN, G. M., McCLOSKEY, D. I. and MITCHELL, J. (1972). Cardiovascular and respiratory responses to changes in central command during isometric exercise at constant muscle tension. *J. Physiol.* **226**, 173–190.

GORDON, J. L., BOWYER, D. E., EVANS, D. W. and MITCHINSON, M. J. (1973). Human platelet reactivity during stressful diagnostic procedures. *J. clin. Path.* **26**, 958–962.

GORDON, T., GARCIA-PALMIERI, M. R., KAGAN, A., KANNEL, W. B. and SCHIFFMAN, J. (1974). Differences in coronary heart disease in Framingham, Honolulu and Puerto Rico. *J. chron. Dis.* **27**, 329–344.

GRAHAM, J. D. P. (1945). "High Blood Pressure After Battle". *Lancet*, **I**, 239–240.

GREENE, W. A., GOLDSTEIN, S. and MOSS, A. J. (1972). Psychosocial aspects of sudden death. *Archs intern. Med.* **129**, 725–731.

GREENFIELD, A. D. M. (1966). Survey of the evidence for active neurogenic vasodilatation in man. *Fed. Proc.* **25**, 1607–1610.

GRIBBIN, B., PICKERING, T. G., SLEIGHT, P. and PETO, R. (1971). Effect of age and high blood pressure on baroreflex sensitivity in man. *Circulation Res.* **29**, 424–431.

GUNN, G. C. and HAMPTON, J. W. (1967). Central nervous system influence on plasma levels of factor VIII activity. *Am. J. Physiol.* **212**, 124–130.

GUNNING, A. J., PICKERING, G. W., ROBB-SMITH, A. H. T. and ROSS RUSSELL, R. (1964). Mural thrombosis of the internal carotid artery and subsequent embolism. *Q. Jl Med.* **33**, 155–195.

GUTHRIE, G. D., GENEST, J., KUCHEL, O., NOWACZYNSKI, W. and BOUCHER, R. (1978). Low-renin hypertension: Classification, mechanisms and therapy. *In* "Hypertension: Mechanisms, Diagnosis and Treatment", pp. 43–49. F. A. Davis, Philadelphia.

GUYTON, A. C. (1978). Essential cardiovascular regulation – the control linkages between bodily needs and circulatory function. *In* "Developments in Cardiovascular Medicine" (C. J. Dickinson and J. Marks, Eds), pp. 265–302. MTP, Lancaster.

GUYTON, A. C., COLEMAN, T. G. and GRANGER, H. J. (1972). Circulation: Overall regulation. *A. Rev. Physiol.* **34**, 13–46.

GUYTON, A. C., COLEMAN, T. G., NORMAN, R. A., HALL, J. E. and YOUNG, D. B. (1976). Overall circulatory control in hypertension. *Aust. N.Z. J. Med.* **6**, Suppl. 2, 72–80.

HACKETT, T. P. and CASSEM, N. H. (1978). Psychologic aspects of rehabilitation after myocardial infarction. *In* "Rehabilitation of the Coronary Patient" (N. K. Wenger and H. K. Hellerstein, Eds), pp. 243–253. Wiley, Chichester.

HAFT, J. I. and FANI, K. (1973). Stress and the induction of intravascular platelet aggregation in the heart. *Circulation*, **48**, 164–169.

HAFT, J. I. and ARKEL, Y. S. (1976). Effect of emotional stress on platelet aggregation in humans. *Chest*, **70**, 501–505.

HALLBÄCK, M. and FOLKOW, B. (1974). Cardiovascular responses to acute mental "stress" in spontaneously hypertensive rats. *Acta physiol. scand.* **90**, 684–698.

HANSEN, J. R., STØA, K. F., BLIX, A. S. and URSIN, H. (1978). Urinary levels of epinephrine and norepinephrine in parachutist trainees. *In* "The Psychobiology of Stress" (H. Ursin, H. Baade and S. Levine, Eds), pp. 63–74. Academic Press, London and New York.

HANSON, J. D., LARSON, M. E. and SNOWDON, L. T. (1976). Effects of control over high intensity noise on plasma cortisol levels in rhesus monkeys. *Behav. Biol.* **16**, 333–340.

HANSSON, L. and HENNING, M. (1978). Negative consequences of blood pressure reduction. *Acta med. scand.* Suppl. 628.

HARBURG, E., ERFURT, J. C., HAUENSTEIN, L. S., CHAPE, C., SCHULL, W. J. and SCHORK, M. A. (1973). Socio-ecological stress, suppressed hostility, skin color, and black–white male blood pressure: Detroit. *Psychosom. Med.* **35**, 276–296.

HARBURG, E., BLAKELOCK, E. H. and ROEPER, P. J. (1979). Resentful and reflective coping with arbitrary authority and blood pressure: Detroit. *Psychosom. Med.* **41**, 189–202.

HARLAN, W. R., OSBORNE, R. K. and GRAYBIEL, A. (1964). Prognostic value of the cold pressor test. *Am. J. Cardiol.* **13**, 832–837.

HARRIS, A. H. and BRADY, J. V. (1977). Long-term studies of cardiovascular control in primates. *In* "Biofeedback: Theory and Research" (G. E. Schwartz and J. Beatty, Eds), pp. 243–264. Academic Press, London and New York.

HARRIS, A. H., GOLDSTEIN, D. C. and BRADY, J. V. (1977). Visceral learning: Cardiovascular conditioning in primates. *In* "Biofeedback and Behavior" (J. Beatty and H. Legewie, Eds), pp. 201–224. Plenum, New York.

HARRIS, A. S., ESTANDIA, A. and TILLOTSON, R. F. (1951). Ventricular fibrillation following cardiac sympathectomy and coronary occlusion. *Am. J. Physiol.* **165**, 505–512.

HARRIS, R. E. (1967). Long-term studies of blood pressure recorded annually, with implications for the factors underlying essential hypertension. *Trans. Ass. Life Insur. med. Dir. Am.* **51**, 130–149.

HAYNES, R. B., SACKETT, D. L., GIBSON, E. S., TAYLOR, D. W., HACKETT, B. C., ROBERTS, R. S. and JOHNSON, A. L. (1976). Improvement of medication compliance in uncontrolled hypertension. *Lancet*, **I**, 1265–1468.

HAYNES, S. G., LEVINE, S., SCOTCH, N., FEINLEIB, M. and KANNEL, W. B. (1978a). The relationship of psychosocial factors to coronary heart disease in the Framingham study. I. Methods and risk factors. *Am. J. Epidemiol.* **107**, 362–383.

HAYNES, S. G., FEINLEIB, M., LEVINE, S., SCOTCH, N. and KANNEL, W. B.

(1978b). The relationship of psychosocial factors to coronary heart disease in the Framingham study. II. Prevalence of coronary heart disease. *Am. J. Epidemiol.* **107**, 384–402.

HEINE, B. and SAINSBURY, P. (1970). Prolonged emotional disturbance and essential hypertension. *Psychother. Psychosom.* **18**, 341–348.

HELLERSTEIN, H. K. and TURELL, D. J. (1964). The mode of death in coronary artery disease – an electrocardiographic and clinicopathological correlation. *In* "Sudden Cardiac Death" (B. Surawicz and E. D. Pellegrino, Eds), pp. 17–31. Grune and Stratton, New York.

HELLERSTEIN, H. K. and FRANKLIN, B. A. (1978). Exercise testing and prescription. *In* "The Rehabilitation of the Coronary Patient" (N. K. Wenger and H. K. Hellerstein, Eds), pp. 149–202. Wiley, Chichester.

HELLMAN, L., NAKADA, F., CURTI, J., WEITZMAN, E., KREAM, J., ROFFWEG, H., ELLMAN, S., FUKUSHIMA, D. and GALLAGHER, T. F. (1970). Cortisol is secreted episodically in man. *J. clin. Endocr. Metab.* **30**, 411–422.

HENNESSEY, J. W., KING, M. G., McCLURE, T. A. and LEVINE, S. (1977). Uncertainty, as defined by the contingency between environmental events, and the adrenocortical response of the rat to electric shock. *J. comp. physiol. Psychol.* **91**, 1447–1460.

HENRY, J. P. (1976). Mechanisms of psychosomatic disease in animals. *Adv. vet. Sci. comp. Med.* **20**, 115–145.

HENRY, J. P. and CASSEL, J. C. (1969). Psychosocial factors in essential hypertension – recent epidemiologic and animal experimental evidence. *J. Epidemiol.* **96**, 171–200.

HENRY, J. P. and STEPHENS, P. M. (1977). "Stress, Health and the Social Environment". Springer-Verlag, New York.

HENRY, J. P., ELY, D. L. and STEPHENS, P. M. (1974). The role of psychosocial stimulation in the pathogenesis of hypertension. *Verh. dt. Ges. Inn. Med.* **80**, 1724–1740.

HENRY, J. P., STEPHENS, P. M. and SANTISTEBAN, G. A. (1975). A model of psychosocial hypertension showing reversibility and progression of cardiovascular complications. *Circulation Res.* **36**, 156–164.

HERD, J. A., KELLEHER, R. T., MORSE, W. H. and GROSE, S. A. (1974). Sympathetic and parasympathetic activity during behavioural hypertension in the squirrel monkey. *In* "Cardiovascular Psychophysiology" (P. A. Obrist, A. H. Black, J. Brener and L. V. DiCara, Eds), pp. 211–225. Aldine, Chicago.

HERMANN, H. J. M., RASSEK, M., SCHAFER, N., SCHMIDT, T. and VON UEXKÜLL, T. (1976). Essential hypertension: Problems, concepts and attempted synthesis. *In* "Modern Trends in Psychosomatic Medicine – 3" (O. W. Hill, Ed.), pp. 260–287. Butterworths, London.

HILTON, S. M. (1963). Inhibition of baroreceptor reflexes on hypothalamic stimulation. *J. Physiol.* **165**, 56P–57P.

HILTON, S. M. (1975). Ways of viewing the central nervous control of the circulation – old and new. *Brain Res.* **87**, 213–219.

HINKLE, L. E., WHITNEY, L. H., LEHMAN, E. W., DUNN, J., BENJAMIN, B., KING, R., PLAKUN, A. and FLEHINGER, B. (1968). Occupation, education and coronary heart disease. *Science*, **161**, 238–246.

HINKLE, L. E., CARVER, S. T. and STEVENS, M. (1969). The frequency of asymptomatic disturbances of cardiac rhythm and conduction in middle-aged men. *Am. J. Cardiol.* **24**, 629–650.

HODAPP, V., WEYER, G. and BECKER, J. (1975). Situational stereotypy in essential hypertensive patients. *J. psychosom. Res.* **19**, 113–122.

HOFER, M. A., WOLFF, C. T., FRIEDMAN, S. B. and MASON, J. W. (1972). A psychoneuroendocrine study of bereavement. Part 1. 17-OHCS excretion. *Psychosom. Med.* **34**, 481–491.

HOFF, E. C. and GREEN, H. D. (1936). Cardiovascular reactions induced by electrical stimulation of the cerebral cortex. *Am. J. Physiol.* **117**, 411–422.

HOFF, E. C., KELL, J. and CARROLL, M. (1963). Effects of cortical stimulation and lesions on cardiovascular function. *Physiol. Rev.* **43**, 68–114.

HOFFMAN, B. F. (1977). Neural influences on cardiac electrical activity and rhythm. *In* "Neural Regulation of the Heart" (W. C. Randall, Ed.), pp. 289–312. Oxford University Press, Oxford.

HOFMAN, A., BOOMSMA, F., SCHALEKAMP, M. A. D. H. and VALKENBURG, H. A. (1979). Raised blood pressure and plasma noradrenaline concentrations in teenagers and young adults selected from an open population. *Br. med. J.* **I**, 1536–1538.

HOKANSON, J. F., DEGOOD, D. E., FORREST, M. S. and BRITTAIN, T. M. (1971). Availability of avoidance behaviours in modulating vascular stress responses. *J. Person. soc. Psychol.* **19**, 60–68.

HOLMBERG, G., LEVI, L., MATHE, A., ROSEN, A. and SCOTT, H. (1965). Comparison of plasma catecholamine levels and the influence of propranolol on peripheral haemodynamic manifestations of emotional stress in labile hypertensives and normal subjects. *Circulation*, **32**, Suppl. 2, 115–121.

HOLMES, T. H. and RAHE, R. H. (1967). The Social Readjustment Rating Scale. *J. Psychosom. Res.* **11**, 213–218.

HOLMES, T. H. and MASUDA, M. (1974). Life change and illness susceptibility. *In* "Stressful Life Events: Their Nature and Effects" (B. S. Dohrenwend and B. P. Dohrenwend, Eds), pp. 45–72. Wiley, Chichester.

HORAN, P. M. and GRAY, B. H. (1974). Status inconsistency, mobility and coronary heart disease. *J. Hlth soc. Behav.* **15**, 300–310.

HORNSTRA, G. and TEN HOOR, F. (1975). The Fitragometer: A new device for measuring platelet aggregation in venous blood of man. *Thromb. Diath. haemorrh.* **34**, 531–544.

HORNSTRA, G. and HADDEMA, F. (1977). Effects of dietary fats on the role of platelets in arterial thromboembolism. *In* "Platelets and Thrombosis" (D. C. B. Mills and F. I. Pareti, Eds), pp. 106–110. Academic Press, London and New York.

HOROWITZ, M., SCHAEFER, C., HIROTO, D., WILNER, N. and LEVIN, B. (1977). Life event questionnaires for measuring presumptive stress. *Psychosom. Med.* **39**, 413–431.

HOUSE, J. S. (1975). Occupational stress as a precursor to heart disease. *In* "Psychological Aspects of Myocardial Infarction and Coronary Care" (W. D. Gentry and R. B. Williams, Eds), pp. 24–36. C. V. Mosby Co, St. Louis.

HOUSE, J. S., MCMICHAEL, A. J., WELLS, J. A., KAPLAN, B. H. and LANDERMAN, L. R. (1979). Occupational stress and health among factory workers. *J. Hlth soc. Behav.* **20**, 139–160.

HOWARD, J. H., CUNNINGHAM, D. A. and RECHNITZLER, P. A. (1976). Health patterns associated with Type A behaviour: A managerial problem. *J. Human Stress,* **2** (1), 24–31.

HUGHES, C. W. and LYNCH, J. J. (1978). A reconsideration of psychological precursors of sudden death in infrahuman animals. *Am. Psychol.* **33**, 419–429.

HUGHES, C. W., STEIN, E. A. and LYNCH, J. J. (1978). Hopelessness-induced sudden death in rats. *J. nerv. ment. Dis.* **166**, 387–401.

IMHOF, P. R., BLATTER, K., FUCCELLA, L. M. and TURRI, M. (1969). Beta-blockade and emotional tachycardia: Radiotelemetric investigations in ski-jumpers. *J. appl. Physiol.* **27**, 366–369.

JACOBS, D. R., ANDERSON, J. T. and BLACKBURN, H. (1979). Diet and serum cholesterol: Do zero correlations negate the relationship? *Am. J. Epidemiol.* **110**, 77–87.

JENKINS, C. D. (1966). Components of the coronary-prone behavior pattern: Their relation to silent myocardial infarction and blood lipids. *J. chron. Dis.* **21**, 191–204.

JENKINS, C. D. (1971). Psychologic and social precursors of coronary disease. *New Engl. J. Med.* **284**, 244–255 and 307–317.

JENKINS, C. D. (1976). Recent evidence supporting psychologic and social risk factors for coronary disease. *New Engl. J. Med.* **294**, 987–994 and 1033–1038.

JENKINS, C. D., ROSENMAN, R. H. and FRIEDMAN, M. (1968). Replicability of rating the coronary-prone behavior pattern. *Br. J. prev. soc. Med.* **255**, 237–244.

JENKINS, C. D., ZYZANSKI, S. J., ROSENMAN, R. H. and CLEVELAND, G. L. (1971). Association of coronary-prone behavior scores with recurrence of coronary heart disease. *J. chron. Dis.* **24**, 601–611.

JENKINS, C. D., ROSENMAN, R. H. and ZYZANSKI, S. J. (1974). Prediction of clinical coronary heart disease by a test for the coronary-prone behavior pattern. *New Engl. J. Med.* **290**, 1271–1275.

JENKINS, C. D., ZYZANSKI, S. J. and ROSENMAN, R. H. (1976). Risk of new myocardial infarction in middle aged men with manifest coronary heart disease. *Circulation,* **53**, 342–347.

JENKINS, C. D., ZYZANSKI, S. J., RYAN, T. J., FLESSAS, A. and TANNENBAUM, S. I. (1977). Social insecurity and coronary-prone type A responses as identifiers of severe atherosclerosis. *J. Cons. clin. Psychol.* **45**, 1060–1067.

JENKINS, C. D., ZYZANSKI, S. J. and ROSENMAN, R. H. (1978). Coronary-prone behavior: One pattern or several? *Psychosom. Med.* **40**, 25–43.

JENNI, M. A. and WOLLERSHEIM, J. P. (1979). Cognitive therapy, stress management training, and the Type A behavior pattern. *Cogn. Ther. Res.* **3**, 61–73.

JOHANSSON, G. and FRANKENHAEUSER, M. (1973). Temporal factors in sympatho-adrenomedullary activity. *Biol. Psychol.* **1**, 63–73.

JOHANSSON, G., ARONSSON, G. and LINDSTRÖM, B. O. (1978). Social psychological and neuroendocrine stress reactions to highly mechanised work. *Ergonomics*, **21**, 583–599.

JOHANSSON, G., JONSSON, L., LANNEK, N., BLOMGREN, L., LINDBURG, P. and POUPA, O. (1974). Severe stress-cardiopathy in pigs. *Am. Heart J.* **87**, 451–457.

JOHNSON, A. L., TAYLOR, D. W., SACKETT, D. L., DUNNETT, C. W. and SHIMIZU, A. C. (1978). Self-recording of blood pressure in the management of hypertension. *CMA Journal*, **119**, 1034–1039.

JOHNSON, J. E. (1975). Stress reduction through sensation information. *In* "Stress and Anxiety" (I. Sarason and C. Spielberger, Eds), vol. 2, pp. 361–378. Wiley, Chichester.

JONSSON, A. and HANSSON, L. (1977). Prolonged exposure to a stressful stimulus (noise) as a cause of raised blood pressure in man. *Lancet*, **I**, 86–87.

JORGENSEN, R. J., BOLLING, D. R., YODER, O. C. and MURPHY, E. A. (1972). Blood pressure studies in the Amish. *Johns Hopkins med. J.* **131**, 329–350.

JULIUS, S. and CONWAY, J. (1968). Hemodynamic studies in patients with borderline blood pressure elevation. *Circulation*, **38**, 282–288.

JULIUS, S. and SCHORK, M. A. (1971). Borderline hypertension—a critical review. *J. chron. Dis.* **23**, 723–754.

JULIUS, S. and ESLER, M. D. (1975). Autonomic nervous cardiovascular regulation in borderline hypertension. *Am. J. Cardiol.* **36**, 685–696.

JULIUS, S. and ESLER, M. D. (Eds) (1976a). "The Nervous System in Arterial Hypertension". Charles Thomas, Springfield, Illinois.

JULIUS, S. and ESLER, M. D. (1976b). Increased central blood volume: A possible pathophysiological factor in mild low-renin essential hypertension. *Clin. Sci.* **51**, 207S–210S.

JULIUS, S., PASCUAL, A., SANNERSTEDT, R. and MITCHELL, C. (1971). Relationship between cardiac output and peripheral resistance in borderline hypertension. *Circulation Res.* **43**, 382–390.

JULIUS, S., ESLER, M. D. and RANDALL, O. S. (1975). Role of the autonomic nervous system in mild human hypertension. *Clin. Sci.* **48**, 243S–252S.

JULIUS, S., QUADIR, H. and GAJENDRAGADKAR, S. (1979). Hyperkinetic state: A precursor of hypertension? A longitudinal study of borderline hypertension. *In* "Mild Hypertension: Natural History and Management" (F. Gross and T. Strasser, Eds), pp. 116–126. Pitman Medical, Bath.

KAGAN, A. R., STERNBY, N. H. and VIHERT, A. M. (1976a). Atherosclerosis of the aorta and coronary arteries in five towns. *Bull. Wld Hlth Org.* **53**, 485–645.

KAGAN, A., POPPER, J., RHOADS, G., TAKEYA, Y., KATO, H., GOODE, G. B. and MARMOT, M. (1976b). Epidemiologic studies of coronary heart disease and stroke in Japanese men living in Japan, Hawaii and California: Prevalence of stroke. *In* "Cerebrovascular Diseases" (P. Scheinberg, Ed.), pp. 267–277. Raven Press, New York.

KAHNEMAN, D., TURSKY, B., SHAPIRO, D. and CRIDER, A. (1969). Pupillary, heart rate and skin resistance changes during a mental task. *J. exp. Psychol.* **79**, 164–167.

KANNEL, W. B. (1976). Epidemiology of cerebrovascular disease. *In* "Cerebral Arterial Disease" (R. Ross Russell, Ed.), pp. 1–23. Churchill Livingstone, Edinburgh.

KANNEL, W. B. and DAWBER, T. R. (1973). Hypertensive cardiovascular disease: The Framingham Study. *In* "Hypertension: Mechanisms and Management" (G. Onesti, K. E. Kim and J. H. Meyer, Eds), pp. 5–23. Grune and Stratton, New York.

KANNEL, W. B., GORDON, T. and SCHWARTZ, M. J. (1971). Systolic versus diastolic blood pressure and risk of coronary heart disease. *Am. J. Cardiol.* **27**, 335–346.

KASL, S. V. (1978). Epidemiological contributions to the study of work stress. *In* "Stress at Work" (C. L. Cooper and R. Payne, Eds), pp. 3–48. Wiley, Chichester.

KASL, S. V. and COBB, S. (1970). Blood pressure changes in men undergoing job loss: A preliminary report. *Psychosom. Med.* **32**, 19–38.

KAWASAKI, T., DeLEA, C. S., BARTTER, F. C. and SMITH, H. (1978). The effect of high-sodium and low-sodium intakes on blood pressure and other related variables in human subjects with idiopathic hypertension. *Am. J. Med.* **64**, 193–198.

KEITH, R. A., LOWN, B. and STARE, F. J. (1965). Coronary heart disease and behavior patterns: An examination of method. *Psychosom. Med.* **27**, 424–434.

KELLEHER, R. J., MORSE, W. H. and HERD, J. A. (1976). A pharmacological analysis of behaviourally induced changes in cardiovascular function in the squirrel monkey. *In* "Behavioural Control and Modification of Physiological Activity" (D. Mostofsky, Ed.), pp. 314–338. Prentice-Hall, New York.

KENIGSBERG, D., ZYZANSKI, S. J., JENKINS, C. D., WARDWELL, W. I. and LICCIARDELLO, A. T. (1974). The coronary-prone behavior pattern in hospitalised patients with and without coronary heart disease. *Psychosom. Med.* **36**, 344–351.

KEYS, A. (1970). Coronary heart disease in seven countries. *American Heart Association Monograph*, 29.

KEZDI, P. (1977). Baroreceptors in normotension. *Prog. Brain Res.* **47**, 35–42.

KITAGAWA, E. M. and HAUSER, P. M. (1973). "Differential Mortality in the US: A Study in Socioeconomic Epidemiology". Harvard University Press, Cambridge, Massachusetts.

KITCHIN, A. H. and POCOCK, S. J. (1977). Prognosis of patients with acute myocardial infarction admitted to a coronary care unit. 1. Survival in hospital. *Br. Heart J.* **39**, 1163–1166.

KITTEL, F., KORNITZER, M., ZYZANSKI, S. J., JENKINS, C. D., RUSTIN, R. and DEGRE, C. (1978). Two methods of assessing the type A coronary-prone behavior pattern in Belgium. *J. chron. Dis.* **31**, 147–156.

KJELDSON, K. (1975). Smoking and carbon monoxide uptake as a risk factor in atherosclerotic cardiovascular disease. *In* "Lipids, Lipoproteins and Drugs" (D. Kritchevsky, R. Paoletti and W. L. Holmes, Eds), pp. 317–321. Plenum Press, New York.

KLEIN, R. F., GARRITY, T. F. and GELEIN, J. (1974). Emotional adjustments and catecholamine excretion during early recovery from myocardial infarction. *J. psychosom. Res.* **18**, 425–435.

KOIZUMI, K. and BROOKS, C. M. (1972). The integration of autonomic system reactions: A discussion of autonomic reflexes, their control and their association with somatic reactions. *Ergebn. Physiol.* **67**, 1–68.

KOLMAN, B. S., VERRIER, R. L. and LOWN, B. (1975). The effects of vagus nerve stimulation upon vulnerability of the canine ventrical. *Circulation*, **52**, 578–585.

KORNER, P. I. (1971). Integrative neural cardiovascular control. *Physiol. Rev.* **51**, 312–367.

KORNER, P. I. (1976). Central control of blood pressure: Implications in the pathophysiology of hypertension. *In* "Regulation of Blood Pressure by the Central Nervous System" (G. Onesti, M. Fernandes and K. E. Kim, Eds), pp. 3–20. Grune and Stratton, New York.

KRANTZ, D. S., GLASS, D. C. and SNYDER, M. L. (1974). Helplessness, stress level, and the coronary-prone behavior pattern. *J. abnorm. Psychol.* **10**, 284–300.

KULLER, L. H., PERPER, J. A. and COOPER, M. C. (1975). Sudden and unexpected death due to arteriosclerotic heart diseases. *In* "Modern Trends in Cardiology III" (M. F. Oliver, Ed.), pp. 292–332. Butterworths, London.

KURTZKE, J. F. (1976). An introduction to the epidemiology of cerebrovascular disease. *In* "Cerebrovascular Diseases" (P. Scheinberg, Ed.), pp. 238–253. Raven Press, New York.

KVETŇANSKÝ, R. and MIKULAJ, L. (1970). Adrenal and urinary catecholamines in rats during adaptation to repeated immobilization stress. *Endocrinology*, **87**, 738–743.

KVETŇANSKÝ, R., McCARTY, R., THOA, N. B., LAKE, C. R. and KOPIN, I. J. (1979). Sympatho-adrenal responses of spontaneously hypertensive rats to immobilization stress. *Am. J. Physiol.* **236**, H457–H462.

LACEY, J. I. (1967). Somatic response patterning and stress: Some reformulations of activation theory. *In* "Psychological Stress—Issues in Research" (M. H. Appley and R. Trumball, Eds), pp. 14–44. Appleton-Century-Crofts, New York.

LACEY, B. C. and LACEY, J. I. (1978). Two way communication between the heart and the brain: Significance of time within the cardiac cycle. *Am. Psychol.* **33**, 99–113.

LAIS, L. T. and BRODY, M. J. (1975). Mechanism of vascular hyperresponsiveness in the spontaneously hypertensive rat. *Circulation Res.* **36**, Suppl. I, 216–222.

LAKE, R. C., ZIEGLER, M. G. and KOPIN, I. J. (1976). Use of plasma norepinephrine for evaluation of sympathetic neuronal function in man. *Life Sci.* **18**, 1315–1326.

LAKE, R. C., ZEIGLER, M. G., COLEMAN, M. and KOPIN, I. J. (1977). Age adjusted plasma norepinephrine levels are similar in normotensives and hypertensives. *New Engl. J. Med.* **296**, 208–209.

LANDABURU, R. H. and CASTELLANOS, D. E. (1973). Further evidence for humoral control of factor VIII plasma levels. *Thromb. diath. Haemorrh.* **30**, 460–470.

LANG, C. M. (1967). Effects of psychic stress on atherosclerosis in the squirrel monkey. *Proc. Soc. exp. Biol. Med.* **126**, 30–34.

LANGER, A. W., OBRIST, P. A. and McCUBBIN, J. A. (1979). Hemodynamic and metabolic adjustments during exercise and shock avoidance in dogs. *Am. J. Physiol.: Heart Circ. Physiol.* **5**, H225–H230.

LANGER, E. J., JANIS, J. L. and WOLFER, J. A. (1975). Reduction of psychological stress in surgical patients. *J. exp. Soc. Psychol.* **11**, 155–165.

LANGFIELD, S. B. (1973). Hypertension: Deficient care in the medically served. *Ann. intern. Med.* **78**, 19–23.

LANGFORD, H. G., WATSON, R.·L. and DOUGLAS, B. N. (1968). Factors affecting blood pressure in population groups. *Trans. Ass. Am. Physns.* **81**, 135–146.

LÁNGOS, J., KVETŇANSKÝ, R., BLAŽIČEK, P., NOVOTNÝ, J., VENCEL, P., BURDIGA, A. and MIKULAJ, L. (1976). Plasma renin activity and dopamine-beta-hydroxylase activity and catecholamine excretion in man during stress. *In* "Catecholamines and Stress" (E. Usdin, R. Kvetňanský and I. J. Kopin, Eds), pp. 567–574. Pergamon Press, Oxford.

LANGOSCH, W. (1976). Personality structure and actual condition of patients with heart disease. *In* "Psychological Approach to the Rehabilitation of Coronary Patients" (U. Stocksmeier, Ed.), pp. 42–48. Springer-Verlag, New York.

LAWLER, J. E., OBRIST, P. A. and LAWLER, K. A. (1975). Cardiovascular function during behavioral stress in dogs. *Psychophysiology*, **12**, 4–11.

LAWLER, J. E., BOTTICELLI, L. and LOWN, B. (1976). Changes in cardiac refractory period during signalled shock avoidance in dogs. *Psychophysiology*, **13**, 373–377.

LAWLER, J. E., BARKER, G. F., HUBBARD, J. W. and ALLEN, M. T. (1980). The effects of conflict on tonic levels of blood pressure in genetically borderline hypertensive rats. *Psychophysiology*, **17**, 363–370.

LAZARUS, R. S. and OPTON, E. M. (1966). The study of psychological stress: A summary of theoretical formulations and experimental findings. *In* "Anxiety and Behaviour" (C. Spielberger, Ed.), pp. 225–262. Academic Press, London and New York.

LAZARUS, R. S. and COHEN, J. B. (1977). Environmental stress. *In* "Human Behavior and Environment" (I. Altman and J. S. Wohlwill, Eds), vol. 2. pp. 90–127. Plenum Press, New York.

LEBOVITS, B. Z., SHEKELLE, R. B., OSTFELD, A. and PAUL, O. (1967). Prospective and retrospective studies of coronary heart disease. *Psychosom. Med.* **29**, 265–272.

LEENEN, F. H. and SHAPIRO, A. P. (1974). Effect of intermittent electric shock on plasma renin activity in rats. *Proc. Soc. exp. Biol. Med.* **146**, 534–538.

LEHMAN, E. W. (1967). Social class and coronary heart disease: A sociological assessment of the medical literature. *J. chron. Dis.* **20**, 381–391.

LETHEBY, B. A., DAVIS, R. and LARSEN, A. E. (1974). Effect of major surgical procedures on plasma and platelet levels of factor VIII. *Thromb. diath. Haemorrh.* **31**, 20–29.

LEVI, L. (1965). Urinary output of adrenalin and noradrenalin during pleasant and unpleasant emotional states. *Psychosom. Med.* **27**, 80–85.

LEVI, L. (1972). Psychological and physiological reactions to psychomotor performance during prolonged and complex stressor exposure. *Acta med. scand.* Suppl. 528, 119–142.

LEVINE, S., GOLDMAN, L. and COOVER, G. D. (1972). Expectancy and the Pituitary-adrenal system. *In* "Physiology, Emotion and Psychosomatic Illness". CIBA Foundation Symposium, pp. 281–296. Associated Scientific Publication, Amsterdam.

LEVINE, S. A. (1963). Benign atrial fibrillation of 40 years duration with sudden death from emotion. *Ann. intern. Med.* **58**, 681–684.

LEVY, L. and HERZOG, A. N. (1974). Effects of population density and crowding on health and social adaptation in the Netherlands. *J. Hlth Soc. Behav.* **15**, 228–240.

LEVY, L. and HERZOG, A. N. (1978). Effects of crowding on health and social adaptation in the city of Chicago. *Urban Ecol.* **3**, 327–354.

LEVY, M. N. (1977). Parasympathetic control of the heart. *In* "Neural Regulation of the Heart" (W. C. Randall, Ed.), pp. 95–129. Oxford University Press, Oxford.

LEVY, R. L., HILLMAN, C. C. and STROUD, W. D. (1944). Transient hypertension: Its significance in terms of later development of sustained hypertension and cardiovascular–renal diseases. *J. Am. med. Ass.* **126**, 829–833.

LEVY, R. L., WHITE, P. D., STROUD, W. D. and HILLMAN, C. C. (1945). Transient tachycardia. *J. Am. med. Ass.* **129**, 585–588.

LEY, P. (1977). Psychological studies of doctor-patient communication. *In* "Contributions to Medical Psychology" (S. Rachman, Ed.), vol. 1, pp. 9–42. Pergamon Press, Oxford.

LIARD, J. F., TARAZI, R. C. and FERRARIO, C. (1976). Hemodynamic effects of stellate ganglion stimulation in conscious dogs. *In* "The Nervous System in Arterial Hypertension" (S. Julius and M. D. Esler, Eds), pp. 151–161. Charles Thomas, Springfield, Illinois.

LIGHT, K. C. and OBRIST, P. A. (1980). Cardiovascular response to stress:

Effects of opportunity to avoid, shock experience and performance feedback. *Psychophysiology*, **17**, 243–252.

LINDVALL, K., ERHARDT, J., LUNDMAN, N., REHMQUIST, N. and SJÖGREN, A. (1979). Early mobilization and discharge of patients with acute myocardial infarction. *Acta med. scand.* **206**, 169–176.

LITTLER, W. A., HONOUR, A. J. and SLEIGHT, P. (1973). Direct arterial pressure and ECG recording during motor car driving. *Br. Med. J.* **II**, 273–277.

LOGAN, W. P. D. (1952). Mortality from coronary and myocardial disease in different social classes. *Lancet*, **I**, 758–759.

LORIMER, A. R., MACFARLANE, P. W., PROVAN, G., DUFFY, T. and LAWRIE, T. D. V. (1971). Blood pressure and catecholamine respőnse to "stress" in normotensive and hypertensive subjects. *Cardiovasc. Res.* **5**, 169–173.

LOTT, G. G. and GATCHEL, R. J. (1978). A multi-response analysis of learned heart rate control. *Psychophysiology*, **15**, 576–581.

LOVEGROVE, T. and THOMPSON, P. (1978). The role of acute myocardial infarction in sudden cardiac death—a statistician's nightmare. *Am. Heart J.* **96**, 711–713.

LOWN, B., VERRIER, R. and CORBALAN, R. (1973a). Psychologic stress and the threshold for repetitive ventricular response. *Science*, **183**, 834–836.

LOWN, B., TYKOCINSKI, M., GARFEIN, A. and BROOKS, P. (1973b). Sleep and ventricular premature beats. *Circulation*, **48**, 691–701.

LOWN, B., TEMTE, J. V., REICH, P., GAUGHIN, C., REGESTEIN, Q. and HAI, H. (1976). Basis for recurring ventricular fibrillation in the absence of coronary heart disease and its management. *New Engl. J. Med.* **294**, 623–629.

LOWN, B., VERRIER, R. L. and RABINOWITZ, S. H. (1977). Neural and psychologic mechanisms and the problem of sudden cardiac death. *Am. J. Cardiol.* **39**, 890–902.

LUDBROOK, J., VINCENT, A. and WALSH, T. A. (1975). Effects of mental arithmetic on arterial pressure and hand blood flow. *Clin. exp. Pharmac. Physiol.* Suppl. 2, 67–70.

LUND-JOHANSEN, P. (1967). Hemodynamics in early essential hypertension. *Acta med. scand.* Suppl. 482, 1–101.

LUND-JOHANSEN, P. (1977). Central haemodynamics in essential hypertension. *Acta med. scand.* Suppl. 606, 35–42.

LUNDBERG, U. (1980). Catecholamine and cortisol excretion under psychologically different laboratory conditions. *In* "Catecholamines and Stress: Recent Progress" (E. Usdin, R. Kvetnansky and I. J. Kopin, Eds). Elsevier, New York.

LUNDBERG, U. and FRANKENHAEUSER, M. (1978). Psychophysiological reactions to noise as modified by personal control over noise intensity. *Biol. Psychol.* **6**, 51–59.

LUNDBERG, U., THEORELL, T. and LIND, E. (1975). Life changes and myocardial infarction: Individual differences in life change scaling. *J. psychosom. Res.* **19**, 27–32.

LYNCH, J. J. (1977). "The Broken Heart." Basic Books, New York.

LYNCH, J. J., FLAHERTY, L., EMRICH, C., MILLS, M. E. and KATCHER, A. (1974). Effect of human contact on the heart activity of curarized patients in a shock-trauma unit. *Am. Heart J.* **88**, 160–169.

MACDOUGALL, J. M., DEMBROSKI, T. M. and MUSANTE, L. (1979). The SI and questionnaire methods of assessing coronary-prone behavior in male and female college students. *J. behav. Med.* **2**, 71–83.

MACKAY, D. M. (1974). The effects of civil war on the health of a rural community in Bangladesh. *J. trop. Med. Hyg.* **77**, 120–127.

MANCIA, G., BACCELLI, G. and ZANCHETTI, A. (1974). Regulation of renal circulation during behavioural changes in the cat. *Am. J. Physiol.* **227**, 536–542.

MANCIA, G., FERRARRI, A., GREGORINI, L., LUDROOK, J. and ZANCHETTI, A. (1978). Baroreceptor control of heart rate in man. *In* "Neural Mechanisms in cardiac arrhythmias" (P. J. Schwartz, A. J. Brown, A. Malliani and A. Zanchetti, Eds), pp. 323–333. Raven Press, New York.

MANN, A. H. (1977). Psychiatric morbidity and hostility in hypertension. *Psychol. Med.* **7**, 653–659.

MANNUCCI, P. M., RUGGERI, Z. M. and GAGNATELLI, G. (1971). Nervous regulation of factor VIII levels in man. *Br. J. Haematol.* **20**, 195–207.

MANUCK, S. B. and GARLAND, F. N. (1979). Coronary-prone behavior pattern, task incentive and cardiovascular response. *Psychophysiology*, **16**, 136–142.

MANUCK, S. B., HARVEY, A. H., LECHLEITER, S. L. and NEAL, K. S. (1978a). Effects of coping on blood pressure responses to threat of aversive stimulation. *Psychophysiology*, **15**, 544–549.

MANUCK, S. B., CRAFT, S. and GOLD, K. J. (1978b). Coronary-prone behavior and cardiovascular response. *Psychophysiology*, **15**, 403–411.

MARKS, R. V. (1967). Factors involving social and demographic characteristics. *Millbank Mem. Fund Q.* **45** (2), 51–108.

MARMOT, M. G. and SYME, S. L. (1976). Acculturation and coronary heart disease in Japanese-Americans. *Am. J. Epidemiol.* **104**, 225–247.

MARMOT, M. G., SYME, S. L., KAGAN, A., KATO, H., COHEN, J. B. and BELSKY, J. (1975). Epidemiologic studies of coronary heart disease and stroke in Japanese men living in Japan, Hawaii and California: Prevalence of coronary and hypertensive heart disease and associated risk factors. *Am. J. Epidemiol.* **102**, 514–525.

MARMOT, M. G., ADELSTEIN, A. M., ROBINSON, N. and ROSE, G. A. (1978). Changing social-class distribution of heart disease. *Br. Med. J.* **II**, 1109–1112.

MARWOOD, J. F. and LOCKETT, M. F. (1977). Stress-induced hypertension in rats. *In* "Stress and the Heart" (D. Wheatley, Ed.), pp. 121–135. Raven Press, New York.

MASON, J. W. (1968). A review of psychoendocrine research on the pituitary adrenal cortical system. *Psychosom. Med.* **30**, 576–607.

MASON, J. W. (1972). A re-evaluation of the concept of "non-specificity" in stress theory. *In* "Principles, Practices and Positions in Neuropsychiatric Research" (J. V. Brady and W. J. H. Nauta, Eds), pp. 323–334. Pergamon Press, Oxford.

MASON, J. W. (1975). Emotions as reflected in patterns of endocrine integration. *In* "Emotions — their Parameters and Measurement" (L. Levi, Ed.), pp. 143–181. Raven Press, New York.

MASON, J. W., BRADY, J. V. and SIDMAN, M. (1957). Plasma 17-hydroxycorticosteroid levels and conditioned behavior in the rhesus monkey. *Endocrinology*, **60**, 741–752.

MASON, J. W., MAHER, J. T., HARTLEY, L. H., MOUGEY, E. H., PERLOW, M. J. and JONES, L. G. (1976). Selectivity of corticosteroid and catecholamine responses to various natural stimuli. *In* "Psychopathology of Human Adaptation" (G. Serban, Ed.), pp. 147–171. Plenum Press, New York.

MASUDA, M. and HOLMES, T. H. (1978). Life events: Perceptions and frequencies. *Psychosom. Med.* **40**, 236–261.

MATHEWS, A. M. and LADER, M. (1971). Evaluation of forearm blood flow as a psychophysiological measure. *Psychophysiology*, **8**, 509–524.

MATTA, R. J., LAWLER, J. E. and LOWN, B. (1976). Ventricular electrical instability in the conscious dog. *Am. J. Cardiol.* **38**, 594–598.

MATTHEWS, K. A. (1978). Assessment and developmental antecedents of the coronary-prone behavior pattern in children. *In* "Coronary-prone Behavior" (T. M. Dembroski, S. M. Weiss, J. L. Shields, S. G. Haynes and M. Feinleib, Eds), pp. 207–215. Springer-Verlag, New York.

MATTHEWS, K. A. and SAAL, F. E. (1978). Relationship of the Type A coronary-prone behavior pattern to achievement, power and affiliation motives. *Psychosom. Med.* **40**, 631–636.

MAYOU, R., WILLIAMSON, B. and FOSTER, A. (1976). Attitudes and advice after myocardial infarction. *Br. med. J.* **I**, 1577–1579.

MAYTHAN, J. C., KLINE, R. L. and CALARESU, F. R. (1977). Effect of stimulation of somatic nerves on the ventricular fibrillation threshold in dogs. *Am. Heart J.* **94**, 731–739.

McCLELLAND, D. C. (1976). Sources of stress and the drive for power. *In* "Psychopathology of Human Adaptation" (G. Serban, Ed.), pp. 247–270. Plenum Press, New York.

McCUBBIN, J. W., GREEN, J. H. and PAGE, I. H. (1956). Baroreceptor function in chronic renal hypertension. *Circulation Res.* **4**, 205–210.

McFARLAND, D. V. and COBB, S. (1967). Causal interpretations from cross-sectional data: An examination of the stochastic processes involved in the relation between a personal characteristic and coronary heart disease. *J. chron. Dis.* **20**, 393–406.

McGILL, H. C. (1968). "The Geographic Pathology of Atherosclerosis". Williams and Wilkins, Baltimore.

McGILL, H. C. (1977). Atherosclerosis: Problems in Pathogenesis. *In* "Atherosclerosis Reviews" (R. Paoletti and A. M. Gotto, Eds), vol. 2, pp. 27–65. Raven Press, New York.

McKenney, J. M., Slining, J. M., Henderson, H. R., Devins, D. and Barr, M. (1973). The effect of clinical pharmacy services on patients with essential hypertension. *Circulation*, **48**, 1104–1111.

Medalie, J. H., Snyder, M., Groen, J. J., Neufeld, H. N., Goldbourt, V. and Riss, E. (1973a). Angina pectoris among 10,000 men: 5 year incidence and univariate analysis. *Am. J. Med.* **55**, 583–594.

Medalie, J. H., Kahn, H. A., Neufeld, H. N., Riss, E. and Goldbourt, V. (1973b). 5 year myocardial infarction incidence–II. Association of single variables to age and birthplace. *J. chron. Dis.* **26**, 329–349.

Meittinen, M., Turpeinen, O., Karvonen, M. J., Elosuo, R. and Paavilainen, E. (1972). Effect of cholesterol-lowering diet on mortality for coronary heart disease and other causes. *Lancet*, **IV**, 835–838.

Mendelson, J., Kubansky, P., Leiderman, P. H., Wexler, D., Dutoit, C. and Solmon, P. (1960). Catecholamine excretion and behaviour during sensory deprivation. *Arch. gen. Psychiat.* **2**, 147–155.

Mettlin, C. (1976). Occupational careers and the prevention of coronary-prone behavior. *Soc. Sci. Med.* **10**, 367–372.

Metzner, H. L., Harburg, E. and Lamphiear, D. E. (1977). Early life social incongruities, health risk factors and chronic disease. *J. chron. Dis.* **30**, 225–245.

Meyer, A. J. and Henderson, J. B. (1974). Multiple risk factor reduction in the prevention of cardiovascular disease. *Prev. Med.* **3**, 225–236.

Meyer, J. S., Deshmukh, V. D. and Welch, K. M. A. (1976). Experimental studies concerned with the pathogenesis of cerebral ischaemia and infarction. *In* "Cerebral Arterial Disease" (R. W. Ross Russell, Ed.), pp. 57–84. Churchill-Livingstone, Edinburgh.

Miall, W. E. (1959). Follow-up study of arterial pressure in the population of a Welsh mining valley. *Br. med. J.* **II**, 1204–1210.

Miall, W. E. and Oldham, P. D. (1963). The hereditary factor in arterial blood pressure. *Br. med. J.* **I**, 75–80.

Miall, W. E. and Chinn, S. (1974). Screening for hypertension: Some epidemiological observations. *Br. med. J.* **III**, 595–600.

Miall, W. E. and Brennan, P. J. (1979). Observations on the natural history of mild hypertension in the control groups of therapeutic trials. *In* "Mild Hypertension: Natural History and Management" (F. Gross and T. Strasser, Eds), pp. 38–46. Pitman Medical, Bath.

Miall, W. E., Kass, E. H., Ling, J. and Stuart, K. L. (1962). Factors affecting arterial pressure in the general population in Jamaica. *Br. med. J.* **II**, 497–506.

Mikhail, Y. and Amin, F. (1969). Intrinsic innervation of the human adrenal gland. *Acta Anat. (Basel)*, **72**, 25–32.

Mikulaj, L., Kvetnansky, R., Murgas, K., Parizkova, J. and Vencel, P. (1976). Catecholamines and corticosteroids in acute and repeated stress. *In* "Catecholamines and Stress" (E. Usdin, R. Kvetňanský and I. J. Kopin, Eds), pp. 445–455. Pergamon Press, Oxford.

MILLAR-CRAIG, M. W., KENNY, D., MANN, S., BALASUBRAMANIAN, V. and RAFTERY, E. B. (1979). Effect of once-daily atenolol on ambulatory blood pressure. *Br. med. J.* **I**, 237–238.

MILLER, D. G., GROSSMAN, Z. D., RICHARDSON, R. L., WISTOW, B. W. and Thomas, F. D. (1978). Effects of signalled versus unsignalled stress on rat myocardium. *Psychosom. Med.* **40**, 432–434.

MILLER, R. A. and SHEKELLE, R. B. (1976). Blood pressure in 10th-grade students. *Circulation,* **54**, 993–1000.

MILLER, R. G., RUBIN, R. T., CLARK, B. R., CRAWFORD, W. and ARTHUR, R. J. (1970). The stress of aircraft carrier landings. 1. Corticosteroid responses in naval aviators. *Psychosom. Med.* **32**, 581–588.

MILLER, S. M. (1979). Controllability and human stress: Method, evidence and theory. *Behav. Res. Ther.* **17**, 287–304.

MISCHEL, W. B. (1968). "Personality and Assessment". Wiley, Chichester.

MITCHELL, J. R. A. and SCHWARTZ, C. J. (1965). "Arterial Disease". Blackwell, Oxford.

MONTAGNER, H., HENRY, J. C., LAMBARDOT, M., BENEDINI, M., BURNOD, J. and NICHOLAS, R. M. (1978). Circadian and weekly rhythms in corticosteroid excretion levels of children as indicators of adaptation to social context. *In* "Human Behaviour and Adaptation" (N. Blurton-Jones and V. Reynolds, Eds), pp. 209–266. Taylor and Francis, London.

MORGAN, T., ADAM, W., GILLIES, A., WILSON, M., MORGAN, G. and CARNEY, G. (1978). Hypertension treated by salt restriction. *Lancet,* **I**, 227–230.

SHEELAN, D. J. (1973). Vigorous exercise in leisure time and the incidence of coronary heart disease. *Lancet,* **I**, 333–340.

MOSS, A. J. and WYNAR, B. (1970). Tachycardia in house officers presenting cases in grand rounds. *Ann. intern. Med.* **72**, 255–256.

MOSS, A. J., VITTANDS, I. and SCHENK, E. A. (1966). Cardiovascular effects of sustained norepinephrine infusions. 1. Hemodynamics. *Circulation Res.* **18**, 596–604.

MULCAHY, R. (1976). The rehabilitation of patients with coronary heart disease: A clinician's view. *In* "Psychological Approach to the Rehabilitation of Coronary Patients" (U. Stocksmeier, Ed.), pp. 52–61. Springer-Verlag, New York.

MURGAS, K. and KVETŇANSKÝ, R. (1973). Effect of septal lesions on adrenal cortical and medullary activity during stress. *In* "Hormones and Brain Function" (K. Lissak, Ed.), pp. 437–441. Plenum Press, New York.

NAGLE, R., MORGAN, D., BIRD, J. and BIRD, J. (1976). Interaction between physical and psychological abnormalities after myocardial infarction. *In* "Psychological Approach to the Rehabilitation of Coronary Patients" (U. Stocksmeier, Ed.), pp. 84–88. Springer-Verlag, New York.

NAISMITH, L. D., ROBINSON, J. F., SHAW, G. B., MACINTYRE, M. M. J. (1979). Psychological rehabilitation after myocardial infarction. *Br. med. J.* **I**, 439–446.

NAKAMOTO, K. (1965). Psychogenic paroxysmal cardiac arrhythmias. *Jap. Circulation J.* **29**. 701–717.

NATHANSON, M. H. (1935). Action of acetyl-beta-methylcholin on ventricular rhythms induced by adrenalin. *Proc. Soc. exp. Biol. Med.* **32**, 1297–1299.

National Heart, Lung and Blood Institute (1977). "Fact Book for Fiscal Year 1977". U.S. Dept Health, Education and Welfare.

NAUGHTON, J. and HELLERSTEIN, H. K., Editors (1973). "Exercise Testing and Exercise Training in Coronary Heart Disease". Academic Press, London and New York.

NEIL-DWYER, G., WALTER, P., CRUICKSHANK, J. M., DOSHI, B. and O'GORMAN, P. (1978). Effect of propranolol and phentolamine on myocardial necrosis after subarachnoid haemorrhage. *Br. med. J.* **II**, 990–992.

NELSON, E. C., STASON, W. B., NEUTRA, R., SOLOMON, H. and McARDLE, P. (1978). Impact of patient perceptions on compliance with treatment for hypertension. *Med. Care*, **16**, 893–906.

NESTEL, P. J. (1969). Blood pressure and catecholamine excretion after mental stress in labile hypertension. *Lancet*, **I**, 692–694.

NEUFELD, A. N., ZIVNER, Z., ELDAR, M. and RABINOWITZ, B. (1978). Sinus bradycardia in acute myocardial infarction. *In* "Neural Mechanisms in Cardiac Arrhythmias" (P. J. Schwartz, A. M. Brown, A. Malliani and A. Zanchetti, Eds), pp. 19–30. Raven Press, New York.

NEWLIN, D. B. and LEVENSON, R. W. (1979). Pre-ejection period: Measuring beta-adrenergic influences upon the heart. *Psychophysiology*, **16**, 546–554.

NEWTON, J. E. O. (1967). Psychogenic vagotonia in a family of Beagle dogs. *Cond. Reflex*, **2**, 302–322.

NEWTON, J. E. O., MURPHREE, O. D. and DYKMAN, J. A. (1970). Sporadic transient atrioventricular block and slow heart rate in nervous pointer dogs. *Cond. Reflex*, **5**, 75–89.

NICOTERO, J. A., BEAMER, V., MOUTSOS, S. E. and SHAPIRO, A. (1968). Effects of propranolol on the pressor response to noxious stimulation in hypertensive patients. *Am. J. Cardiol.* **22**, 657–666.

NORMAN-TAYLOR, W. and REES, W. H. (1963). Blood pressure in three New Hebrides communities. *Br. J. prev. soc. Med.* **17**, 141–144.

NOTH, R. H. and MULROW, P. J. (1976). Serum dopamine-beta-hydroxylase as an index of sympathetic nervous system activity in man. *Circulation Res.* **38**, 2–5.

OBERMAN, A., LANE, N. E., HARLAN, W. R., GRAYBIEL, A. and MITCHELL, R. E. (1967). Trends in systolic blood pressure in the thousand aviator cohort over a twenty-four year period. *Circulation*, **36**, 812–822.

OBRIST, P. A. (1976). The cardiovascular-behavioral interaction—as it appears today. *Psychophysiology*, **13**, 95–107.

OBRIST, P. A. and LIGHT, K. C. (1979). Heart rate reactivity to stress as a predictor of systolic blood pressure lability. *Psychophysiology*, **16**, 195.

OBRIST, P. A., HOWARD, J. L., LAWLER, J. E., SUTTERER, J. R., SMITHSON, K. W. and MARTIN, P. L. (1972). Alterations in cardiac contractility during classical aversive conditioning in dogs: Methodological and theoretical implications. *Psychophysiology*, **9**, 246–261.

OBRIST, P. A., LAWLER, J. E., HOWARD, J. L., SMITHSON, K. W., MARTIN, P. L. and MANNING, J. (1974). Sympathetic influences on the heart in humans—effects on contractility and heart rate of acute stress. *Psychophysiology*, **11**, 405–427.

OBRIST, P. A., GAEBELEIN, C. T., TELLER, E. S., LANGER, A. W., GRIGNOLO, A., LIGHT, K. C. and McCUBBIN, J. A. (1978). The relationship among heart rate, carotid dp/dt and blood pressure in humans as a function of the type of stress. *Psychophysiology*, **15**, 102–115.

OLDRIDGE, N. B., WICKS, J. R., HANLEY, C., SUTTON, J. R. and JONES, N. (1978). Noncompliance in an exercise rehabilitation program for men who have suffered a myocardial infarction. *Can. med. Ass. J.* **188**, 361–364.

OLIVER, M. (1976). Dietary cholesterol, plasma cholesterol and coronary heart disease. *Br. Heart J.* **38**, 214–218.

OLIVER, M. (1978). A co-operative trial in the primary prevention of ischaemic heart disease using clofibrate. *Br. Heart J.* **14**, 1069–1118.

OSTFELD, A. and D'ATRI, D. A. (1977). Rapid sociocultural change and high blood pressure. *Adv. psychosom. Med.* **9**, 20–37.

PADMOVATI, S. and GUPTA, S. (1959). Blood pressure studies in rural and urban groups in Delhi. *Circulation*, **19**, 395–405.

PAFFENBARGER, R. D. and WING, A. L. (1969). Characteristics in youth predisposing to fatal stroke in later years. *Lancet*, **I**, 753–754.

PAFFENBARGER, R. D., THORNE, M. C. and WING, A. L. (1968). Chronic disease in former college students, VIII: Characteristics in youth predisposing to hypertension in later years. *Am. J. Epidemiol.* **88**, 25–32.

PAGE, L. B. (1976). Epidemiologic evidence on the etiology of human hypertension and its possible prevention. *Am. Heart J.* **91**, 527–534.

PAGE, L. B., DAMON, A. and MOELLERING, R. C. (1974). Antecedents of cardiovascular disease in six Solomon Island societies. *Circulation*, **49**, 1132–1146.

PALMBLAD, J., BLOMBACK, M., EGBERG, N., FRÖBERG, J., KARLSSON, C. and LEVI, L. (1977). Experimentally induced stress in man: Effects on blood coagulation and fibrinolysis. *J. psychosom. Res.* **21**, 87–92.

PALKOVITS, M. and ZABORSZKY, L. (1977). Neuroanatomy of central cardiovascular control. *Prog. Brain Res.* **47**, 9–34.

PANCHERI, P., BELLATERRA, M., MATTEOLI, S., CRISTOFARI, M., POLIZZI, C. and PULETTI, M. (1978). Infarct as a stress agent: Life history and personality characteristics of improved vs not-improved patients after severe heart attack. *J. Human Stress*, **4** (1), 16–22.

PARKES, C. M. and BROWN, R. J. (1972). Health after bereavement: A controlled study of young Boston widows and widowers. *Psychosom. Med.* **34**, 449–461.

PARKES, C. M., BENJAMIN, B. and FITZGERALD, R. G. (1969). Broken heart: A statistical study of increased mortality among widowers. *Br. med. J.* **I**, 740–743.

PATEL, C. (1975). Yoga and biofeedback in the management of "stress" in hypertensive patients. *Clin. Sci.* **48**, 141–145.

PATEL, C. (1976). Reduction of serum cholesterol and blood pressure in hypertensive patients by behaviour modification. *Jl. R. Coll. Gen. Pract.* **26**, 211–215.

PATEL, C. and NORTH, W. R. S. (1975). Randomised controlled trial of Yoga and biofeedback in management of hypertension. *Lancet*, **II**, 93–99.

PATEL, C., MARMOT, M., TERRY, D., CARRUTHERS, M. and SEVER, P. Coronary risk factor reduction through biofeedback-aided relaxation and meditation. Unpublished manuscript.

PAUL, O. (1971). Risks of mild hypertension: A 10 year report. *Br. Heart J.* **33**, Suppl. 116–121.

PAULUS, P. B., McCAIN, G. and COX, V. C. (1978). Death rates, psychiatric commitments, blood pressure, and perceived crowding as a function of institutional crowding. *Envir. Psychol. nonverb. Behav.* **3**, 107–116.

PENROSE, R. J. J. (1972). Life events before subarachnoid haemorrhage. *J. psychosom. Res.* **16**, 329–333.

PERLMAN, R. L. and CHALFIE, M. (1977). Catecholamine release from the adrenal medulla. *Clinics Endocrin. Metab.* **6**, 551–576.

PERLOW, M. J., KOROUM, F., BRAUN, D. and WYATT, R. J. (1979). Adrenergic and dopaminergic responses to chronic chair restraint in the rhesus monkey. *Psychosom. Med.* **41**, 139–145.

PERRY, H. M. and SMITH, W. McF. (Eds) (1978). Mild hypertension: To treat or not to treat. *Ann. N.Y. Acad. Sci.* **304**.

PERSKI, A. and ENGEL, B. T. (1980). The role of behavioral conditioning in the cardiovascular adjustment to exercise. *Biofeedback Self-regulation*, **5**, 91–104.

PETERFY, G. and PINTER, E. J. (1973). Some physiological aspects of emotional stress. *In* "Hormones and Brain Function" (K. Lissak, Ed.), pp. 459–474. Plenum Press, New York.

PETERSON, J. E., KEITH, R. A. and WILCOX, A. (1962). Hourly changes in serum cholesterol concentration: Effects of anticipation of stress. *Circulation*, **25**, 798–803.

PICKERING, G. W. (1961). "The Nature of Essential Hypertension". Churchill, London.

PICKERING, G. W. (1968). "High Blood Pressure", 2nd Edition. Churchill, London.

PICKERING, T. G. and GORHAM, G. (1975). Learned heart-rate controlled by a patient with a ventricular parasystolic rhythm. *Lancet*, **I**, 252–253.

PICKERING, T. G. and MILLER, N. E. (1977). Learned voluntary control of heart rate and rhythm in two subjects with premature ventricular contractions. *Br. Heart J.* **39**, 152–159.

PICKERING, T. G. and SLEIGHT, P. (1977). Baroreceptors and hypertension. *Prog. Brain Res.* **47**, 43–60.

Pooling Project Research Group (1978). Relation of blood pressure, serum cholesterol, smoking habit, relative weight and ECG abnormalities to incidence of major coronary events: Final report of the Pooling Project. *J. chron. Dis.* **31**, 201–306.

PRICE, K. P., LOTT, G., FIXLER, D. E. and BROWNE, R. H. (1979). Cardiovascular responses to stress in adolescents with elevated blood pressures. *Psychosom. Med.* **41**, 74.

PRIOR, I., STANHOPE, J., EVANS, J. and SALMOND, C. (1974). The Tokelau Island Migrant Study. *Int. J. Epidemiol.* **3**, 225–232.

PROVOOST, A. P., BOHUS, B. and DE JONG, W. (1977). Differential influence of neonatal sympathectomy on the development of DOCA-salt and spontaneous hypertension in the rat. *Prog. Brain Res.* **47**, 417–424.

PURVES, M. J. (1978). Do vasomotor nerves significantly regulate cerebral blood flow? *Circulation Res.* **43**, 485–493.

RAAB, W. (1968). Correlated cardiovascular adrenergic and adrenocortical responses to sensory and mental annoyances in man. *Psychosom. Med.* **30**, 809–818.

RABKIN, S. W., MATHEWSON, F. A. L. and HSU, P. (1977). Relation of body weight to development of ischaemic heart disease in a cohort of young North American men after a 26-year observation period: The Manitoba study. *Am. J. Cardiol.* **39**, 452–458.

RAHE, R. H. and ARTHUR, R. J. (1967). Life events surrounding illness onset. *J. psychosom. Res.* **11**, 341–345.

RAHE, R. H. and PASSIKIVI, J. (1971). Psychosocial factors and myocardial infarction—II. An outpatient study in Sweden. *J. psychosom. Res.* **15**, 33–39.

RAHE, R. H., RUBIN, R. T., GUNDERSON, L. K. and ARTHUR, R. J. (1971). Psychologic correlates of serum cholesterol in man—a longitudinal study. *Psychosom. Med.* **33**, 399–410.

RAHE, R. H., RUBIN, R. T. and ARTHUR, R. J. (1974a). The three investigators study. Serum uric acid, cholesterol and cortisol variability during stresses of everyday life. *Psychosom Med.* **36**, 258–268.

RAHE, R. H., ROMO, M., BENNETT, L. and SILTANEN, P. (1974b). Recent life changes, myocardial infarction and abrupt coronary deaths. *Archs intern. Med.* **133**, 221–228.

RAHE, R. H., ARAJÄRVI, H., ARAJÄRVI, S., PUNSAR, S. and KARVONEN, M. J. (1976). Recent life change and coronary heart disease in east versus west Finland. *J. psychosom. Res.* **20**, 431–437.

RANDALL, D. C. and HASSON, D. M. (1977). A note on ECG changes observed during Pavlovian conditioning in a rhesus monkey following coronary arterial occlusion. *Pavlov. J. biol. Sci.* **12**, 229–231.

RANDALL, D. C., KAYE, M. P., RANDALL, W. C., BRADY, J. V. and MARTIN, K. H. (1976). Response of primate heart to emotional stress before and after cardiac denervation. *Am. J. Physiol.* **230**, 988–995.

RANDALL, D. C., HASSON, D. M. and BRADY, J. V. (1979). Conditional cardiovascular response to shock before and after coronary arterial occlusion. *Am. J. Physiol.* **236**, H273–H279.

RAW, M. (1977). The psychological modification of smoking. *In* "Contributions to Medical Psychology" (S. Rachman, Ed.), vol. 1, pp. 189–210. Pergamon Press, Oxford.

REICHENBACH, D. D., MOSS, N. S. and MEYER, F. (1977). Pathology of the heart in sudden cardiac death. *Am. J. Cardiol.* **39**, 865–872.

REIS, D. J., GAUTHIER, P. and NATHAN, M. A. (1976). Hypertension, adrenal catecholamine release, pulmonary edema and behavioral excitement elicited from the anterior hypothalamus in rat. *In* "Catecholamines and Stress" (E. Usdin, R. Kvetňanský and I. J. Kopin, Eds), pp. 195–206. Pergamon Press, Oxford.

REIS, D. J., DOBA, N., SNYDER, D. W. and NATHAN, M. (1977). Brain lesions and hypertension: Chronic lability and elevation of arterial pressure produced by electrolytic lesions and 6-hydroxy-dopamine treatment of nucleus tractus solitarii in rat and cat. *Prog. Brain Res.* **47**, 169–188.

REISEN, E., ABEL, R., MODAN, M., SILVERBERG, D. S., ELIAHAU, H. and MODAN, B. (1978). Effect of weight loss without salt restriction on the reduction of blood pressure in overweight hypertensive patients. *New Engl. J. Med.* **298**, 1–6.

REISER, M. F., BRUST, A. A. and FERRIS, E. B. (1951). Life situations, emotions and the course of patients with hypertension. *Psychosom. Med.* **13**, 133–139.

REYNOLDS, R. C. (1974). Community and occupational influences in stress at Cape Kennedy: Relationships to heart disease. *In* "Stress and the Heart" (R. S. Eliot, Ed.), pp. 33–49. Futura, New York.

RICHARD, J. (1976). Epidemiology of hypertension and stroke in European and Mediterranean countries. *In* "Hypertension and Stroke Control", pp. 60–79. WHO, Geneva.

RICHARDSON, P., STELLA, A., LEONETTI, G., BARTORELLI, A. and ZANCHETTI, A. (1974). Mechanisms of renal release of renin by electrical stimulation of the brainstem in the cat. *Circulation Res.* **34**, 425–434.

RICHTER, C. P. (1957). On the phenomenon of sudden death in animals and man. *Psychosom. Med.* **19**, 191–198.

RIESS, W. F., WERDEGER, D. and SOKOLOW, M. (1967). Blood pressure responses to daily life events. *Trans. Ass. Life Insur. med. Dir. Am.* **51**, 116–129.

ROBINSON, B. F. (1967). Relation of heart rate and systolic blood pressure to the onset of pain in angina pectoris. *Circulation,* **35**, 1073–1083.

ROBINSON, J. O. (1964). A possible effect of selection on the test scores of a group of hypertensives. *J. psychosom. Res.* **8**, 239–243.

ROMO, M., SILTANEN, P., THEORELL, T. and RAHE, R. H. (1974). Work behaviour, time urgency and life dissatisfactions in subjects with myocardial infarction: A cross cultural study. *J. psychosom. Res.* **18**, 1–8.

ROSE, K. D. (1974). The post coronary patient as a spectator sportsman. *In* "Stress and the Heart" (R. S. Eliot, Ed.), pp. 207–218. Futura, New York.

ROSENMAN, R. H. (1978). The interview method of assessment of the coronary-prone behavior pattern. *In* "Coronary-prone Behavior" (T. M. Dembroski, S. M. Weiss, J. L. Shields, S. G. Haynes and M. Feinleib, Eds), pp. 55–70. Springer-Verlag, New York.

ROSENMAN, R. H. and FRIEDMAN, M. (1974). Neurogenic factors in pathogenesis of coronary heart disease. *Med. Clins. N. Am.* **58**, 269–279.

ROSENMAN, R. H., FRIEDMAN, M., STRAUS, R., JENKINS, C. D., ZYZANSKI, S. J. and WURM, M. (1964). A predictive study of coronary heart disease: The Western Collaborative Group Study. *J. Am. med. Ass.* **189**, 15–22.

ROSENMAN, R. H., BRAND, R. J., JENKINS, C. D., FRIEDMAN, M., STRAUS, R. and WURM, M. (1975). Coronary heart disease in the Western Collaborative Group Study: Final follow-up experience of $8\frac{1}{2}$ years. *J. Am. med. Ass.* **233**, 872–877.

ROSENMAN, R. H., BRAND, R. J., SHOLTZ, R. I. and FRIEDMAN, M. (1976). Multivariate prediction of coronary heart disease during $8\frac{1}{2}$ year follow-up in the Western Collaborative Group Study. *Am. J. Cardiol.* **37**, 903–910.

ROSKIES, E., SPEVACK, M., SURKIS, A., COHEN, C. and GILMAN, S. (1978). Changing the coronary-prone (Type A) behavior pattern in a non-clinical population. *J. behav. Med.* **1**, 201–216.

ROSKIES, E., KEARNEY, H., SPEVACK, M., SURKIS, A., COHEN, C. and GILMAN, S. (1979). Generalizability and durability of treatment effects in an intervention program for coronary-prone (Type A) responses. *J. behav. Med.* **2**, 195–207.

ROSS, A. and STEPTOE, A. (1980). Attenuation of the diving reflex in man by mental stimulation. *J. Physiol.* **302**, 387–393.

ROSS, J., HIGGINSON, L., FRANKLIN, D. and TONIOKE, H. (1978). Beta-adrenergic blockade in experimental myocardial ischaemia and infarction: Effects on regional myocardial function and dysrhythmias. *In* "Neural Mechanisms in Cardiac Arrhythmias" (P. Schwartz, A. M. Brown, A. Malliani and A. Zanchetti, Eds), pp. 401–418. Raven Press, New York.

ROSS RUSSELL, R. W. (1975). How does blood pressure cause stroke. *Lancet*, **II**, 1283–1285.

ROTHFELD, B., PARE, W. P., VARADY, A., ISOM, K. and KARMEN, A. (1973). The effects of environmental stress on cholesterol synthesis and metabolism. *Biochem. Med.* **7**, 292–298.

ROWE, M. J., NEILSON, J. M. M. and OLIVER, M. J. (1975). Control of ventricular arrhythmias during myocardial infarction by antilipolytic treatment using a nicotinic acid analogue. *Lancet*, **I**, 295–300.

ROWLAND, K. (1977). Environmental events predicting death for the elderly. *Psychol. Bull.* **84**, 349–372.

RUBIN, R. T., RAHE, R. H., ARTHUR, R. J. and CLARK, B. R. (1969). Adrenal cortical activity changes during underwater demolition team training. *Psychosom. Med.* **31**, 553–564.

RUDOLFF, G. D. M. (1955). Clinical blood pressure in anxiety. *J. ment. Sci.* **101**, 893–894.

RUSKIN, A., BEARD, O. W. and SCHAFFER, R. (1948). Blast hypertension. *Am. J. Med.* **4**, 228–236.

RUSSEK, H. I. and ZOHMAN, B. L. (1958). Relative significance of heredity, diet and occupational stress in coronary heart disease of young adults. *Am. J. med. Sci.* **235**, 266–275.

RUSSEK, H. I. and RUSSEK, L. G. (1976). Is emotional stress an etiologic factor in coronary heart disease. *Psychosom. Med.* **17**, 63–67.

RUSSEK, H. I. and RUSSEK, L. G. (1977). Behavior patterns and emotional stress in the etiology of coronary heart disease: Social and occupational aspects. *In* "Stress and the Heart" (D. Wheatley, Ed.), pp. 1–13. Raven Press, New York.

SACKETT, D. L., HAYNES, R., GIBSON, E., HACKETT, B., TAYLOR, W., ROBERTS, R. and JOHNSON, A. (1975). Randomised clinical trial of strategies for improving medication compliance in primary hypertension. *Lancet*, **1**, 1205–1207.

SACKETT, D. L., TAYLOR, D. W., HAYNES, R. B., JOHNSON, A. L., GIBSON, E. S. and ROBERTS, R. S. (1979). Compliance with therapeutic regimen. *In* "Mild Hypertension: Natural History and Management" (F. Gross and T. Strasser, Eds), pp. 309–327. Pitman Medical, Bath.

SAFAR, M. E., WEISS, Y. A., LEVENSON, J. A., LONDON, G. M. and MILLIEZ, P. L. (1973). Haemodynamic study of 85 patients with borderline hypertension. *Am. J. Cardiol.* **31**, 315–319.

SAFAR, M. E., KAMIENIECKA, H. A., LEVENSON, J. A., DIMITRIU, V. M. and PAULEAU, N. F. (1978). Haemodynamic factors and Rorschach testing in borderline and sustained hypertension. *Psychosom. Med.* **40**, 620–630.

SALES, S. M. and HOUSE, J. (1971). Job dissatisfaction as a possible risk factor in coronary heart disease. *J. chron. Dis.* **23**, 861–874.

SAMPSON, L. D., FRANCIS, J. S. and SCHNEIDERMAN, N. (1974). Selective autonomic blockade: Effects upon classical conditioning of heart rate and lever-lift suppression in rabbits. *J. comp. physiol. Psychol.* **87**, 953–962.

SAPIRA, J. D. and SHAPIRO, A. P. (1966). Studies in man on the relationship of adrenergic correlates to pressor responsivity. *Circulation*, **34**, 226–241.

SASSENRATH, E. N. (1970). Increased adrenal responsiveness related to social stress in rhesus monkey. *Horm. Behav.* **1**, 238–298.

SCHENK, E. A. and MOSS, A. J. (1966). Cardiovascular effects of sustained norepinephrine infusions. 2: Morphology. *Circulation Res.* **18**, 605–615.

SCHEUER, J. and TIPTON, C. (1977). Cardiovascular adaptations to physical training. *A. Rev. Physiol.* **39**, 221–251.

SCHERWITZ, L., BERTON, K. and LEVENTHAL, H. (1977). Type A assessment and interaction in the behavior pattern interview. *Psychosom. Med.* **39**, 229–240.

SCHERWITZ, L., BERTON, K. and LEVENTHAL, H. (1978). Type A behavior, self-involvement and cardiovascular response. *Psychosom. Med.* **40**, 593–609.

SCHMITT, F. O. and WORDEN, F. G. (Eds) (1979). The neurosciences: Fourth study program. M.I.T. Press, Cambridge, Massachusetts.

SCHRAMM, L. P., ANDERSON, D. E. and RANDALL, D. (1975). Renal blood flow changes during aversive conditioning in the dog. *Experientia*, **31**, 71–73.

SCHUCKER, B. and JACOBS, D. R. (1977). Assessment of behavioral risk for coronary disease by voice characteristics. *Psychosom. Med.* **39**, 219–228.

SCOTCH, N. A. (1963). Sociocultural factors in the epidemiology of Zulu hypertension. *Am. J. publ. Hlth,* **53**, 1205–1213.

SEGERS, M. J., GRAULICH, P. and MERTENS, C. (1974). Relations psycho-biocliniques dans un group de coronariens: Étude preliminaire. *J. psychosom. Res.* **18**, 307–313.

SELIGMAN, M. E. P. (1975). Chronic fear produced by unpredictable electric shock. *J. comp. physiol. Psychol.* **66**, 402–411.

SELYE, H. (1976). "The Stress of Life", 2nd ed. McGraw-Hill, New York.

SELYE, H. and BAJUSZ, E. (1959). Conditioning by corticoids for the production of cardiac lesions with noradrenaline. *Acta Endocr.* **30**, 183–187.

SHAPER, A. G. (1962). Cardiovascular studies in the Samburu tribe of Northern Kenya. *Am. Heart J.* **63**, 437–442.

SHAPIRO, A. P. and HORN, P. W. (1955). Blood pressure, plasma pepsinogen and behaviour in cats subjected to experimental production of anxiety. *J. nerv. ment. Dis.* **122**, 222–231.

SHAPIRO, A. P. and MELHADO, J. (1957). Factors affecting development of hypertensive vascular disease after renal injury in rats. *Proc. Soc. exp. Biol. Med.* **96**, 619–623.

SHAPIRO, A. P., MOUTSOS, S. E. and KRIFCHER, E. (1963). Patterns of pressor response to noxious stimuli in normal, hypertensive and diabetic subjects. *J. clin. Invest.* **42**, 1890–1898.

SHEKELLE, R. B., OSTFELD, A. M. and PAUL, O. (1969). Social status and incidence of coronary heart disease. *J. chron. Dis.* **22**, 381–394.

SHEKELLE, R. B., SCHOENBERGER, J. A. and STAMLER, J. (1976). Correlates of the JAS type A behavior pattern score. *J. chron. Dis.* **29**, 381–394.

SHERRY, S. (1977). The role of the platelet in thrombosis. *In* "Platelets and Thrombosis" (D. C. B. Mills and F. I. Pareti, Eds), pp. 111–114. Academic Press, London and New York.

SHIBATA, H. and HATANO, S. (1979). A salt restriction trial in Japan. *In* "Mild Hypertension: Natural History and Management" (F. Gross and T. Strasser, Eds), pp. 147–160. Pitman Medical, Bath.

SHORT, D. (1975). A policy for hypertension. *Br. Heart J.* **37**, 893–896.

SIDMAN, M., MASON, J. P., BRADY, J. V. and THACH, J. (1962). Quantitative relations between avoidance behavior and pituitary-adrenocortical activity. *J. exp. Analysis Behav.* **5**, 353–362.

SIMON, A. C., SAFAR, M. E., WEISS, Y. A., LONDON, G. M. and MILLIEZ, P. L. (1977). Baroreflex sensitivity and cardiopulmonary blood volume in normotensive and hypertensive patients. *Br. Heart J.* **39**, 799–805.

SIMPSON, M. T., OLEWINE, D. A., JENKINS, C. D., RAMSAY, F. H., ZYZANSKI, S. J., THOMAS, G. and HAMES, C. G. (1974). Exercise-induced catecholamines and platelet aggregation in the coronary-prone behavior pattern. *Psychosom. Med.* **36**, 476–487.

SINGER, J. E., LUNDBERG, U. and FRANKENHAEUSER, M. (1978). Stress on the train: A study of urban commuting. *In* "Advances in Environmental Psychology" (A. Baum, J. E. Singer and S. Valins, Eds), vol. 1, pp. 41–56. Lea, Hillsdale.

SINGER, M. T. (1974). Engagement-involvement: A central phenomenon in psychophysiological research. *Psychosom. Med.* **36**, 1–17.

SIRTORI, C., RICCI, G. and GIORINI, S. (Eds) (1975). "Diet and Atherosclerosis". Plenum Press, New York.

SLEIGHT, P. (1975). Neural control of the cardiovascular system. *In* "Modern Trends in Cardiology — III" (M. F. Oliver, Ed.), pp. 1–43. Butterworths, London.

SLUSHER, M. A. and HYDE, J. E. (1966). Effect of diencephalic and midbrain stimulation on ACTH levels in unrestrained cats. *Am. J. Physiol.* **210**, 103–108.

SMIRK, F. H. (1957). "High Arterial Pressure". Blackwell, Oxford.

SMITH, E. B. and SLATER, R. S. (1973). Lipids and low density lipoproteins in intima in relation to its morphological characteristics. *In* "Atherogenesis: Initiating Factors". CIBA Foundation Symp. 12. pp. 39–52. Elsevier, Amsterdam.

SMITH, G. P. (1973). Adrenal hormones and emotional behavior. *In* "Progress in Physiological Psychology" (E. Stellar and J. M. Sprague, Eds), vol. 5, pp. 299–351. Academic Press, New York and London.

SOKOLOW, E. I. and VOLKOVA, V. I. (1977). An investigation into the influence of psychological-emotional stress on the changes in coagulating properties of the blood in patients with hypertensive disease. *Soviet Med.* **I**, 29–33.

STAMLER, J. (1978). Lifestyles, major risk factors, proof and public policy. *Circulation*, **58**, 3–20.

STAMLER, J., STAMLER, R. and PULLMAN, R. N. (Eds) (1967). "The Epidemiology of Hypertension: Proceedings of an International Symposium". Grune and Stratton, New York.

STAMLER, J., STAMLER, B., RIEDLINGER, W., ALGERA, G. and ROBERTS, R. (1976). Hypertension screening of 1 million Americans. *J. Am. med. Ass.* **235**, 2299–2306.

STEPTOE, A. (1976). Blood pressure control: A comparison of feedback and instructions using pulse wave velocity measurements. *Psychophysiology*, **13**, 528–536.

STEPTOE, A. (1977a). Psychological methods in the treatment of hypertension: A review. *Br. Heart J.* **39**, 587–593.

STEPTOE, A. (1977b). Blood pressure control with pulse wave velocity feedback: Methods of analysis and training. *In* "Biofeedback and Behavior" (J. Beatty and H. Legewie, Eds), pp. 355–368. Plenum Press, New York.

STEPTOE, A. (1977c). Voluntary blood pressure reductions measured with pulse transit time: Training conditions and reactions to mental work. *Psychophysiology*, **14**, 492–498.

STEPTOE, A. (1978a). New approaches to the management of essential hypertension with psychological techniques. *J. psychosom. Res.* **22**, 339–354.

STEPTOE, A. (1978b). The regulation of blood pressure reactions to taxing conditions using pulse transit time feedback and relaxation. *Psychophysiology*, **15**, 429–438.

STEPTOE, A. (1979a). Biofeedback: Experimental research and clinical applications. *In* "Psychosomatics and Biofeedback" (W. H. G. Wolters and G. Sinnema, Eds), pp. 11–25. Bohn, Scheltema and Holkema, Utrecht.

STEPTOE, A. (1979b). Cardiovascular reactivity and its management with psychological techniques. *In* "Research in Psychology and Medicine" (D. J. Oborne, M. M. Gruneberg and D. R. Eiser, Eds), vol. 1, pp. 191–198. Academic Press, London and New York.

STEPTOE, A. (1980a). "Blood Pressure". *In* "Techniques in Psychophysiology" (P. Venables and I. Martin, Eds), pp. 247–273. Wiley, Chichester.

STEPTOE, A. (1980b). Stress and medical disorders. *In* "Contributions to Medical Psychology" (S. Rachman, Ed.), vol. 2, pp. 55–77. Pergamon Press, Oxford.

STEPTOE, A. and ROSS, A. (1980a). Psychophysiological reactivity and the prediction of cardiovascular disorders. *J. psychosom. Res.* In press.

STEPTOE, A. and ROSS, A. (1980b). Voluntary control of cardiovascular reactions to demanding mental tasks. Submitted for publication.

STEPTOE, A., MATHEWS, A. M. and JOHNSTON, D. (1974). The learned control of differential temperature in the human earlobes. *Biol. Psychol.* **1**, 237–242.

STEPTOE, A., SMULYAN, H. and GRIBBIN, B. (1976). Pulse wave velocity and blood pressure: Calibration and applications. *Psychophysiology*, **13**, 488–493.

STERN, M. J., PASCALE, L. and ACKERMAN, A. (1977). Life adjustment after myocardial infarction. *Arch. intern. Med.* **137**, 1680–1685.

STERNBACH, R. A. (1968). "Pain – a Psychophysiological Analysis". Academic Press, New York and London.

STEVENSON, I. P., DUNCAN, C. H., WOLF, S., RIPLEY, H. S. and WOLFF, H. G. (1949). Life situations, emotions and extrasystoles. *Psychosom. Med.* **11**, 257–272.

STOCKSMEIER, U. (Ed.) (1976). "Psychological Approach to the Rehabilitation of Coronary Patients". Springer-Verlag, Berlin.

STONE, R. and DELEO, J. (1976). Psychotherapeutic control of hypertension. *New Engl. J. Med.* **294**, 80–84.

STOREY, P. B. (1968). The precipitation of subarachnoid haemorrhage. *J. psychosom. Res.* **13**, 175–182.

STOUT, C., MORROW, J., BRANDT, E. and WOLF, S. (1964). Unusually low incidence of death from myocardial infarction in an Italian-American community in Pennsylvania. *J. Am. med. Ass.* **188**, 845–849.

STRØMME, S. B., WIKEBY, P. C., BLIX, A. S. and URSIN, H. (1978). "Additional Heart Rate". *In* "The Psychobiology of Stress" (H. Ursin, E. Baade and S. Levine, Eds), pp. 83–89. Academic Press, London.

SUINN, R. M. and BLOOM, L. J. (1978). Anxiety management training for pattern A behaviour. *J. Behav. Med.* **1**, 25–35.

SURWIT, R., SHAPIRO, D. and GOOD, M. I. (1978). Comparison of cardiovascular biofeedback, neuromuscular biofeedback and meditation in the treatment of borderline essential hypertension. *J. cons. clin. psychol.* **46**, 252–263.

SYME, S. L. and TORFS, C. P. (1978). Epidemiologic research in hypertension : A critical appraisal. *J. Human Stress*, **4**(3), 43–48.

SYME, S. L., BORHANI, N. O. and BUECHLEY, R. W. (1966). Cultural mobility and coronary heart disease in an urban area. *Am. J. Epidemiol.* **82**, 334–346.

SZKLO, M., TONASCIA, J. and GARDIS, L. (1976). Psychosocial factors and the risk of myocardial infarction in white women. *Am. J. Epidemiol.* **103**, 312–320.

TAGGART, P. and CARRUTHERS, M. (1971). Endogenous hyperlipidaemia induced by emotional stress of racing driving. *Lancet*, **I**, 363–366.

TAGGART, P., GIBBONS, P. and SOMERVILLE, W. (1969). Some effects of motor car driving on the normal and abnormal heart. *Br. med. J.* **IV**, 130–134.

TAGGART, P., HEDWORTH-WHITTY, R., CARRUTHERS, M. and GORDON, P. D. (1976). Observations on ECG and plasma catecholamines during dental procedures : The forgotten vagus. *Br. med. J.* **II**, 787–789.

TAGGART, P., CARRUTHERS, M., JOSEPH, S., KELLY, H. B., MARCONICHELAKIS, J., NOBLE, P., O'NEILL, G. and SOMERVILLE, W. (1979). ECG changes resembling myocardial ischaemia in asymptomatic men with normal arteriograms. *Br. Heart J.* **41**, 214–225.

TAGUCHI, J. and FRIES, E. D. (1974). Partial reduction of blood pressure and prevention of complications in hypertension. *New Engl. J. Med.* **291**, 329–331.

TALBOTT, E., KULLER, L. H., DETRE, K. and PERPER, J. (1977). Biologic and psychosocial risk factors of sudden death from coronary disease in white women. *Am. J. Cardiol.* **39**, 858–864.

TARAZI, R. C., IBRAHIM, M., DUSTAN, H. P. and BRAVO, E. L. (1976). Use of systolic time intervals in studying hypertension. *Aust. N.Z. J. Med.* **6**, Suppl. 2, 8–14.

TAYLOR, C. B., FARQUHAR, J. W., NELSON, E. and AGRAS, S. (1977). Relaxation therapy and high blood pressure. *Arch. gen. Psychiat.* **34**, 339–342.

TECCE, J. J., FRIEDMAN, S. B. and MASON, J. W. (1966). Anxiety, defensiveness and 17-hydroxycorticosteroid excretion. *J. nerv. ment. Dis.* **141**, 549–554.

THACKRAY, R. I. and PEARSON, P. W. (1968). Stress, heart rate and performance. *Perc. Motor Skills*, **27**, 651–658.

THEORELL, T. (1976). Selected illnesses and somatic factors in relation to two psychosocial stress indices—a prospective study on middle-aged construction building workers. *J. psychosom. Res.* **20**, 7–20.

THEORELL, T. and ÅKERSTEDT, T. (1976). Day and night work : Changes in cholesterol, uric acid, glucose and potassium in serum and in circadian patterns of urinary catecholamine excretion. *Acta med. scand.* **200**, 47–53.

THEORELL, T. and FLODERUS-MYRHED, B. (1977). "Workload" and risk of myocardial infarction—a prospective psychosocial analysis. *Int. J. Epidemiol.* **6**, 17–21.

THEORELL, T. and LIND, E. (1973). Systolic blood pressure, serum cholesterol, and smoking in relation to sociological factors and myocardial infarction. *J. psychosom. Res.* **17**, 327–332.

THEORELL, T. and RAHE, R. H. (1971). Psychosocial factors and myocardial infarction — 1. An inpatient study in Sweden. *J. psychosom. Res.* **15**, 25–31.

THEORELL, T. and RAHE, R. H. (1975). Life change events, ballistocardiography and coronary death. *J. Human Stress*, **1**(3), 18–24.

THEORELL, T., LIND, E., FRÖBERG, J., KARLSSON, C. and LEVI, L. (1972). A longitudinal study of 21 subjects with coronary heart disease: Life changes, catecholamine excretion and related biochemical reactions. *Psychosom. Med.* **34**, 505–516.

THEORELL, T., BLUNK, D. and WOLF, S. (1974). Emotions and cardiac contractility as reflected in ballistocardiographic recordings. *Pavl. J. Biol. Sci.* **9**, 65–75.

THEORELL, T., LIND, E. and FLODERUS, B. (1975). Relationship of disturbing life changes and emotions to the early development of myocardial infarction and other serious illnesses. *Int. J. Epidemiol.* **4**, 281–293.

THEORELL, T., OLSSON, A. and ENGHOLM, G. (1977). Concrete work and myocardial infarction. *Scand. J. Work environ. Hlth*, **3**, 144–153.

THIEL, H. G., PARKER, D. and BRUCE, T. A. (1973). Stress factors and the risk of myocardial infarction. *J. psychosom. Res.* **17**, 43–57.

THOMAS, C. B. and GREENSTREET, R. L. (1973). Psychobiological characteristics in youth as predictors of 5 disease states: Suicide, mental illness, hypertension, coronary heart disease and tumor. *Johns Hopkins med. J.* **132**, 16–43.

THOMAS, G. W., LEDINGHAM, J., BEILIN, L. J. and STOTT, A. N. (1976). Reduced plasma renin activity in essential hypertension: Effects of blood pressure, age and sodium. *Clin. Sci. molec. Med.* **51**, 185S–188S.

THOMPSON, D. D. and PITTS, R. F. (1952). Effects of alterations of renal arterial pressure on sodium and water excretion. *Am. J. Physiol.* **168**, 490–499.

THOMPSON, P. L. and LOWN, B. (1972). Sequential R/T pacing to expose electrical instability in the ischaemic ventricle. *Clin. Res.* **20**, 401–405.

TIBBLIN, G. (1969). The men born in 1913 study. *Pehr. Dubb. J.* **3**, 8–13.

TIMIO, M., GENTILI, S. and PEDE, S. (1979). Free adrenaline and noradrenaline excretion related to occupational stress. *Br. Heart J.* **42**, 471–474.

TORGERSEN, S. and KRINGLEN, E. (1971). Blood pressure and personality. A study of the relation between intra-pair differences in systolic blood pressure and personality in monozygotic twins. *J. psychosom. Res.* **15**, 183–191.

TÖRÖK, E. (1979). The beginnings of hypertension: Studies in childhood and adolescence. *In* "Mild Hypertension: Natural History and Management" (F. Gross and T. Strasser, Eds), pp. 67–80. Pitman Medical, Bath.

TRULSON, M. E. (1977). Role of glucocorticoids in abnormal grooming behaviour in cats with pontile or frontal neocortical lesions. *J. comp. physiol. Psychol.* **91**, 761–769.

TSENG, W. (1967). Blood pressure and hypertension in an agricultural and a fishing population. *Am. J. Epidemiol.* **86**, 513–525.

UHLEY, H. N., FRIEDMAN, M. (1959). Blood lipids, clotting and coronary atherosclerosis in rats exposed to a particular form of stress. *Am. J. Physiol.* **197**, 396–398.

ULRYCH, M. (1969). The haemodynamics of mental activity. *Clin. Sci. molec. Med.* **36**, 453–461.

ULRYCH, M., FROHLICH, E., DUSTAN, H. and PAGE, I. (1968). Immediate haemodynamic effects of beta-adrenergic blockade with propranolol in normotensive and hypertensive man. *Circulation*, **37**, 411–416.

URSIN, H., BAADE, E. and LEVINE, S. (Eds) (1978). "The Psychobiology of Stress". Academic Press, London and New York.

VANDER, A. J., HENRY, J. P., STEPHENS, P. M., KAY, L. L. and MOUW, D. (1978). PRA in psychosocial hypertension of CBA mice. *Circulation Res.* **42**, 496–502.

VAN DIJL, H. (1974). Activity and job responsibility as measured by judgement behaviour in myocardial infarction patients. *Psychother. Psychosom.* **24**, 126–128.

VAN DIJL, H. (1977). The A/B typology according to Friedman and Rosenman and an effort to test some of the characteristics by means of a psychological test (RSL or BUL). *J. psychosom. Res.* **22**, 101–109.

VAN TOLLER, C. and TARPY, E. A. (1974). Immunosympathectomy and avoidance behavior. *Psychol. Bull.* **81**, 132–137.

VASSALLE, M., LEVINE, M. J. and STUCKEY, J. H. (1968). On the sympathetic control of ventricular automaticity: The effects of stellate ganglion stimulation. *Circulation Res.* **23**, 249–255.

VATNER, S. F. (1978). Effects of exercise and excitement on mesenteric and renal dynamics in conscious, unrestrained baboons. *Am. J. Physiol.* **234**, H210–H214.

VERGROESEN, A. J. (1975). Influence of dietary fatty acids on blood lipids. *In* "Blood and Arterial Wall in Atherogenesis and Arterial Thrombosis" (J. G. A. J. Hautvast, R. J. J. Hermus and F. Van Der Haar, Eds), pp. 128–132. E. J. Brill, Leiden.

VERRIER, R. L. and LOWN, B. (1978). Sympathetic-parasympathetic interactions and ventricular electrical stability. *In* "Neural Mechanisms in Cardiac Arrhythmias" (P. J. Schwartz, A. M. Brown, A. Malliani and A. Zanchetti, Eds), pp. 75–85. Raven Press, New York.

VERRIER, R. L., CALVERT, A. and LOWN, B. (1974). Effect of acute blood pressure elevation on the ventricular fibrillation threshold. *Am. J. Physiol.* **226**, 893–897.

VERRIER, R. L., CALVERT, A. and LOWN, B. (1975). Effect of posterior hypothalamic stimulation on ventricular fibrillation threshold. *Am. J. Physiol.* **228**, 923–927.

VETTER, N. J., ADAMS, W., STRANGE, R. C. and OLIVER, M. F. (1974). Initial metabolic and hormonal responses to acute myocardial infarction. *Lancet*, **I**, 284–288.

VICTOR, R., MAINARDI, A. and SHAPIRO, D. (1978). Effects of biofeedback and voluntary control procedures on heart rate and perception of pain during the cold pressor test. *Psychosom. Med.* **40**, 216–225.

VON EIFF, A. W. and PEIKARSKI, C. (1977). Stress reactions of normotensives and hypertensives and the influence of female sex hormones on blood pressure regulation. *Prog. Brain Res.* **47**, 289–299.

VON HOLST, D. (1972a). Renal failure as the cause of death in Tupaia Belangeri exposed to persistent social stress. *J. comp. Physiol.* **78**, 236–273.

VON HOLST, D. (1972b). Die Funktion der Nebennieren männlicher Tupaia Belangeri. *J. comp. Physiol.* **78**, 289–306.

WADE, J. G., LARSON, C. P., HICKEY, P. F., EHRONFELD, W. K. and SEVERINGHAUS, J. W. (1970). The effect of carotid endarterectomy on carotid chemoreceptor and baroreceptor function in man. *New Engl. J. Med.* **282**, 828–829.

WAKIM, K. G., SLAUGHTER, O. and CLAGETT, O. T. (1948). Studies on the blood flow in the extremities in cases of coarctation of the aorta: Determination before and after excision of the coarctate region. *Proc. Mayo Clinic*, **23**, 347–358.

WALD, N., HOWARD, S., SMITH, P. G. and KJELDSON, K. (1973). Association between atherosclerotic diseases and carboxyhaemoglobin levels in tobacco smokers. *Br. med. J.* **I**, 761–765.

WALDRON, I., ZYZANSKI, S. J., SHEKELLE, R. B., JENKINS, C. D. and TANNEBAUM, S. (1977). The coronary-prone behavior pattern in employed men and women. *J. Human Stress*, **3**(4), 2–18.

WALL, P. D. and DAVIS, G. D. (1951). Three cerebral cortical systems affecting autonomic function. *J. Neurophysiol.* **14**, 507–517.

WALLIN, B. C., DELIUS, W. and HAGBARTH, K-E. (1973). Comparison of sympathetic nerve activity in normotensive and hypertensive subjects. *Circulation Res.* **33**, 9–21.

WALTON, K. W. (1975). Factors affecting lipoprotein deposition in the arterial wall. *In* "Blood and Arterial Wall in Atherogenesis and Arterial Thrombosis" (J. G. A. J. Hautvast, R. J. J. Hermus and F. Van Der Haar, Eds), pp. 79–86. E. J. Brill, Leiden.

WARDWELL, W. I. and BAHNSON, C. B. (1973). Behavioral variables and myocardial infarction in the southeastern Connecticut heart study. *J. chron. Dis.* **26**, 447–461.

WARHEIT, G. J. (1974). Occupation: A key factor in stress at the Manned Space Center. *In* "Stress and the Heart" (R. S. Eliot, Ed.), pp. 51–65. Futura, New York.

WEINER, H. (1979). "The Psychobiology of Essential Hypertension". Elsevier, New York.

WEINSTEIN, M. C. and STASON, W. B. (1976). "Hypertension: A Policy Perspective". Harvard University Press, Cambridge, Massachusetts.

WEISS, J. M. (1970). Somatic effects of predictable and unpredictable shock. *Psychosom. Med.* **32**, 397–408.

WEISS, T. and ENGEL, B. T. (1971). Operant conditioning of heart rate in patients with premature ventricular contractions. *Psychosom. Med.* **33**, 301–321.

WEISS, Y. A., SAFAR, M. E., LONDON, G. M., SIMON, A. C., LEVENSON, J. A. and MILLIEZ, P. M. (1978). Repeat haemodynamic determinations in borderline hypertension. *Am. J. Med.* **64**, 382–387.

WENGER, N. K. (Ed.) (1978). "Exercise and the Heart". F. A. Davis, Philadelphia.

WENGER, N. K. and HELLERSTEIN, H. K. (Eds) (1978). "Rehabilitation of the Coronary Patient". Wiley, Chichester.

WERDEGAR, D., SOKOLOW, M. and PERLOFF, D. E. (1967). Portable recordings of blood pressure: A new approach to assessments of the severity and prognosis of hypertension. *Trans. Ass. Life Insur. med. Dir. Am.* **51**, 93–115.

WHEELER, E. D., WHITE, P. D. and REED, W. (1950). Neurocirculatory asthenia (anxiety neurosis, effort syndrome, neurasthenia): 20 year follow-up study of 173 patients. *J. Am. med. Ass.* **142**, 878–889.

WHITEHEAD, W. E., BLACKWELL, B., DE SILVA, H. and ROBINSON, A. (1977). Anxiety and anger in hypertension. *J. psychosom. Res.* **21**, 383–389.

WIKSTRAND, J., BERGLUND, G., WILHELMSEN, L. and WALLENTIN, I. (1976). Noninvasive assessment of the heart in the hypertensive. *Aust. N.Z. J. Med.* **6**, Suppl. 2, 1–7.

WILHELMSEN, L., SANNE, H., ELMFELDT, D. (1975). A controlled trial of physical training after myocardial infarction. *Prev. Med.* **4**, 491–496.

WILHELMSEN, L., TIBBLIN, G., ELMFELDT, D., WEDEL, A. and WERKÖ, L. (1977). Coffee consumption and coronary heart disease in middle-aged Swedish men. *Acta med. scand.* **201**, 547–552.

WILHELMSSON, C., VEDIN, J. A., WILHELMSEN, L., TIBBLIN, G. and WERKÖ, L. (1974). Reduction of sudden deaths after myocardial infarction by treatment with alprenolol. *Lancet*, **II**, 1157–1166.

WILLIAMS, R. B., BITTKER, T. E., BUCHSBAUM, M. S. and WYNNE, L. (1975). Cardiovascular and neurophysiologic correlates of sensory intake and rejection 1. Effect of cognitive tasks. *Psychophysiology*, **12**, 427–433.

WILLIAMS, R. B., FRIEDMAN, M., GLASS, D. C., HERD, J. A. and SCHNEIDER-MAN, N. (1978). Section summary: Mechanisms linking behavioural and pathophysiological processes. *In* "Coronary-prone Behavior" (T. M. Dembroski, S. Weiss, J. L. Shields, S. G. Haynes and M. Feinleib, Eds), pp. 119–128. Springer-Verlag, New York.

WILLIAMS, R. B., EICHELMAN, B. S. and NG, L. K. Y. (1979). The effects of peripheral chemosympathectomy and adrenalectomy upon blood pressure responses of the rat to footshock under varying conditions: Evidence for behavioural effects on patterning of sympathetic nervous system responses. *Psychophysiology*, **16**, 89–93.

WOLF, S. (1967). The bradycardia of the dive reflex – a possible mechanism of sudden death. *Cond. Reflex*, **2**, 88–95.

WOLF, S. (1978). Psychophysiological influences on the dive reflex in man. *In* "Neural Mechanisms in Cardiac Arrhythmias" (P. J. Schwartz, A. J.

Brown, A. Malliani and A. Zanchetti, Eds), pp. 237–250. Raven Press, New York.

WOLF, S., PFEIFFER, J., RIPLEY, H., WINTER, O. and WOLFF, H. (1948). Hypertension as a reaction pattern to stress: Summary of experimental data on variations in blood pressure and renal blood flow. *Arch. intern. Med.* **58**, 1056–1076.

WOLF, S., CARDON, P. V., SHEPARD, E. M. and WOLFF, H. G. (1955). "Life Stress and Essential Hypertension". Williams and Wilkins, Baltimore.

WOLF, S., McCABE, W. R., YAMAMOTO, J., ADSETT, C. and SCHOTSTAEDT, W. (1962). Changes in serum lipids in relation to emotional stress during rigid control of diet and exercise. *Circulation,* **26**, 379–387.

WOLFF, C., FRIEDMAN, S., HOFER, M. and MASON, J. (1964). Relationship between psychological defences and mean urinary 17-OHCS excretion rates. *Psychosom. Med.* **26**, 576–591.

WOODMAN, D. D., HINTON, J. W. and O'NEILL, M. T. (1978). Plasma catecholamines, stress and aggression in maximum security patients. *Biol. Psychol.* **6**, 147–154.

ZANCHETTI, A. (1976). Hypothalamic control of the circulation. *In* "The Nervous System in Arterial Hypertension" (S. Julius and M. D. Esler, Eds), pp. 397–429. Charles Thomas, Springfield.

ZANCHETTI, A., STELLA, A. and DAMPNEY, R. (1977). Central and reflex control of renin release. *Prog. Brain Res.* **47**, 397–407.

ZBROZYNA, A. W. (1976). Renal vasoconstriction in naturally elicited fear and its habituation in baboons. *Cardiovasc. Res.* **10**, 295–300.

ZYZANSKI, S. J. (1978). Coronary-prone behavior and coronary heart disease: Epidemiological observations. *In* "Coronary-prone Behavior" (T. M. Dembroski, S. M. Weiss, J. L. Shields, S. G. Haynes and M. Feinleib, Eds), pp. 25–40. Springer-Verlag, New York.

ZYZANSKI, S. J., JENKINS, C. D., RYAN, T. J., FLESSAS, A. and EVERIST, M. (1976). Psychologic correlates of coronary angiographic findings. *Arch. intern. Med.* **136**, 1234–1237.

Additional references

BALI, L. R. (1979). Long-term effect of relaxation on blood pressure and anxiety levels of essential hypertensive males: A controlled study. *Psychosom. Med.* **41**, 637–646.

COLERIDGE, H. M. and COLERIDGE, J. C. G. (1980). Cardiovascular afferents involved in regulation of peripheral vessels. *A. Rev. Physiol.* **42**, 413–427.

DIMSDALE, J. E. and MOSS, J. (1980). Plasma catacholamines in stress and exercise. *J. Am. med. Ass.* **243**, 340–342.

FRANCIS, K. T. (1979). Psychologic correlates of serum indicators of stress in man: A longitudinal study. *Psychosom. Med.* **41**, 617–628.

FRIEDMAN, M. (1979). The modification of Type A behaviour in post-infarction patients. *Am. Heart J.* **97**, 551–560.

HAYNES, S. G., FEINLEIB, M. and KANNEL, W. B. (1980). The relation of psychosocial factors to coronary heart disease in the Framingham Study III. 8-year incidence of coronary heart disease. *Am. J. Epidemiol.* **111**, 37–58.

HILTON, S. M. and SPYER, K. M. (1980). Central nervous regulation of vascular resistance. *A. Rev. Physiol.* **42**, 399–411.

HILTON, S. M., SPYER, K. M. and TIMMS, R. J. (1979). The origin of the hind limb vasodilatation evoked by stimulation of the motor cortex in the cat. *J. Physiol.* **287**, 545–557.

KORNITZER, M., DE BACKER, G., DRAMAIX, M. and THILLY, C. (1980). The Belgian heart disease prevention project. Modification of the coronary risk profile in an industrial population. *Circulation*, **61**, 18–25.

KRANTZ, D. S., SANMARCO, M. I., SELVESTER, R. H. and MATTHEWS, K. A. (1979). Psychological correlates of progression of atherosclerosis in men. *Psychosom. Med.* **41**, 467–476.

LEBLANC, J., CÔTÉ, J., JOBIN, M. and LABRIE, A. (1979). Plasma catecholamine and cardiovascular responses to cold and mental activity. *J. appl. Physiol.: Respirat. environ. Exercise Physiol.* **47**, 1207–1211.

LUNDBERG, U. and FORSMAN, L. (1979). Adrenal-medullary and adrenal-cortical responses to understimulation and overstimulation: Comparison between type A and type B persons. *Biol. Psychol.* **9**, 79–89.

MEYER, A. J., NASH, J. D., MCCALISTER, A. L., MACCOBY, N. and FARQUHAR, J. W. (1980). Skills training in a cardiovascular health education campaign. *J. Cons. clin. Psychol.* **48**, 129–142.

MULTIPLE risk factor intervention trial (MRFIT) (1976). *J. Am. Med. Ass.* **235**, 825–827.

OSTER, K. A. (1980). Duplicity in a committee report on diet and coronary heart disease. *Am. Heart J.* **99**, 409–412.

PUSKA, P., TUOMILEHTO, J., SALONEN, J., NEITTOANMÄKI, L., MAKI, J., VIRTAMO, J., NISSINEN, A., KOSKELA, K. and TAKALO, T. (1979). Changes in coronary risk factors during comprehensive five-year community programme to control national cardiovascular diseases (North Karelia project). *Br. med. J.* **II**, 1173–1178.

WEIDNER, G. and MATTHEWS, K. (1978). Reported physical symptoms elicited by unpredictable events and the Type A coronary-prone behaviour pattern. *J. Person. soc. Psychol.* **36**, 1213–1220.

Subject Index